D1639455

THE YEAR IN RESPIRATORY MEDICINE 2004

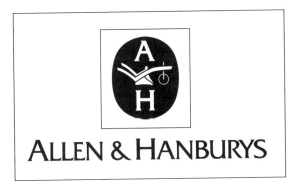

Provided as an
educational service to medicine by
Allen & Hanburys

THE YEAR IN RESPIRATORY MEDICINE

2004

**R FERGUSSON, A HILL, T MACKAY,
P REID, J SIMPSON**

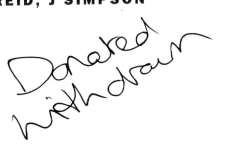

CLINICAL PUBLISHING
OXFORD

Distributed worldwide by
CRC Press

Boca Raton   London   New York   Washington, DC

Clinical Publishing

an imprint of Atlas Medical Publishing Ltd

Oxford Centre for Innovation
Mill Street, Oxford OX2 0JX, UK

Tel: +44 1865 811116
Fax: +44 1865 251550
Web: www.clinicalpublishing.co.uk

Distributed by:

CRC Press LLC
2000 NW Corporate Blvd
Boca Raton, FL 33431, USA
E-mail: orders@crcpress.com

CRC Press UK
23–25 Blades Court
Deodar Road
London SW15 2NU, UK
E-mail: crcpress@itps.co.uk

A catalogue record for this book is available from the British Library

ISBN 1 904392 31 8
ISSN 1477-8114

**The publisher makes no representation, express or implied, that the dosages in this book are correct.
Readers must therefore always check the product information and clinical procedures with the
most up-to-date published product information and data sheets provided by the manufacturers and
the most recent codes of conduct and safety regulations. The authors and the publisher do not accept
any liability for any errors in the text or for the misuse or misapplication of material in this work**

Project manager: Carolyn Newton
Typeset by Footnote Graphics Ltd, Warminster, Wiltshire, UK
Printed in Spain by Fisa-Escudo de Oro SA, Barcelona

Contents

Contributors

RON FERGUSSON, MD, FRCPE, Respiratory Medicine Unit,
Western General Hospital, Edinburgh, UK

ADAM HILL, MD, FRCPE, Department of Respiratory Medicine,
Royal Infirmary, Edinburgh, UK

TOM MACKAY, BSc (Hons), MB ChB, FRCPE, Department of Respiratory
Medicine, Royal Infirmary, Edinburgh, UK

PETER REID, MD, FRCPE, Respiratory Medicine Unit, Western General
Hospital, Edinburgh, UK

JOHN SIMPSON, PhD, FRCPE, MRC/University of Edinburgh Centre for
Inflammation Research, Medical School, Edinburgh, UK

Foreword

Respiratory diseases continue to be one of the most, if not *the*, most important causes of morbidity and mortality across the world. A recent review of the incidence of respiratory diseases in Europe has shown that the UK has the greatest number of deaths due to lung cancer in any European country. It has the highest incidence of chronic obstructive pulmonary disease (COPD) and a very high occurrence of tuberculosis, pneumonia and sleep apnoea. These are all topics covered in this edition of *Year in Respiratory Medicine*.

Following the lines of last year's volume, *Year in Respiratory Medicine 2004* focuses on the key topics of asthma, COPD, infection and lung cancer, but adds sections on pulmonary fibrosis, tuberculosis, mesothelioma and obstructive sleep apnoea. The contents of the book are not only relevant to the UK, but to the rest of the world; the more that can be done to draw attention to these important respiratory diseases, the better.

Year in Respiratory Medicine 2004 contains a large number of significant papers, which are reviewed, summarised and then commented upon by the authors. These expert summaries provide an enjoyable method of reading and sifting through the plethora of available information. This format is an extremely useful method of learning for individuals who are hard pressed to know where to do their academic reading. As a previous editor of *Thorax*, I introduced The Year in Review to the journal as an annual supplement each August. These have now stopped and these current volumes of *Year in Respiratory Medicine* follow the same principle of reviewing key papers in important fields and providing expert comment.

The topics are extremely clearly presented and are equally suitable for specialists, generalists and trainees alike. It is appropriate that the book confines itself in the main to the common diseases within respiratory medicine and highlights both the progress in research and the shortcomings in the management of important diseases. Evidence-based volumes provide all of us with the ammunition to take forward the quest for obtaining increased funding and government support within respiratory medicine that is currently so lacking. Treatment of many disorders highlighted in this volume could probably be improved with better funding and further research.

The authors are to be congratulated on the hard work they have put into producing this extremely valuable textbook, which will certainly keep the reader up to date.

Professor Stephen G Spiro, MD, FRCP
Professor of Respiratory Medicine
University College London Hospitals NHS Trust
London, UK

Part I

Asthma

Asthma

P REID

Introduction

Asthma is a common reason for consultation in primary care and is an important component of the workload of most respiratory physicians. It affects all age groups and, consequently, makes a significant impact on the costs borne by healthcare providers and society as a whole.

The diagnostic term embraces a complex syndrome in which a number of different phenotypes exist. Thus, the presentation and natural history of asthma is highly variable. Epidemiological studies are beginning to home in on factors that may be linked to the appearance or persistence of the disease, but causation is likely to represent a highly complex interaction between genetic and environmental influences. Nevertheless, certain themes consistently appear in the medical literature and the repeated rigorous testing of these is likely to provide useful information in the not too distant future.

Whatever the triggers, an intricate inflammatory response ensues in the airways. Heightened bronchoconstriction to a range of stimuli results in the classical symptoms of cough, shortness of breath and wheeze. Fortunately increased understanding of the pivotal role of inflammation in this process has focused the emphasis of therapy on inhaled corticosteroid therapy. These agents have consistently proved superior to other agents, providing prompt resolution of symptoms, attenuated airway hyper-responsiveness and a reduction in exacerbations. Improved understanding of the therapeutic ratio of these agents has concentrated awareness on the need for managing patients on the optimal therapeutic dose. Thus, we need more information on how to step down therapy and assess medication requirements.

The development of long-acting β_2 agonists has represented a significant advance for those patients who remain symptomatic despite reasonable doses of inhaled steroids and more information continues to appear on the complementary role of these two drug classes. The launch of the leukotriene receptor antagonists was followed by a number of small studies aimed at establishing the potential benefit of this new class of drug in asthma sufferers. These have been followed by larger studies that bring some clarity as to the positioning of these agents in our therapeutic strategy. Many patients with asthma seek information on the use of non-pharmacological therapies such as breathing techniques, but unfortunately limited information is available. All of these efforts need to be coupled with improved methods of educating patients and encouraging self-directed care.

Despite optimal medical management a significant minority of patients continue to experience severe persistent asthma. Further research is needed into the mechanisms and trigger factors that are important in this particular group of patients, hopefully leading to improvements in management.

Finally, asthma presents as a medical emergency and it behoves any practising 'front-door' physician to be conversant with the principles of management. Failure to evaluate the severity of acute attacks is one of the factors that contribute to the ongoing and regrettable toll of asthma death.

The world of medical publishing has become increasingly competitive. Good studies are meticulously planned and a substantial amount of work invested into the recruitment and follow-up of the patients. Good researchers are becoming increasingly professional and highly dedicated individuals. Choosing a selection of the published work from any year is a largely subjective task and to some extent reflects the bias of the author. The papers I have chosen represent a difficult choice from the many more papers that have substantially increased our knowledge and advanced the care of patients. As before, I have tried to give precedence to those papers published in leading medical journals and attempt to reflect some of the themes that are currently receiving most 'air play' at asthma meetings. In so far as possible I have used the comment sections for distilling the major points made by the authors in the discussion sections of their papers, but on occasion I have added my own thoughts. Finally, as always, you will see that good research answers some questions, but proposes many others. Enjoy!

1

Epidemiology and disease causation

Introduction

The rapid rise in the prevalence of asthma, particularly over a relatively short time frame, suggests that environmental rather than genetic factors are important in the development and/or the persistence of the disease. This has focused a significant body of effort into epidemiological research programmes that may identify causative factors. It is hoped that some of these may be potentially modifiable.

Several broad themes have emerged from this research and the most widely popularized has been the hygiene hypothesis, which has been adapted from observations on hay fever |1|. This attempts to explain the attribution of the rising prevalence of asthma to the increasingly hygienic Western lifestyle that is accompanied by a lack of infections in childhood. The hygiene hypothesis has been bolstered by an immunological model of asthma suggesting a bias towards T cells that mediate the immunological reactions against parasites and allergic phenomena and a reduction in those that mediate cellular immunity to bacteria and viruses. T helper (Th) cells are thought to orchestrate the asthmatic inflammatory response and are believed to differentiate into two relatively distinct subsets: Th1 and Th2 cells. Th 2 lymphocytes predominantly secrete cytokines, such as interleukin-4 (IL-4), IL-5 and IL-13, that direct the immune system towards an allergic type of response. Th1 lymphocytes preferentially secrete interferon-γ (IFN-γ) and IL-2, which are important in fighting viral and bacterial infections. The Th cell polarity of the newborn infant is predominantly skewed to Th2 cell function, but as it matures and encounters a variety of infectious insults post-partum a shift in the polarity of the T cells occurs towards Th1 cell responses. Thus, by growing up in a more hygienic environment the infant fails to be exposed to bacterial and viral infections and the polarity of the Th cells remains skewed towards Th2 cells. The infant is therefore at risk of developing allergic diseases such as asthma.

The increasingly cosseted and centrally heated environment of our homes encourages the growth of the house dust mite, which is one of the major factors linked to the development of atopy and asthma. Other indoor allergens may also play key roles and a substantial amount of research has been focused on the role of household pets such as cats and dogs |2–6|. Investigators have also examined potential influences from outdoor settings such as the protective influence of farming environments |7–9|.

The importance of diet has been examined by a number of teams, particularly concentrating on foodstuffs likely to be important in the regulation of the immune system or inflammatory processes |**10,11**|. Closely allayed to diet is the role of obesity in the developing world. This is a major public health problem in its own right, but may be linked to the appearance of asthma through a number of possible mechanisms |**12–14**|. There is also widespread public concern regarding the quality of our air, particularly in cities and towns with high levels of traffic pollution, raising concern that exhaust and diesel fumes may cause or aggravate asthma |**15–17**|.

Although genetic changes are unlikely to account for the rise in asthma, it is highly probable that genetic factors influence its development through complex interactions with the environment. Maternal history appears to be particularly important in governing the response of the individual to many of the exposures investigated |**6**|. The discovery of key target genes such as ADAM33 and others will hopefully begin to unlock the mysteries of the interaction between environmental factors and the host in initiating or perpetuating the disease state |**18**|.

Association between antenatal cytokine production and the development of atopy and asthma at age 6 years
Macaubas C, de Klerk NH, Holt BJ, *et al. Lancet* 2003; **362**: 1192–7

B ACKGROUND. The interaction between the immune system and allergen encountered shortly after birth is in part determined by the degree of immune competence attained at birth and the rate at which the immune system matures. The factors governing the development of the immune system during this critical period are poorly understood, but may be regulated by the production of cytokines by the fetoplacental unit. The aim of this study was to investigate associations between cytokine production at birth measured in cord blood and the subsequent development of atopy and asthma in later childhood.

INTERPRETATION. The authors found an inverse relation between cord-blood concentrations of IL-4, IFN-γ and tumour necrosing factor-α (TNF-α) and the risk of asthma, atopy or both at the age of 6 years, thereby suggesting that cytokine production within the fetoplacental unit may influence disease susceptibility. They also noted that maternal smoking was associated with the development of wheeze and, thus, identify a potentially modifiable target.

Comment

This study was drawn from a large community-based birth cohort and was not selected with reference to any asthma or atopy variables. A comprehensive data set was collected including parental atopy, maternal smoking history, pregnancy complications, various indices of growth including infant birth weight, method of delivery and indicators of fetal distress. Cord blood was sampled at birth and then stored for later analysis. The children were followed prospectively and around their

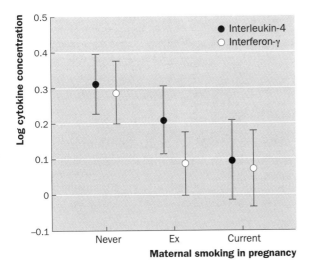

Fig. 1.1 Maternal smoking and cord-blood concentrations of IL-4 and IFN-γ. Error bars indicate 95% CI. Source: Macaubas *et al.* (2003).

sixth birthday were assessed for respiratory outcome by parental questionnaire and allergy skin tests. There were few dropouts.

The main finding from the study was an inverse relationship between the cord blood cytokines IL-4, IFN-γ and TNF-α and the risk of asthma, atopy or both at the age of 6 years. The authors employed a technique known as propensity score adjustment for assessing the likelihood of casual relationships. This score replaces all known confounding variables and risk factors with a single composite score that provides a summary of the collection. The independent effects of each variable of interest are then assessed |**19,20**|. This showed that these findings were independent from known antenatal or perinatal factors. The authors were also able to demonstrate a dose–response relationship between cord blood concentrations of IL-4 and IFN-γ and maternal smoking (Fig. 1.1).

Given that IFN-γ is traditionally viewed as a Th1 cytokine and IL-4 as a Th2 cytokine, these results do not fit neatly into currently held views on the Th1/Th2 model of allergic disease. However, the authors pointed out that previous studies have suggested that the development of atopy is associated with decreased production of both Th1 and Th2 cytokines |**21**|. In addition, it should also be remembered that the Th1/Th2 paradigm is likely to represent an oversimplification |**22**|.

The authors also reported that maternal smoking was associated with an increased risk of wheeze at 6 years (odds ratio [OR] = 1.85 and 95% confidence interval [CI] = 1.09–3.15) and they found that ex-smokers and current smokers had significantly less IFN-γ in their cord blood than non-smokers. The relationship between maternal smoking and the development of wheeze is consistent with other studies and carries an important public health message, particularly as smoking remains common in many women of childbearing age |**23,24**|. In this paper the authors suggested that a possible link between smoking and disease may be explained by its influence on placental trophoblast production of cytokines as has been demonstrated *in vitro* |**25**|.

Association of consumption of products containing milk fat with reduced asthma risk in pre-school children: the PIAMA birth cohort study

Wijga AH, Smit HA, Kerkhof M, *et al. Thorax* 2003; **58**: 567–72

BACKGROUND. This study reports data from the natural history arm of the Prevention and Incidence of Asthma and Mite Allergy (PIAMA) Study, which facilitated a prospective examination of the relationship between food consumption and asthma symptoms in pre-school children. Data collected on food consumption at the age of 2 years were related to the prevalence of asthma symptoms reported at age 3 years.

INTERPRETATION. The frequent consumption of products containing milk fat in pre-school children is associated with a reduced risk of asthma symptoms.

Comment

The PIAMA Study was devised with two arms: a placebo-controlled intervention arm that investigated the impact of mite-impermeable mattress covers and a second arm that was not subject to intervention and designed to allow the natural history of asthma to be investigated. This paper by Wijga *et al.* reports data from the natural history arm of the PIAMA Study. The children studied in this paper were born between July 1996 and October 1997 and included 472 allergic and 2819 non-allergic mothers.

The investigators found that the frequent consumption of products containing milk fat (full cream milk, milk products and butter) was associated with a reduced risk of reporting asthma symptoms at the age of 3 years. They also reported protection from frequent consumption of brown bread. The estimates of the effects of milk fat and brown bread on asthma and wheeze were of the same order of magnitude as the effects of the established risk factors, such as parental allergy and being male.

In order to facilitate the collection of data they employed a short and user-friendly questionnaire that had been validated in other studies |**26**|. The authors defined exposure in terms of the frequency of consumption of different foods and drinks, but they were not able to provide information on portion sizes, total energy or nutrient intake. As food intake is likely to be related to other indicators of lifestyle they acknowledged that they could not exclude the possibility that other important associations between food consumption and asthma symptoms had not been detected. However, whilst a healthy lifestyle may be true of brown bread consumption, foods containing a high content of milk fat are not typically viewed as being associated with a healthy lifestyle. It is interesting that they did not report an association with fruits and vegetables, as identified by other investigators |27|. They suggested that this may have been due to inadequate identification of these foods in their questionnaire, but raised the possibility that the role of antioxidants is age related and less important in younger children.

The study may have limitations in applicability to the wider population. The dropouts were small in number, but only 56% of the potential study population participated and the recruitment under-represented smoking parents and those with only primary school education. Nevertheless, the adjusted regression analysis did not indicate that the observed associations were influenced by parental education or smoking. Although standard methods were used for assessing the prevalence of asthma and wheeze, the authors acknowledged that most children who wheeze in infancy do not develop asthma in later life and accepted that misclassification was possible |28,29|.

In large epidemiological studies the results may be influenced by reverse causation, that is to say that the apparent protection from asthma by milk products merely represented the avoidance of milk products by children who had a recognized allergy to cow's milk and who were already recognized to be at increased risk of developing allergy and asthma. To avoid this the authors excluded 64 children with known allergy to cow's milk. The authors also identified a potential for inverse causation. They included 27 children (<1%) who avoided cow's milk and in these children a parental allergy was more common. Thus, it is possible that parental allergy may have influenced the decision whether or not to supply cow's milk to the child. However, the number was small so any potential effect was likely to be minimal.

In the discussion the authors also draw attention to other studies that support to their findings, including many that have examined links between brown bread, milk and other dairy products and asthma. They suggest that various components of these diets such as fatty acids, antioxidants and other micronutrients may provide possible mechanisms for this association and, interestingly, they also suggest that the influence of diet may differ according to the age of the individual studied.

Pet keeping in childhood and adult asthma and hay fever: European Respiratory Health Survey

Svanes C, Heinrich J, Jarvis D, *et al. J Allergy Clin Immunol* 2003; **112**: 289–300

BACKGROUND. It remains uncertain whether exposure to pets in early life protects or promotes allergic disease. This paper reported data from the European Community Respiratory Health Study and examined the relationship between keeping pet cats, dogs or birds during childhood and the subsequent development of asthma.

INTERPRETATION. The effect of pet keeping varied according to the type of pet, the allergic sensitization of the individual and the wider environmental exposure to the allergen.

Comment

Exposure to pets in early life has traditionally been felt to be causally associated with the development of atopy and asthma. However, recent data have suggested that exposure to certain pets, particularly cats and farm animals, may protect against the development of atopy and asthma |4–8,30,31|. The literature has become confusing, but this paper by Svanes *et al.* is a welcome addition. They reported data from a random sample of at least 1500 men and 1500 women aged 20–44 years. This analysis included data from 1991 to 1993 for 18 530 subjects from 36 centres, representing 16 countries, of which 13 932 subjects (75%) provided tests for the measurement of specific immunoglobulin E (IgE). Information on pet keeping, symptoms and potential confounding variables was obtained by an interviewer-led questionnaire.

The study reported some interesting demographic details. Sixty-one per cent of the study population had kept pets in childhood and 41% currently kept pets. Interestingly, a history of either asthma or allergy in parents and siblings did not seem to influence the decision to keep pets. This observation does not support the theory that families with allergy will avoid purchasing pets and perhaps refutes the concern that reverse causation is a potential confounding factor in studies on pet ownership. However, the authors also reminded us that there was little focus on allergen avoidance during the period when these children were born (1945–1972) and this may be a more appropriate explanation for their finding.

Smokers were more likely to keep pets than non-smokers and people from large families were more likely to keep cats or dogs in childhood, but less likely to do so as adults. Women were more likely to keep cats in both childhood and adulthood. Childhood cats were more common in earlier birth cohorts, whereas children in later birth cohorts were more likely to keep birds.

The study made some interesting observations on the relationship between cat ownership and the development of asthma. It suggested that keeping a cat in childhood was associated with asthma only in atopic subjects. However, the association was highly heterogenous and inversely related to the prevalence of pet cats kept during childhood. Cat ownership in subjects who grew up in an area with a relatively low prevalence of cats was associated with an increased risk of developing adult asthma. Thus, when the prevalence of cats was less than 40%, the OR for adult asthma was 1.84 (95% CI = 1.31–2.57), but when the prevalence of cat ownership was greater than 60% the risk of asthma was not increased (OR = 0.98 and 95% CI = 0.73–1.33). The OR when the prevalence of cats was between 40 and 60% was 1.33 (95% CI = 1.10–1.61).

The relationship between dogs and the development of respiratory symptoms appeared to be related to the presence of atopy. Keeping a dog in childhood appeared to protect atopic individuals against the development of adult hay fever. However, in non-atopic subjects keeping a dog appeared to be associated with more respiratory symptoms in adulthood. These relationships were consistent across the different centres.

Ownership of pet birds during childhood was found to increase the risk of adult respiratory symptoms independent of allergic disposition and these relationships were consistent across the different centres.

That the literature in this area is confusing probably reflects the likelihood that interactions between animal exposure and the development of atopy and asthma are going to be complex. However, this study adds to the evidence that contact with animals in early life does influence the development of the immune system and the airways and forms a basis for contemplating interventional studies aimed at addressing this issue.

Day care attendance in early life, maternal history of asthma and asthma at the age of 6 years

Celedón JC, Wright RJ, Litonjua AA, *et al. Am J Respir Crit Care* 2003; **167**: 1239–43

BACKGROUND. The authors of this study had previously reported that day care attendance in early life was associated with an increased risk of doctor-diagnosed respiratory illnesses in the first year of life but a decreased total serum IgE level at age 2 years. This paper reported the association between day care attendance in the first year of life and asthma and wheezing in the first 6 years of life.

INTERPRETATION. Day care attendance in the first year of life was significantly associated with decreased odds of recurrent wheezing and eczema at the age of 6 years. The main finding was that a maternal history of asthma is an important determinant of the relation between day care-related exposures and the development of childhood asthma.

Comment

Day care attendance in early life has been shown to confer protection against atopy, wheeze and asthma in later childhood |**32,33**|. This paper extended the observations

from the Home Allergens and Asthma Prospective Birth Cohort Study of children
with a history of asthma, hay fever or allergies in at least one parent and explored the
hypothesis that a maternal history of asthma may influence the relationship between
day care and the development of asthma.

Day care attendance in the first year of life was inversely associated with the appearance of eczema (OR = 0.3 and 95% CI = 0.1–0.8) among all the study participants

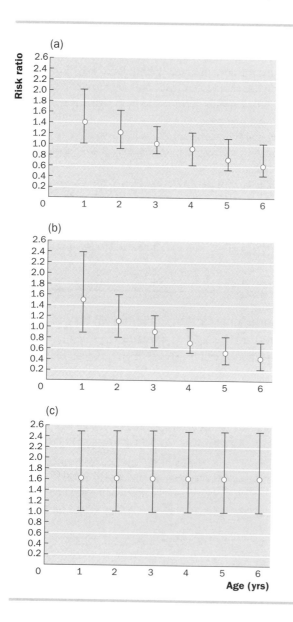

and did not appear to be influenced by maternal history. However, the authors did find that the relationship between day care and the development of asthma was subject to the presence of a maternal history of asthma. Day care attendance in early life was associated with a decreased risk of asthma (OR = 0.3 and 95% CI = 0.1–0.7) and recurrent wheezing (OR = 0.3 and 95% CI = 0.1–0.9) at the age of 6 years and a decreased risk of any wheezing after the age of 4 years only in children without a maternal history of asthma. Day care attendance in early life among children with a maternal history of asthma had no protective effect on asthma or recurrent wheezing at the age of 6 years, but was associated with an increased risk of wheezing in the first 6 years of life (Fig. 1.2).

Definitions of day care may vary. In this study day care was classified as home (at the day care provider's residence), non-residential (not provided at someone else's home) and mixed. Day care was also classified according to the number of children attending with the study participant. However, neither the type of day care nor the number of children attending day care significantly influenced the relationship between day care attendance and asthma, recurrent wheezing or eczema.

In *Year in Respiratory Medicine 2003* (*YIRM 2003*) I included a paper by the same authors reporting that the risk of wheezing associated with exposure to cats appeared to be determined by the presence of a history of allergy in the mother but not the father |6|. Taken together these papers do suggest that a maternal history is important and represents an area for further research. It would be interesting to see the results of a study where the offspring of mothers with asthma were randomized to attend day care or not.

In line with the hygiene hypothesis it has been suggested that attending day care may render the child more likely to contract a greater number of infectious illnesses |34–37|. As I reviewed last year in *YIRM 2003*, children who experienced two or more episodes of runny nose before the age of 1 year were less likely to have physician-diagnosed asthma at 7 years or wheeze. They were also less likely to be atopic before the age of 5 years. Reporting one or more viral infections of the herpes type in the first 3 years of life was inversely associated with asthma at age 7 years |38|.

Fig. 1.2 (a) Adjusted risk ratio of wheezing between the ages of 1 and 6 years for children who attended day care in the first year of life compared with children without exposure to day care in the first year of life. Risk ratios were adjusted for sex, household income, maternal history of asthma, having at least one doctor-diagnosed lower respiratory illness in the first year of life, recurrent nasal catarrh, and bottle feeding before sleep time in the first year of life. (b) Adjusted risk ratio of wheezing between the ages of 1 and 6 years among children without maternal history of asthma who attended day care in the first year of life compared with children without maternal history of asthma without exposure to day care in the first year of life. Risk ratios were adjusted for sex, household income, and having at least one doctor-diagnosed lower respiratory illness in the first year of life. (c) Adjusted risk ratio of wheezing between the ages of 1 and 6 years among children with maternal history of asthma who attended day care in the first year of life compared with children with maternal history of asthma without exposure to day care in the first year of life). Source: Celedón *et al.* (2003).

The authors considered whether the relationship between lower respiratory tract infections in the first year of life and the appearance of asthma at age 6 years might reflect reverse causation, i.e. the risk that the observed finding may be attributed to the fact that children who are asthmatic may be predisposed to lower respiratory tract infections in early life. A further possibility could be that some childhood respiratory infections, such as respiratory syncytial virus, appear to be associated with the later development of asthma |39|.

Urban traffic and pollutant exposure related to respiratory outcomes and atopy in a large sample of children

Nicolai T, Carr D, Weiland SK, *et al. Eur Respir J* 2003; **21**: 956–63

BACKGROUND. This study was designed for determining the relationship between vehicle traffic counts and estimated pollutant levels at the place of residence and reported respiratory symptoms, doctor diagnoses, measured allergic sensitization and respiratory function in a large random sample of children. Random samples of schoolchildren (*n* = 7509) (response rate 83.7%) were studied using the International Study of Asthma and Allergies in Childhood (ISAAC) phase II protocol with skin prick tests, the measurement of specific IgE and lung function. Traffic exposure was assessed via traffic counts and by an emission model that predicted soot, benzene and nitrogen dioxide.

INTERPRETATION. High vehicle traffic density close to the home was related to respiratory complaints such as cough, wheeze and current asthma in children. The authors also found an association between exposure to heavy road traffic and allergic sensitization in a small subgroup additionally exposed to environmental tobacco smoke. High traffic-related air pollution was associated with asthma and cough, but not with allergic sensitization.

Comment

Although there have been considerable improvements in air pollution following reductions in the burning of fossil fuels, there have also been increases in the levels of the pollutants such as ozone, nitrogen dioxide and sulphur dioxide. Thus, air quality remains an important public health issue |40|. Ozone is a secondary pollutant that is derived from the photochemical oxidation of nitrogen dioxide in the presence of sunlight. The development of physician-diagnosed asthma has been associated with playing activity sport in an environment with a high ozone concentration and exposure to ozone has been shown to enhance airway hyper-reactivity in response to house dust mite allergen challenge in children undertaking exercise |41,42|. Nitrogen dioxide and sulphur dioxide have been shown to cause increases in airway hyper-reactivity in the laboratory and have therefore been linked to concerns that peaks in pollution associated with traffic congestion may contribute to exacerbations of asthma.

This study by Nicolai *et al.* followed a population-based design with recruitment of random samples from school classes in two age groups: school beginners aged 5–7 years and school children of the fourth grade aged 9–11 years.

The study population was impressively large. Rather than rely on self-reported exposure the authors employed a computer-based geographical information system for estimating exposure to traffic fumes based on average daily traffic counts. The sum of traffic counts of all street segments within 50 m of the child's home was used for characterizing traffic exposure for an individual child. Further details on their model are provided in a related paper [43]. They suggested that some misclassification of exposure was possible as traffic counts were only available for street segments with greater than 4000 vehicles per day and therefore did not include small side streets.

The authors defined current wheeze, asthma, hay fever and atopic dermatitis on epidemiological grounds. Atopic sensitization was assessed by skin prick tests and serum-specific IgE. A random subsample of the children aged 9–11 years underwent pulmonary function testing including assessment of airway hyper-responsiveness. The participation rates for the allergy tests were lower than for the questionnaire (69.5% skin prick tests), but, except for a slightly higher prevalence of hay fever, there were no significant differences in outcomes or traffic exposure between those for whom skin test data were available and those for whom they were not. This is unlikely to have biased the reported findings.

The main finding from this study was that high levels of traffic exposure were associated with cough, asthma and wheeze in all children. They did not find a relationship between high traffic volume and atopy except in children who were also exposed to environmental tobacco smoke. Cough was associated with soot, benzene and nitrogen dioxide exposure, current asthma with soot and benzene exposure and current wheeze with benzene and nitrogen dioxide exposure.

The questionnaire included potential confounding factors: nationality, family history of atopy, number of siblings, environmental tobacco smoke exposure and parental education as a marker of socio-economic status. Children living close to streets with heavy traffic were from families of lower socio-economic status and were more often exposed to environmental tobacco smoke. There was no evidence of effect modification when the effect of traffic counts on outcomes was stratified for socio-economic status. However, as Munich has no areas of obvious social deprivation, the authors accepted that confounding could not be completely excluded. It is also possible that misclassification of socio-economic status had occurred as this was extrapolated from data on parental education. Interestingly, a Dutch study assessing children living close to a busy motorway showed an effect on asthma only in children with low-to-medium socio-economic status [44].

There was evidence of effect modification when considering environmental tobacco smoke. Among children with environmental tobacco smoke exposure, traffic volume was significantly associated with current asthma and positive skin prick tests to pollen. The cross-sectional design of the study precluded a detailed discussion on causation, but the results are consistent with other studies that have been published and there was some evidence of a dose–response relationship. Certainly among children with environmental tobacco smoke exposure traffic volume was significantly associated with current asthma and positive skin prick tests to pollen. A dose–response effect was observed. The effect of traffic in children without environmental tobacco smoke exposure was significant for cough only. Possible mechanisms have been suggested including the observation that traffic-related pollutants may alter the antigenicity of pollen |45–47|.

Conclusion

A significant and impressive body of epidemiological research continues to be published on asthma and the studies reviewed this year continue to interest and stimulate debate about the mechanisms that underpin the rise in the prevalence of asthma. At present such links as have been described remain largely speculative and it remains difficult to advise individual patients in the consulting room. Nevertheless, they are very interesting and provide a platform for testing a variety of hypotheses. Macaubas *et al.* tackled influences that may act during pregnancy and highlight the potential importance of targeting smoking cessation in pregnant women. The PIAMA Study investigators provide interesting information on the potential role of the diet consumed by children and Svanes *et al.* contribute a substantial amount of information on the topical area of pet exposure. The study by Celedón *et al.* focused attention on the interaction between the environment and genes by exploring the influence of maternal history on the outcome following exposure to day care. Nicolai *et al.* provide information on the role of environmental pollution from traffic and its potential to influence the expression of asthma.

The principle of these studies is that the authors attempted to link an exposure with an outcome, in this case the development of asthma or a surrogate for asthma. The authors attempted to control for background characteristics between the outcome group and the control group, as would be the case in a randomized controlled trial. They then attempted to speculate on the possible links between the two.

When reading these papers it is worth reminding ourselves that the conclusions drawn from observational studies are not always consistent with the results from subsequent randomized, controlled trials |48|. Notable accounts in the medical literature include the influence of hormone replacement therapy (HRT) on the risk of coronary heart disease (CHD) and the influence of diet on lung cancer. Observational studies have suggested that HRT was associated with a reduced risk of CHD, but a randomized, controlled trial failed to support this observation |49,50|. Data from an observational study suggested that dietary carotenoids may reduce the risk of lung cancer, but a subsequent randomized, controlled trial exploring the use of β-carotene was associated with an 18% increase in lung cancer |51,52|. *Caveat emptor!*

References

1. Strachan DP. Hay fever, hygiene and household size. *BMJ* 1989; **299**: 1259–60.

2. Augusto A, Litonjua A, Sparrow D, Weiss ST, O'Connor GT, Long AA, Ohman JL. Sensitisation to cat allergen is associated with asthma in older men and predicts new-onset airway hyperresponsiveness. *Am J Respirat Crit Care Med* 1997; **156**: 23–7.

3. Noretjojo K, Dimich-Ward H, Obata H, Manfreda J, Chan-Yeung M. Exposure and sensitisation to cat dander: asthma and asthma-like symptoms among adults. *J Allergy Clin Immunol* 1999; **104**: 941–7.

4. Custovic A, Hallam CL, Simpson BM, Craven M, Simpson A, Woodcock A. Decreased prevalence of sensitisation to cats with high exposure to cat allergen. *J Allergy Clin Immunol* 2001; **108**: 537–9.

5. Platts-Mills T, Vaughan J, Squillace S, Woodfolk J, Sporik R. Sensitisation, asthma and a modified Th2 response in children exposed to cat allergen: a population-based cross-sectional study. *Lancet* 2001; **357**: 752–6.

6. Celedón JC, Litonjua AA, Ryan L, Platts-Mills T, Weiss ST, Gold DR. Exposure to cat allergen, and wheezing in first 5 years of life. *Lancet* 2002; **360**: 781–2.

7. Leynaert B, Neukirch C, Jarvis D, Chinn S, Burney P, Neukirch F. Does living on a farm during childhood protect against asthma, allergic rhinitis, and atopy in childhood? *Am J Respir Crit Care Med* 2001; **164**: 1829–34.

8. Reidler J, Braun-Fahrländer C, Eder W, Schreuer M, Waser M, Maisch S, Carr D, Schierl R, Nowak D, Von Mutius E and the ALEX Study Team. Exposure to farming in early life and development of asthma and allergy: a cross-sectional study. *Lancet* 2001; **358**: 1129–33.

9. Sears MR, Greene JM, Willan AR, Taylor DR, Flannery EM, Cown JO, Herbison GP, Poulton R. Long-term relation between breastfeeding and development of atopy and asthma in young adults. *Lancet* 2002; **360**: 901–7.

10. Kalliomäki M, Salminen S, Arvilommi H, Kero P, Koskinen P, Isolauri E. Probiotics in primary prevention of atopic disease: a randomised placebo controlled trial. *Lancet* 2001; **357**: 1076–9.

11. Shaheen SO, Sterne JAC, Thompson RL, Songhurst CE, Margetts BM, Burney PGJ. Dietary antioxidants and asthma in adults: population based case–control study. *Am J Respir Crit Care* 2001; **164**: 1823–8.

12. Celedón JC, Palmer LJ, Litonjua AA, Weiss ST, Wang B, Fang Z, Xu X. Body mass index and asthma in adults in families of subjects with asthma in Anqing, China. *Am J Respir Crit Care Med* 2001; **164**: 1835–40.

13. Castro-Rodriguez JA, Holberg CJ, Morgan WJ, Wright AL, Martinez FD. Increased incidence of asthmalike symptoms in girls who become overweight or obese during the school years. *Am J Respir Crit Care Med* 2001; **163**: 1344–9.

14. Tantisira KG, Weiss ST. Complex interactions in complex traits: obesity and asthma. *Thorax* 2001; **56** (Suppl II): ii64–74.

15. McConnell R, Berhane K, Gilliland F, London SJ, Islam T, Gauderman WJ, Avol E, Margolis HG, Peters JM. Asthma in exercising children exposed to ozone: a cohort study. *Lancet* 2002; **359**: 386–91.

16. Brunekreef B, Sunyer J. Asthma, rhinitis and air pollution: is traffic to blame? *Eur Respir J* 2003; **21**: 913–15.

17. Venn AJ, Lewis SA, Cooper M, Hubbard R, Briton J. Living near a main road and the risk of wheezing illness in children. *Am J Respir Crit Care Med* 2001; **164**: 2177–80.

18. Van Eerdwegh P, Little RD, Dupuis J, Del Mastro RG, Falls K, Simon J, Torrey D, Pandit S, McKenny J, Braunschweiger K, Walsh A, Liu Z, Hayward B, Folz C, Manning SP, Bawa A, Saracino L, Thackston M, Benchekroun Y, Capparell N, Wang M, Adair R, Feng Y, Dubois J, Fitzgerald MG, Huang H, Gibson R, Allen KM, Pedan A, Danzig MR, Umland SP, Egan RW, Cuss FM, Rorke S, Clough JB, Holloway JW, Holgate ST, Keith TP. Association of the ADAM33 gene with asthma and bronchial hyperresponsiveness. *Nature* 2002; **418**: 426–30.

19. Holberg CJ, Halonen M. Cytokines, atopy and asthma. *Lancet* 2003; **362**: 1166–7.

20. Rubin D. Estimating causal effects from large data sets using propensity scores. *Ann Intern Med* 1997; **127**: 757–63.

21. Holt PG, Clough JB, Holt BJ, Baron-Hay MJ, Ross AH, Robertson BW, Thomas WR. Genetic risk for atopy is associated with delayed postnatal maturation of T-cell competence. *Clin Exp Allergy* 1992; **22**: 1093–9.

22. Salvi S, Babu KS, Holgate ST. Is asthma really due to a polarised T cell response toward a helper T cell type 2 phenotype? *Am J Respir Crit Care Med* 2001; **164**: 1343–6.

23. Stick SM, Burton PR, Gurrin L, Sly PD, LeSouef PN. Effects of maternal smoking during pregnancy and a family history of asthma on respiratory function in newborn infants. *Lancet* 1996; **348**: 1060–4.

24. Hoo A, Matthias H, Dezateux C, Costeloe K, Stocks J. Respiratory function among preterm infants whose mothers smoke during pregnancy. *Am J Respirat Crit Care Med* 1998; **158**: 700–5.

25. Ouyang Y, Virasch N, Hao P, Aubrey MT, Mukerjee N, Bierer BE, Freed BM. Suppression of human IL-1β, IL-2, IFN, and TNF production by cigarette smoke extracts. *J Allergy Clin Immunol* 2000; **106**: 280–7.

26. Willet W. Reproducibility and validity of food frequency questionnaires. In: Willet W (ed). *Nutritional Epidemiology*, 2nd edn. Oxford: Oxford University Press, 1998: 101–47.

27. Shaheen SO, Sterne JAC, Thompson RL, Songhurst CE, Margetts BM, Burney PGJ. Dietary antioxidants and asthma in adults: population based case–control study. *Am J Respir Crit Care* 2001; **164**: 1823–8.

28. Martinez FD, Wright AL, Taussig LM, Holberg CJ, Halonen M, Morgan WJ. Asthma and wheezing in the first 6 years of life. The Group Health Medical Associates. *N Engl J Med* 1995; **332**: 133–8.

29. Phelan PD, Robertson CF, Olinsky A. The Melbourne Asthma Study: 1964–1999. *J Allergy Clin Immunol* 2002; **109**: 189–94.

30. Perzanowski MS, Ronmark E, Platts-Mills TA, Lundback B. Effect of car and dog ownership on sensitisation and development of asthma among preteenage children. *Am J Respir Crit Care Med* 2002; **166**: 696–702.

31. Litonjua AA, Milton DK, Celedón JC, Ryan L, Weiss ST, Gold DR. A longitudinal analysis of wheezing in young children: the independent effects of early life exposure to house dust endotoxin, allergens, and pets. *J Allergy Clin Immunol* 2002; **110**: 781–2.

32. Ball TM, Castro-Rodriguez JA, Griffith KA, Holberg CJ, Martinez FD, Wright AL. Siblings, day-care attendance, and the risk of asthma and wheezing during childhood. *N Engl J Med* 2000; **343**: 538–43.

33. Kramer U, Heinrich J, Wjst M, Wichmann HE. Age of entry to day nursery and allergy in later childhood. *Lancet* 1999; **353**: 450–4.

34. Marbury MC, Maldonado G, Walker L. Lower respiratory illness, recurrent wheezing, and day care attendance. *Am J Respir Crit Care Med* 1997; **155**: 156–61.

35. Celedón JC, Litonjua AA, Weiss ST, Gold DR. Day care attendance in the first year of life and illnesses of the upper and lower respiratory tract in children with a familial history of atopy. *Pediatrics* 1999; **104**: 495–500.

36. Celedón JC, Litonjua AA, Ryan L, Weiss ST, Gold DR. Day care attendance, respiratory tract illnesses, wheezing, asthma, and total serum IgE level in early childhood. *Arch Pediatr Adolesc Med* 2002; **156**: 241–5.

37. Nafstad P, Hagen J, Oie L, Magnus P, Jouni JK. Day care centres and respiratory health. *Pediatrics* 1999; **103**: 753–8.

38. Illi S, von Mutius E, Lau S, Bergmann R, Niggemann B, Sommerfeld C, Wahn U, MAS Group. Early childhood infectious disease and the development of asthma up to school age: a birth cohort study. *BMJ* 2001; **322**: 390–5.

39. Stein RT, Sherrill D, Morgan WJ, Holberg CJ, Halonon M, Taussig LM, Wright AL, Martinez FD. Respiratory syncytial virus in early life and risk of wheeze and allergy by age 13 years. *Lancet* 1999; **354**: 541–5.

40. Koren HS. Associations between criteria air pollutants and asthma. *Environ Health Perspect* 1995; **103**(Suppl): 235–42.

41. McConnell R, Berhane K, Gilliland F, London SJ, Islam T, Gauderman WJ, Avol E, Margolis HG, Peters JM. Asthma in exercising children exposed to ozone: a cohort study. *Lancet* 2002; **359**: 386–91.

42. Kehrl HR, Peden DB, Ball B, Folinsbee LJ, Horsman D. Increased specific airway reactivity of persons with mild allergic asthma after 7.6 hours of exposure to 0.16 ppm ozone. *J Allergy Clin Immunol* 1999; **104**: 1198–204.

43. Carr D, Von Ehrenstein O, Weiland S, Wagner C, Wellie O, Nicolai T, von Mutius E. Modelling annual benzene, toluene, NO_2, and soot concentrations on the basis of road traffic characteristics. *Environ Res* 2002; **90**: 111–18.

44. Van Vilet P, Knape M, De Hartog J, Janssen N, Harssema H, Brunekreef B. Motor vehicle exhaust and chronic respiratory symptoms in children living near freeways. *Environ Res* 1997; **74**: 122–32.

45. Emberlin J. Interaction between air pollutants and aero-allergens. *Clin Exp Allergy* 1995; **25**(Suppl 3): 33–9.

46. Knox RB, Suphioglu C, Taylor P, Desai R, Watson HC, Peng JL, Bursill LA. Major grass pollen allergen Lol p 1 binds to diesel exhaust particles: implications for asthma and air pollution. *Clin Exp Allergy* 1997; **27**: 246–51.

47. Behrendt H, Becker WM, Fritsche C, Sliwa-Tomczok W, Tomczok J, Friedrichs KH, Ring J. Air pollution and allergy: experimental studies on modulation of allergen release from pollen by air pollutants. *Int Arch Allergy Immunol* 1997; **113**: 69–74.

48. Davey Smith G, Ebrahim S. Data dredging, bias or confounding: they can all get you into the *BMJ* and the Friday papers. *BMJ* 2002; **325**: 1437–8.

49. Stampfer MJ, Colditz GA. Estrogen replacement therapy and coronary heart disease: a quantitative assessment of the epidemiologic evidence. *Prevent Med* 1991; **20**: 47–63.

50. Beral V, Banks F, Reeves G. Evidence from randomised trials on the long-term effects of hormone replacement therapy. *Lancet* 2002; **360**: 942–4.

51. Willet WC. Vitamin A and lung cancer. *Nutr Rev* 1990; **48**: 201–11.

52. Alpha-tocopherol, Beta-carotene Cancer Prevention Study Group. The effect of vitamin E and beta-carotene on the incidence of lung cancer and other cancers in male smokers. *N Engl J Med* 1994; **330**: 1029–35.

2

The course and prognosis of asthma

Introduction

The reporting of large prospective studies is essential for providing information on the course and prognosis of asthma. Such information is clearly important to patients and their carers, but also assists with the identification of factors that may be associated with perpetuation of the disease process. In *Year in Respiratory Medicine 2003* (*YIRM 2003*) I included papers illustrating that asthma in childhood was more common in boys and carried a favourable prognosis if it persisted for less than 5 years |1|. However, it is recognized that abnormalities of lung function, including airway hyper-reactivity, may persist during remission and herald the relapse of asthma in later life |2–4|. I also included a cross-sectional study reporting the persistence of airway inflammation during clinical remission |5|. Asthma appearing post-puberty is more common in women and tends to be persistent |1,6|. This year I include two studies that have enrolled patients from large birth cohorts that provide further insight into this subject.

Fortunately an increased understanding of the inflammatory nature of asthma leading to an emphasis on the use of inhaled corticosteroid therapy has meant that, for the majority of patients, asthma control is relatively straightforward. Nevertheless, an important minority of patients continue to experience severe persistent asthma. These patients typically use more medication (including high doses of inhaled steroids), use more healthcare services and experience a low quality of life. Perhaps even more importantly they appear to be at increased risk of asthma death |7|. This year I have included several papers that focus on this important subgroup of patients attempting to identify the factors that are associated with this particular form of the disease.

Longitudinal study of childhood wheezy bronchitis and asthma: outcome at age 42

Horak E, Lanigan A, Roberts M, *et al. BMJ* 2003; **326**: 422–3

BACKGROUND. The authors wished to determine whether the prognosis of asthma was related to the severity of childhood symptoms and used data from a large

Table 2.1 Distribution of asthma and lung function in participants aged 42 years according to the severity of asthma at age 7 or 10

Symptoms age 7	No. (%) at age 42					Lung function at age 42		
	No recent asthma ($n = 199$)	Infrequent asthma ($n = 58$)	Frequent asthma ($n = 76$)	Persistent asthma ($n = 70$)	Total ($n = 403$)	No. measured ($n = 267$)	FEV$_1$/FVC (95% CI)	Mean % of predicted FEV$_1$ (95% CI)
Mild wheezy bronchitis	40 (66)	12 (20)	9 (15)	0	61	40	80 (79–82)	109 (103–114)
Wheezy bronchitis	50 (57)	13 (15)	16 (18)	9 (10)	88	62	79 (76–81)	102 (98–106)
Asthma	28 (29)	19 (19)	27 (28)	24 (24)	98	70	75* (73–77)	95* (92–99)
Severe asthma	8 (11)	9 (13)	20 (29)	33 (47)	70	42	70* (67–74)	85* (78–91)
Control	73 (85)	5 (6)	4 (5)	4 (5)	86	53	80 (78–82)	104 (101–108)

FEV$_1$, forced exploratory volume in 1 second; FVC, forced vital capacity.
* P <0.001 compared with controls.
Source: Horak et al. (2003).

longitudinal study (The Melbourne Epidemiological Study of Childhood Asthma) for reporting outcome data at age 42 years.

INTERPRETATION. The distribution of severity at age 42 years had not changed from that at age 35 years. The proportion of cases with no recent asthma increased steadily from 20% at age 14 years to 40% at age 42 years. Most children with intermittent symptoms associated with respiratory tract infections had complete resolution of symptoms in adult life. Participants who had asthma aged 7 years had reduced lung function at age 42 years (Table 2.1).

A longitudinal, population-based, cohort study of childhood asthma followed to adulthood

Sears MR, Greene JM, Willan AR, *et al. N Engl J Med* 2003; **349**: 1414–22

BACKGROUND. The outcome of childhood asthma remains unclear and such studies that have been reported have included carefully selected cohorts that may not reflect the breadth of asthma seen in the general population. The aim of this study was to report the outcome of asthma from a large, unselected, population-based cohort recruited in Dunedin, New Zealand.

INTERPRETATION. More than one in four children with wheeze reported persistence or relapse of asthma in adulthood. The factors predicting persistence or relapse included sensitization to house dust mites, airway hyper-responsiveness, female sex, smoking and an early age of onset (Fig. 2.1).

Comment

These studies provide important information on the prognosis of wheeze and asthma in childhood. The Melbourne Epidemiological Study of Childhood Asthma recruited children aged 7 years and then followed them through adolescence and adulthood. They classified their subjects as controls (children who had never wheezed), mild wheezy bronchitis (less than five episodes of wheeze associated with respiratory tract infection), wheezy bronchitis (five or more episodes of wheeze associated with respiratory tract infection), asthma (wheeze not associated with respiratory tract infection) and severe asthma (onset of symptoms at less than 3 years, persistent symptoms aged 10 years and a barrel chest deformity or forced expiratory volume in 1 s:forced vital capacity [FEV$_1$:FVC] ratio ≤50%).

The authors found that the pattern of asthma during childhood provided important information on the outcome. Children with intermittent symptoms of wheezy bronchitis by and large reported resolution of their symptoms and displayed normal lung function. Indeed, the proportion of cases with no recent asthma increased from 20% aged 14 years to 40% aged 42 years, but had not changed appreciably from data reported at the age of 35 years [8]. Thus, this paper provided grounds for optimism for most patients with childhood wheeze. In line with other studies, the presence of

Age at assessment (yr)   **Classification**

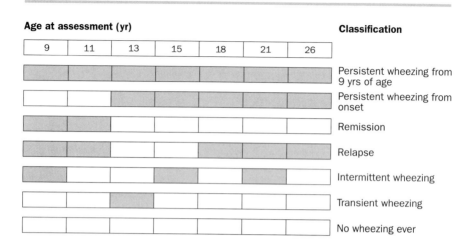

Fig. 2.1 Patterns of wheezing (shaded bars) in childhood reported by study members or their parents illustrating definitions of persistent wheezing, remission, relapse, intermittent wheezing, transient wheezing and no wheezing ever. Source: Sears *et al.* (2003).

asthma in childhood was associated with a greater likelihood of persistence into adulthood and reduced lung function at age 42 years.

The Dunedin Multidisciplinary Health and Development Study was a longitudinal investigation of health and behaviour in a complete birth cohort. Study members were born in Dunedin between April 1972 and March 1973 and represented the full range of socio-economic status in New Zealand's South Island. The children recruited to the study were subject to a detailed follow-up that included periodic respiratory questionnaires and lung function measurements. Airway hyperresponsiveness to methacholine, atopy and responsiveness to bronchodilators were also assessed at various time points (Table 2.2). This paper presented data from this cohort followed into adulthood and provided valuable data into the risk factors that are associated with persistence or relapse of childhood asthma and pulmonary function outcomes (Table 2.3).

Wheeze was very common, being reported at some time by 72.6% of the cohort. The authors suggested that this might represent an overestimate from the true sample as only 613 study members provided study data at every assessment and this group had a higher prevalence of respiratory symptoms than those who did not. They considered but discounted bias due to the longitudinal design of their study, as their results were broadly similar to a cross-sectional study performed elsewhere in New Zealand |9|. Thus, wheeze in childhood may be common, but is usually transient.

Symptoms of as ˙   ed in over one-third of those who reported wheezing. Approximately hal   d persistent symptoms from childhood and the other

Table 2.2 Characteristics of study members with different patterns of wheezing*

Characteristic	Wheezing pattern						P for trend†
	Persistent from onset	Relapse	Remission	Intermittent	Transient	Never wheezed	
	Per cent (number of study members with data)						
Male sex	44.9 (89)	53.9 (76)	53.3 (92)	51.7 (58)	48.5 (130)	56.0 (168)	—
Smoking at 18 yr	40.5 (89)	35.5 (76)	31.5 (92)	37.9 (58)	30.8 (130)	14.9 (168)	—
Smoking at 26 yr	46.1 (89)	43.4 (76)	35.9 (92)	43.1 (58)	32.3 (130)	19.6 (168)	—
Father smoked when study member was a child	39.8 (88)	56.6 (76)	54.4 (92)	62.1 (58)	50.0 (130)	44.1 (168)	—
Mother smoked when study member was a child	37.1 (89)	40.8 (76)	46.7 (92)	50.0 (58)	36.9 (130)	38.7 (168)	—
Positive skin test for house dust mite allergen at 13 yr	55.7 (88)	54.9 (71)	35.6 (87)	30.4 (56)	23.3 (129)	12.7 (166)	<0.001
Positive skin test for cat allergen at 13 yr	28.4 (88)	26.8 (71)	21.8 (87)	14.3 (56)	7.8 (129)	4.2 (166)	<0.001
Positive skin test for house dust mite allergen at 21 yr	77.5 (80)	73.9 (69)	64.8 (88)	55.6 (54)	54.8 (124)	43.2 (162)	<0.001
Positive skin test for cat allergen at 21 yr	53.8 (80)	47.8 (69)	35.2 (88)	24.1 (54)	18.6 (124)	11.7 (162)	<0.001
$PC_{20} \leq 8$ mg/ml or BDR $\geq$10% at 9 yr	42.5 (87)	43.1 (72)	23.9 (92)	15.5 (58)	5.6 (126)	3.6 (165)	<0.001
$PC_{20} \leq 8$ mg/ml or BDR $\geq$10% at any assessment from 9–21 yr	52.8 (89)	56.6 (76)	31.5 (92)	27.6 (58)	8.6 (128)	7.2 (167)	<0.001
FEV_1 at 26 yr (% of predicted)	96.6 (85)	95.7 (76)	100.6 (89)	103.7 (58)	102.5 (126)	105.6 (161)	<0.001
FEV_1:FVC at 26 yr (%)‡	78.0 (86)	79.1 (76)	83.1 (89)	82.2 (58)	83.4 (126)	83.7 (162)	<0.001
Firstborn	41.6 (89)	32.9 (76)	32.6 (92)	34.5 (58)	36.2 (130)	43.5 (168)	—
Breast-fed $\geq$4 wk	57.3 (89)	52.6 (76)	59.8 (92)	37.9 (58)	49.2 (130)	51.2 (168)	—

* PC_{20} denotes the concentration of methacholine causing a 20% decrease in the forced expiratory volume in one second (FEV_1), BDR the response of FEV_1 to a bronchodilator (increase from baseline), and FVC the forced vital capacity.
† The trend is across categories of frequency from persistent from onset to never wheezed.
‡ FEV_1 (% of predicted) was based on a prediction formula from New Zealand population and was measured without the use of a bronchodilator.
Source: Sears et al. (2003).

Table 2.3 Odds ratios for factors predicting persistence of wheezing from onset to the age of 26 years or relapse by the age of 26 years*

Model	Persistence		Relapse	
	OR (95% CI)	P value	OR (95% CI)	P value
Univariate				
PC_{20} or BDR at 9 yr	4.32 (2.64–7.06)	<0.001	6.82 (3.89–11.95)	<0.001
$PC_{20} \leq 8$ mg/ml at any assessment from 9–15 yr	4.24 (2.64–6.79)	<0.001	6.93 (4.07–11.77)	<0.001
$PC_{20} \leq 8$ mg/ml or BDR at any assessment to 21 yr	4.13 (2.59–6.59)	<0.001	7.22 (4.29–12.17)	<0.001
Positive skin test for house dust mite allergen at 13 yr	3.38 (2.12–5.37)	<0.001	4.17 (2.49–7.01)	<0.001
Positive skin test for cat allergen at 13 yr	2.81 (1.65–4.79)	<0.001	3.27 (1.78–6.03)	<0.001
Smoking at 21 yr	2.05 (1.30–3.24)	0.002	1.84 (1.11–3.04)	0.02
Father smoked when study member was a child	0.63 (0.40–1.00)	0.05	1.29 (0.79–2.11)	0.31
Mother smoked when study member was a child	0.84 (0.53–1.37)	0.46	0.98 (0.60–1.61)	0.93
Family history of wheezing	1.44 (0.92–2.27)	0.11	1.59 (0.98–2.60)	0.06
Age at onset of wheezing†	0.97 (0.94–1.01)	0.11	0.87 (0.83–0.91)	<0.001
Female sex	1.37 (0.87–2.16)	0.17	0.95 (0.58–1.55)	0.84
Multivariate (significant factors only)				
$PC_{20} \leq 8$ mg/ml or BDR >10% at any assessment from 9–21 yr	3.00 (1.71–5.26)	<0.001	3.03 (1.65–5.55)	<0.001
Positive skin test for house dust mite allergen at 13 yr	2.41 (1.42–4.09)	0.001	2.18 (1.18–4.00)	0.01
Female sex	1.71 (1.04–2.82)	0.03	–	–
Smoking at 21 yr	1.84 (1.13–3.00)	0.01	–	–
Age at onset wheezing†	–	–	0.89 (0.85–0.94)	<0.001

* The odds ratio (OR) for persistence of wheezing is for the comparison with all other study members except those who never reported wheezing. The OR for relapse is for the comparison with all other study members except those with persistent wheezing and those who never reported wheezing. CI denotes confidence interval, PC_{20} the concentration of methacholine causing a 20-percent decrease in the forced expiratory volume in one second (FEV_1), and BDR the response of the FEV_1 to a bronchodilator (increase from base line).
† The OR was calculated for persistence or relapse per year of increase in the age at onset (i.e., a later age at onset was protective).
Source: Sears *et al.* (2003).

half appeared to have suffered a relapse. Relapse appeared to be more likely when the onset of asthma had been at an early age. Indeed, a 10-year later age at onset reduced the risk of relapse by 69%.

Both studies provided important information on the outcome of lung function in patients with a history of childhood wheeze and asthma. In the study reported by Horak *et al.* most children with severe asthma reported symptoms that persisted into adulthood and these individuals had significant reductions in lung function, while Sears *et al.*'s study provided information suggesting that the impairment in lung function observed in some adult asthmatic patients may be evident during childhood and persist. Lung function was first measured at the age of 9 years and those patients with persistently abnormal lung function throughout childhood also displayed reduced lung function in adulthood. This is known as tracking. Greater impairment in lung function was reported in those with airway hyper-responsiveness and in those treated with inhaled corticosteroids, but the authors suggested the latter observation is likely to represent confounding by severity, with the use of inhaled corticosteroids reflecting greater disease severity.

These papers extend the findings from a large UK study that reported the presence of reduced lung function in adult asthmatic patients who reported a history of persistent wheeze throughout childhood and adolescence [10]. In the study by Sears *et al.* there was no difference in the rate of decline of lung function, although this has been reported in other studies [11]. A similar study from Aberdeen, UK, reported the 25-year follow-up of 455 subjects randomly collected from a community survey and found that those who had suffered from asthma in childhood had significantly lower FEV_1 (% predicted) values than children who wheezed only in the presence of infection and children with no history of respiratory illness [12]. The lowest values were reported from patients with a history of persistent symptoms. However, the authors have recently written to the *British Medical Journal* World Wide Web site reporting that further follow-up showed that those with a history of wheezy bronchitis in childhood had a decline in FEV_1 similar to those with childhood asthma [13].

Sears *et al.* also provided a strong public health message with regard to cigarette smoking, which unfortunately remains common in young people in Western society, particularly so in young women. In common with other studies, smoking at 21 years of age was associated with both persistent wheezing and relapse of wheezing [14].

Persistent wheeze at age 26 years was associated with a higher prevalence of sensitivity to house dust mites and cat allergen and lower lung function measurements compared to those whose wheeze did not persist or relapse. However, the highest odds ratio (OR) of either persistence or relapse was associated with the presence of airway hyper-reactivity between the ages of 9 and 21 years. This observation reinforces observations made by others that airway hyper-reactivity is an important adverse prognostic indictor [15,16].

Thus, in summary, the persistence of asthma appears to be associated with allergy to house dust mites, smoking, airway hyper-responsiveness and being female. The factors predicting relapse include allergy to house dust mites, airway hyper-responsiveness and an early age of onset.

Exposure and sensitization to indoor allergens: association with lung function, bronchial reactivity and exhaled nitric oxide measures in asthma

Langley SJ, Goldthorpe S, Craven M, Morris J, Woodcock A, Custovic A.

J Allergy Clin Immunol 2003; **112**: 362–8

BACKGROUND. Animal models have suggested that chronic exposure to allergens to which they are sensitized leads to chronic airway inflammation and structural airway wall remodelling |17,18|. The authors speculated that chronic exposure to allergens over long periods of time might lead to irreversible airway obstruction and severe airway hyper-reactivity. They therefore set out to explore the relationship between allergen exposure in the home and its interaction with sensitization on asthma control and severity in adults. The authors measured pulmonary function, exhaled nitric oxide and airway hyper-reactivity. They performed home visits and assessed allergen exposure by sampling vacuumed dust for the allergens Der p 1, Fel d 1 and Can f 1.

INTERPRETATION. Patients with asthma who are sensitized and exposed to an allergen they encounter in their own home have a more severe form of the asthma as assessed by FEV_1, exhaled nitric oxide and airway hyper-reactivity.

Comment

The formation of circulating immunoglobulin E (IgE) antibodies to allergens appears to be important to the expression of the asthmatic phenotype |19|. Indeed, atopy has been recognized as a risk factor with a strong influence on the emergence of persistent asthma |20|. House dust mites are a major source of allergens and significant exposure in sensitized individuals is recognized in the development of asthma with those exposed to the highest levels reporting more severe disease |21|. The principal allergenic component is the protease Der p 1, which is found in their faeces. Other important allergens include exposure to pets, particularly cats (Fel d 1) and dogs (Can f 1).

This study was designed for exploring the possible role between exposure to sensitizing allergens and the level of asthma severity. The authors recruited patients with physician-diagnosed asthma from both primary and secondary care and examined the relationship between the severity of asthma, as judged by pulmonary function, airway hyper-reactivity and exhaled nitric oxide and exposure to house dust mites, cats and dogs. They divided their subjects into four groups on the basis of sensitization and exposure.

1. Not sensitized and not exposed to any study allergens.
2. Sensitized but not exposed to any study allergens.
3. Not sensitized but exposed to any study allergens.
4. Sensitized and exposed to one or more study allergen.

Table 2.4 Analysis of pulmonary function in relation to allergen sensitization and exposure status

	Mean GM (95% CI)				Overall ANOVA	S/E vs all other subgroups Linear contrast	2-sample t test
	NS/NE	S/NE	NS/E	S/E			
FEV$_1$ % predicted	(n = 21) 92.9 (85.2–100.6)	(n = 73) 86.9 (81.9–92.0)	(n = 61) 90.8 (85.9–95.7)	(n = 118) 83.7 (79.6–87.7)	F(3269) = 2.2; P = 0.086	t(269) = 2.4; P = 0.018	t(271) = 2.2; P = 0.029; mean = 83.7 vs 89.3; mean difference = 5.6; 95% CI = 0.6–10.6
PD$_{20}$	(n = 15) 0.70 (0.29–1.72)	(n = 47) 0.54 (0.32–0.90)	(n = 31) 1.03 (0.53–1.97)	(n = 65) 0.25 (0.16–0.37)	F(3154) = 5.7; P = 0.001 S/E significantly lower than NS/E	t(154) = 3.8; P = <0.001	t(156) = 3.8; P = <0.001; GM = 0.25 vs 0.70; mean ratio difference = 2.9; 95% CI = 1.6–4.8
eNO	(n = 20) 6.8 (4.9–9.4)	(n = 59) 11.2 (9.2–13.6)	(n = 57) 7.8 (6.1–9.9)	(n = 104) 12.9 (10.9–15.3)	F(3236) = 6.3; P = 0.001 S/E significantly higher than NS/E and NS/NE	t(236) = 3.7; P = <0.001	t(238) = 3.3; P = 0.001; GM = 12.9 vs 8.9; mean ratio difference = 0.7; 95% CI = (0.6–0.9)

Source: Langley et al. (2003).
GM, geometric mean; NS/NE, not sensitized and not exposed; S/NE, sensitized but not exposed; NS/E, not sensitized but exposed; S/E, sensitized and exposed; ANOVA, analysis of variance; eNO, exhaled nitric oxide.

They found that subjects in the group that was sensitized and exposed to one or more study allergen had a significantly lower percentage predicted FEV_1, greater bronchial hyper-reactivity and higher exhaled nitric oxide values (Table 2.4). Examining individual allergens they found that patients who were both sensitized and exposed to house dust mites displayed greater airway hyper-reactivity and higher exhaled nitric oxide. Subjects who were both sensitized and exposed to cat allergen displayed significantly lower pulmonary function and greater airway hyper-reactivity and exhaled nitric oxide. Those who were sensitized and exposed to dog allergen displayed significant differences in airway hyper-reactivity and exhaled nitric oxide, but not lung function.

Endogenous nitric oxide is detectable in exhaled breath and appears to be important in the regulation of airway tone. Levels of measurable endogenous nitric oxide are increased in patients with asthma and this is believed to be because the airway epithelium in patients with asthma shows enhanced expression of the genes that up-regulate nitric oxide |22,23|. As a marker it does appear to be biologically relevant as increases in endogenous nitric oxide are observed following allergen challenge and the levels of endogenous nitric oxide appear to correlate with the level of sputum eosinophilia and the degree of airway hyper-reactivity |24,25|. Therapy with inhaled corticosteroids decreases endogenous nitric oxide |26|.

Although this paper strengthens the links between sensitization, exposure and the expression of disease, studies demonstrating that reduction or avoidance of allergens are associated with clinically relevant improvements are lacking. High altitude, as a means of mite avoidance, has been shown to be associated with improvements in clinical parameters, lung function and inflammation |27,28|. Last year I included a paper examining the effect of mite-impermeable mattress covers, which, despite reducing house dust mite levels in bedding, did not lead to clinically relevant improvements in asthma control |29| and this year I have included a paper by Woodcock *et al.* (from the same group as this study) with similarly disappointing results |30| (see Chapter 3).

The ENFUMOSA cross-sectional European multicentre study of the clinical phenotype of chronic severe asthma

European Network for Understanding Mechanisms of Severe Asthma Study Group. *Eur Respir J* 2003; **22**: 470–7

BACKGROUND. Severe asthma accounts for approximately 10% of the asthmatic population, but has a major impact on morbidity and healthcare costs. The European Network for Understanding Mechanisms of Severe Asthma (ENFUMOSA) was established in order to investigate the mechanisms that underpin severe disease. This paper reported the findings from the first cross-sectional analysis and compared clinical, physiological and laboratory measures in subjects with severe asthma and a similar sized cohort of patients whose asthma was controlled by low to moderate doses of inhaled corticosteroids.

INTERPRETATION. The clinical and physiological characteristics of severe asthma suggest that it may be a different disease. It is more common in women, particularly when overweight and it appears that infection may be a more important trigger factor than allergy.

Comment

Patients with severe persistent asthma are fortunately a minority, but represent an important subgroup of patients who continue to experience ongoing symptoms and frequent exacerbations |7|. They make a significant contribution to asthma-related health expenditure |31|. However, little is known about the mechanisms that contribute to severe persistent asthma. Atopy has been recognized as an important factor with regard to the persistence of childhood asthma and, as we have seen from the above discussion (Langley *et al.*), may be related to the presence of more severe asthma in adult life |32|. Nevertheless, asthma is a heterogeneous condition and it is likely that mechanisms other than atopy may be relevant. We are already aware that patients with aspirin-sensitive asthma display a severe and persistent form of the disease |33|.

The ENFUMOSA Study Group consists of twelve European centres that have developed a common methodology for the reporting of patients with severe asthma with the aim of beginning to characterize and unravel the mechanisms leading to severe persistent disease. They enrolled patients under the age of 45 years of age who had a diagnosis of asthma that was verified by a specialist and was accompanied by evidence of variable airways obstruction in the previous 5 years. Asthma severity was then classified according to their regular inhaled corticosteroid dose and the number of exacerbations experienced in the previous year. Inclusion in the severe asthma group required one asthma exacerbation in the previous year despite treatment with ≥1200 μg/day beclomethasone or budesonide or equivalent (or 500 μg/day fluticasone or equivalent). An exacerbation was defined as either the initiation of a course of oral corticosteroid therapy in those on regular inhaled corticosteroid treatment or a temporary increase in the dose of oral corticosteroids in those requiring maintenance systemic corticosteroids.

The patients were characterized by a thorough clinical examination recording skin prick tests to a range of allergens. Further assessment included detailed pulmonary function tests including the measurement of spirometry, bronchodilator reversibility, lung volumes and gas transfer. A battery of blood tests included IgE and arterial samples. Patients provided samples of induced sputum, exhaled breath and urine for analysis of inflammatory markers.

A total of 321 patients were recruited comprising 163 with severe and 158 with mild to moderate asthma. The duration of asthma was the same in both groups, but in multiple linear regression analysis severe asthma was associated with female sex (OR = 2.69 and 95% confidence interval [CI] = 1.62–4.49), perennial symptoms (OR = 2.9 and 95% CI = 1.8–4.5) and exacerbations during the autumn (OR = 2.42 and 95% CI = 1.19–4.94). Negative associations were found for mother's history of atopy and a history of allergic rhinitis.

The finding that severe asthma was more common in females was consistent across all participating regions. This raises the possibility that severe asthma is sex related and identifies an area of further investigation. A further interesting observation was that the women with severe asthma had a greater body mass index (BMI) than women with mild to moderate asthma. We are already aware that weight gain (particularly in women) is associated with the development of asthma. In a prospective study of 85 911 women enrolled in the Nurses' Health Study, the relative risk of incident asthma was 2.7 (95% CI = 2.3–3.1) for women with a BMI of $\geq$30 kg/m^2 compared with those with a BMI of between 20.0 and 22.4 kg/m^2 [34]. A further study published in 2001 followed a cohort of 4547 African-American and white adults (18–30 years) participating in the Coronary Artery Risk Development in Young Adults Study [35] and in *YIRM 2003* I included a longitudinal study from Spanish authors reporting that females who became overweight between the ages of 6 and 13 years were more likely to develop new asthma symptoms [36]. Why this should be so remains unclear, but it represents an important public health message and is a potentially modifiable risk factor [37,38].

Atopy was inversely related to asthma severity with the geometric mean total serum IgE being 109 (95% CI = 85–139 units) in patients with severe asthma compared to 148 (95% CI = 118–188 units) in patients with mild to moderate asthma. In a multiple linear regression model controlling for the number of positive skin prick tests, age and sex, the serum total IgE was not associated with asthma severity. The authors raised the possibility that infections (particularly fungal, viral and atypical organisms) rather than allergy may be more important in patients with severe asthma.

The lung function tests in patients with severe asthma displayed a lower baseline FEV_1, lower FEV_1:FVC ratio, a significantly reduced vital capacity and an increased residual volume (RV). There was a trend towards an increased RV: total lung capacity (TLC) ratio and a marginally reduced gas transfer (K_{CO}). They were slightly hypoxic and hypocapnic at rest. Patients had been excluded if they had a smoking history of more than five pack years (one pack year = 20 cigarettes per day for one year) and if they had started smoking before the diagnosis of their asthma, making confounding by chronic obstructive pulmonary disease (COPD) unlikely, so this finding supports the concerns that patients with severe asthma develop fixed airflow limitation.

The study also provides insight into the inflammatory reaction in patients with severe asthma. Analysis of induced sputum showed that patients with severe asthma had a greater number of neutrophils, but there was no difference in the number or proportion of eosinophils or other leukocytes. This is interesting from two points. In the first instance it raises the possibility of corticosteroid resistance [39]. Assuming that these patients were adherent with therapy, the persisting eosinophilia and indeed exhaled nitric oxide and urinary excretion of leukotriene E_4 suggests an ongoing inflammatory response. The second highlights the observations by others that have questioned the role of the eosinophil in severe asthma [40,41]. The finding of elevated sputum neutrophils may reflect a relative increase as corticosteroids artificially increase the number by promoting eosinophil apoptosis and inhibiting neutrophil apoptosis |42,43|. However, there is increasing recognition of the role of neutrophils in asthma, particularly in those patients with more severe disease |44–46|. The neutrophil contains an array of proteases and reactive oxygen species that could initiate injury and repair processes within the airway. In *YIRM 2003* I included a paper reporting an association between sputum neutrophils and reduced FEV_1 |47|.

The trigger factors for worsening asthma also displayed a sex bias: sinusitis, the pre-menstrual period, aspirin intake, exercise and the work environment were important for females, while in male patients physical exercise, stress and aspirin intake were identified. Aspirin appears as a trigger factor for both sexes and has been reported to be a trigger factor in approximately 10% of asthma patients depending on which diagnostic criteria are applied |48|. It is recognized to be associated with a chronic persistent course and is associated with near-fatal attacks. These patients display increased production of cysteinyl leukotrienes despite corticosteroid therapy |49–51|. The elevated levels of urinary leukotriene E_4 reported in this paper are consistent with this and raise the possibility that leukotriene receptor antagonists may be beneficial in these patients. So far there is little evidence for this but further studies are awaited |52|.

The study was observational and pragmatic in nature and was not an epidemiological survey of representative populations in each country. It was also a cross-sectional study and as such it is not appropriate to make assumptions regarding causation. Nevertheless, it is clearly an important first step in prompting research into this very important group of patients.

Predictors of therapy-resistant asthma: outcome of a systematic evaluation
Heaney LG, Conway E, Kelly C, *et al. Thorax* 2003; **58**: 561–6

BACKGROUND. The majority of asthmatic patients can be controlled on moderate doses of inhaled corticosteroids. However, approximately 5% of asthmatics are apparently refractory to high doses of inhaled corticosteroids. These patients experience substantial morbidity and contribute to a sizeable proportion of asthma-related health expenditure. They are also an important risk group for asthma death. In this study the authors employed a systematic evaluation of these patients in order to identify the factors contributing to poor control and identify predictors of therapy-resistant asthma.

INTERPRETATION. Co-morbidity is common in therapy-resistant asthma, but no more so than in asthmatic patients who respond to therapy. However, the treatment of identified co-morbidity has little impact on asthma-related quality of life.

Comment

The European Respiratory Society Task Force on Difficult Asthma has recommended that such patients should undergo a period of assessment and evaluation in order to identify and whenever possible modify any factors likely to contribute to poor control. The factors to consider include an appraisal of inhaler technique and an assessment of adherence to the agreed prescriptions. It is also appropriate to identify and, if possible, remove any aggravating factors in the home or work environment and then to search for complications of asthma or concomitant disease including psychosocial problems. Physicians should be alert to the possibility of dysfunctional breathing and recognize that a minority of individuals probably have true corticosteroid resistance.

In this paper the authors identified 73 patients referred to a specialist asthma clinic for assessment of difficult asthma, defined as persisting symptoms due to asthma despite high-dose inhaled corticosteroid therapy (2000 μg of beclomethasone, 1600 μg of budesonide or 1000 μg of fluticasone) in combination with a long-acting β_2 agonist and the requirement for either maintenance systemic steroids or at least two rescue courses of steroids during a follow-up period of 12 months and despite trials of other add-on therapies. The authors then performed a thoroughly comprehensive systematic evaluation that included an inhaler assessment, skin prick testing, chest radiography, spirometry with reversibility, urinalysis, a standardized battery of blood tests and induced sputum. They assessed health status with the use of an asthma-related quality of life score and the Hospital Anxiety Questionnaire. Specialists from ear nose and throat surgery and psychiatry assessed patients with a view to the identification of co-morbidity. The patients also underwent detailed pulmonary function tests, a high-resolution computed tomography (HRCT) scan of the thorax, oesophageal pH monitoring and dual emission X-ray absorptiometry. The services of a social worker were provided if deemed appropriate. As part of their management the patients were instructed on performing peak flow records and maintaining an asthma diary and they received a written self-management plan based on the British Thoracic Society guidelines |53|. Management also included an advice on allergen avoidance sheet for atopic patients.

The authors identified 34 of the 73 patients who completed the assessment as having therapy-resistant asthma, while 39 responded to therapy (non-therapy-resistant asthma). They assessed these patients for characteristics that were associated with each phenotype and found that the patients with therapy-resistant asthma had a greater period of instability, a higher dose of inhaled steroids at referral, more rescuer steroid use and a lower best percentage FEV_1. Employing multivariate logistic regression analysis three variables emerged as key predictive features of therapy-resistant asthma: an inhaled steroid dose >2000 μg of beclomethasone dipropionate equivalent, a presenting pre-bronchodilator FEV_1 <70% predicted and previous specialist referral. The presence of all three variables gave rise to a 93% chance of having therapy-resistant asthma and the absence of all was associated with an 8% chance (Table 2.5). The authors are currently exploring the prospective power of these variables for determining positive and negative predictive values.

The authors identified a range of co-morbid conditions in 34% of the total group. However, with the exception of osteoporosis, they did not find that any of these were more common in patients with therapy-resistant asthma than non-therapy-resistant

Table 2.5 Probability of therapy-resistant asthma (TRA) when different prognostic factors were present at presentation

Inhaled steroid >2000 μg BDP equivalent	Presenting FEV₁ <70% predicted	Previous specialist referral	Probability of TRA
×	×	×	0.08
×	×	✔	0.27
×	✔	×	0.29
✔	×	×	0.44
×	✔	✔	0.62
✔	×	✔	0.76
✔	✔	×	0.78
✔	✔	✔	0.93

✔ = variable present; × = variable absent.
Source: Heaney *et al.* (2003)

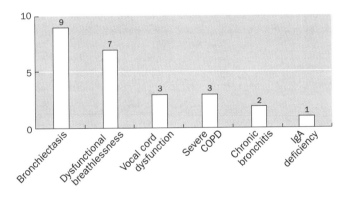

Fig. 2.2 Additional diagnoses causing respiratory symptoms in 73 sequential referrals to a difficult asthma service. Twenty-five of the 73 subjects (34%) had an additional diagnosis. IgA, immunoglobulin A. Source: Heaney *et al.* (2003).

asthma patients. Oesophageal reflux, upper airway disease and psychiatric morbidity were common and of similar prevalence in both groups. In common with other studies on patients with severe asthma the authors found reduced lung function |54,55|. The cross-sectional design of this study precluded determination of causation, so it is not possible to say whether these patients had had low lung function from childhood or whether this represented a consequence of therapy-resistant asthma.

Sputum eosinophil counts were only present in 31 of the 73 patients and they reported that a number of patients could not tolerate the induction procedure or failed to provide an adequate sample. However, they did not find that sputum eosinophilia was associated with therapy-resistant asthma. In the light of the findings by the ENFUMOSA Study Group and others it would be interesting to report data on sputum neutrophilia.

This study reminds us that it is important to identify other contributing factors in patients with difficult asthma, but at what cost? For many practitioners and, indeed, many specialist centres this exhaustive assessment would be neither practical nor feasible within cost restraints. It would be interesting to see an economic analysis of the data.

Systematic assessment of difficult to treat asthma
Robinson DR, Campbell DA, Durham SR, Pfeffer J, Barnes PJ, Chung KF.
Eur Respir J 2003; **22**: 478–83

B A C K G R O U N D . **The aim of this study was to perform a comprehensive systematic evaluation of patients whose asthma appeared poorly controlled despite treatment with high doses of inhaled corticosteroids in order to determine how often difficult to treat asthma is due to intractable asthma, misdiagnosis and non-adherence with therapy of psychiatric problems.**

I N T E R P R E T A T I O N . Systematic evaluation identifies alternative and/or additional diagnoses including psychiatric illness or non-concordance with therapy in a significant number of patients.

Comment
In this study the authors took a pragmatic approach to the definition of difficult asthma including any patient referred to their hospital with such a diagnostic label. They defined difficult asthma as symptomatic asthma despite high-dose inhaled corticosteroid therapy (>1000 µg/day beclomethasone dipropionate or equivalent) and long-acting β_2 agonist or theophylline treatment or patients treated with long-term (>3 months) oral corticosteroid treatment for asthma.

The authors evaluated 100 sequential patients (92 from hospital chest clinics and eight from primary care). Assessment was performed during a 4-day stay in a minimal dependency ward. Two consultant respiratory physicians, an ear nose and throat surgeon and a psychiatrist reviewed each patient. The patient's history, examination and treatment were recorded on a standardized questionnaire. The St George's Respiratory Questionnaire and General Health Questionnaire were completed. Atopy was assessed by skin prick tests to a range of allergens and measurement of serum IgE. Further blood tests included measuring the patients' *Aspergillus preciptins*, serum cortisol and prednisolone levels. Detailed pulmonary function tests and an HRCT scan were also performed (Fig. 2.3).

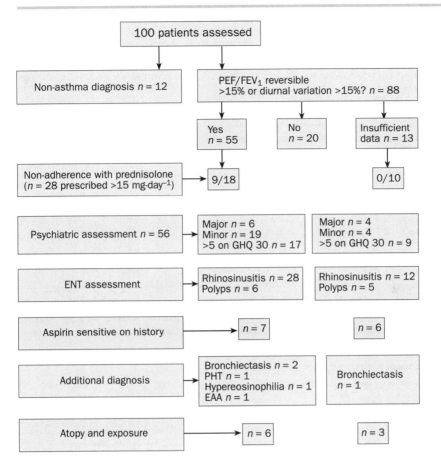

Fig. 2.3 Flow chart showing the numbers of patients in each category. GHQ, General Health Questionnaire; PHT, pulmonary hypertension; EAA, extrinsic allergic alveolitis. Source: Robinson *et al.* (2003).

Table 2.6 Diagnoses in patients without asthma

Chronic obstructive pulmonary disease	6
Emphysema (α_1-antitrypsin deficient)	1
Cystic fibrosis	1
Cardiomyopathy	1
Obliterative bronchiolitis	1
Respiratory muscle incoordination	1
Severe anxiety and vocal cord dysfunction	1

Source: Robinson *et al.* (2003).

The authors found that the diagnosis of asthma was incorrect in twelve patients, the most common alternative diagnosis being COPD (Table 2.6). The authors then divided the remaining patients into those with confirmed asthma and those with unconfirmed asthma on the basis of the presence or absence of reversibility. Fifty-five of these patients displayed reversible airflow narrowing or peak flow variability and 20 did not.

The study highlighted that non-compliance with therapy is common, being found in 50% of the patients prescribed >15 mg/day prednisolone. Corticosteroid resistance was not formally assessed and a systematic trial of high-dose oral corticosteroids was not part of the evaluation.

Over one-half of their patients had rhinosinusitis. This is important to identify, as treatment of upper airway disease has been shown to improve asthma control [58]. They also identified continued exposure to pets in eleven sensitized individuals and a history of aspirin sensitivity in 13 patients. Interestingly, the total IgE was normal in a number of patients with atopy and the authors suggested that it might not be a useful screening tool.

Lung function was found to be normal in four patients with unconfirmed asthma, but the authors felt that two of these patients had brittle asthma and two had major psychiatric morbidity. The authors also highlighted the possibility that assessing patients for hyperventilation syndrome may be a useful modification for further studies.

Conclusion

The papers selected in this chapter have added to our understanding of the natural history of wheeze and asthma from childhood. For the most part, childhood wheeze, although common, does appear to be associated with a favourable prognosis in adult life. The persistence of asthma may be associated with several characteristics including onset at a young age, sensitivity to house dust mites, airway hyper-reactivity, being female and cigarette smoking. Reassuringly, although more patients may be developing asthma later in life, the control of the disease appears to be improving and only a minority of patients experience severe persistent asthma. The papers from Langley *et al.*, the ENFUMOSA Study Group, Heaney *et al.* and Robinson *et al.* provide information on the value of a thorough and systematic evaluation of these patients and will provide valuable data on which to base further studies.

References

1. De Marco R, Locatelli F, Cerveri I, Bugiani M, Marinoni A, Giammanco G. Incidence and remission of asthma: a retrospective study on the natural history of asthma. *J Allergy Clin Immunol* 2002; **110**: 228–35.

2. Kerrebijn KF, Fioole AC, Van Bentveld RD. Lung function in asthmatic children after a year or more without symptoms or treatment. *BMJ* 1978; **1**: 886–8.

3. Gruber W, Eber E, Steinbrugger B, Modl M, Weinhandl E, Zach MS. Atopy, lung function and bronchial hyperresponsiveness in symptom-free paediatric asthma patients. *Eur Respir J* 1997; **10**: 1041–5.

4. Panhuysen CIM, Vonk JM, Koëter GH, Schouten JP, Van Altena R, Bleeker ER, Postma DS. Adult patients may outgrow their asthma: a 25 year follow-up study. *Am J Respir Crit Care* 1997; **155**: 1267–72.

5. Van den Toon LM, Overbeek SE, De Johgste JC, Leman K, Hoogsteden HC, Prins J-B. Airway inflammation is present during clinical remission of atopic asthma. *Am J Respir Crit Care Med* 2001; **164**: 2107–13.

6. Xuan W, Marks GB, Toelle BG, Belousova E, Peat JK, Berry G, Woolcock AJ. Risk factors for onset and remission of atopy, wheeze and airway hyperresponsiveness. *Thorax* 2002; **57**: 104–9.

7. Barnes PJ, Woolcock AJ. Difficult asthma. *Eur Respirat J* 1998; **12**: 1209–18.

8. Oswald H, Phelan PD, Lanigan A, Hibbert M, Bowes G, Olinsky A. Outcome of childhood asthma in mid-adult life. *BMJ* 1994; **309**: 95–6.

9. Sears MR, Lewis S, Herbison GP, Robson B, Flannery EM, Holdaway MD, Pearce N, Crane J, Silva PA. Comparison of reported prevalences of recent asthma in longitudinal and cross-sectional studies. *Eur Respir J* 1997; **10**: 51–4.

10. Strachan DP, Griffiths JM, Johnston IDA, Anderson HR. Ventilatory function in British adults after asthma or wheezing illness at age 0–35. *Am J Respir Crit Care Med* 1996; **154**: 1629–35.

11. Lange P, Parner J, Vestbo J, Schnohr P, Jensen G. A 15-year follow-up study of ventilatory function in adults with asthma. *N Engl J Med* 1998; **339**: 1194–200.

12. Godden DJ, Ross S, Abdalla M, McMurray D, Douglas A, Oldman D, Friend JA, Legge JS, Douglas JG. Outcome of wheeze in childhood. Symptoms and pulmonary function 25 years later. *Am J Respir Crit Care Med* 1994; **149**: 106–12.

13. Edwards CA, Osman LM, Godden DJ, Douglas JG. Wheezy bronchitis in childhood—a distinct clinical entity with lifelong significance. Available on-line at www.bmj.com. eletter/326/7386/422

14. Strachan DP, Butland BK, Anderson HR. Incidence and prognosis of asthma and wheezing illness from early childhood to age 33 in a national British cohort. *BMJ* 1996; **312**: 1195–9.

15. Xu X, Rijcken B, Schouten JP. Airway hyperresponsiveness and development and remission of chronic respiratory symptoms in adults. *Lancet* 1997; **350**: 1431–4.

16. Xuan W, Marks GB, Toelle BG, Belousova E, Peat JK, Berry G, Woolcock AJ. Risk factors for onset and remission of atopy, wheeze and airway hyperresponsiveness. *Thorax* 2002; 57: 104–9.

17. Palmans E, Kips JC, Pauwels RA. Prolonged allergen exposure induces structural airway changes in sensitised rats. *Am J Respir Crit Care Med* 2000; 161: 627–35.

18. Palmans E, Pauwels RA, Kips JC. Repeated allergen exposure changes collagen composition in airways of sensitised brown Norway rats. *Eur Respir J* 2002; 20: 280–5.

19. Burrows B, Martinez FD, Halonen M, Barbee RA, Cline MG. Association of asthma with serum IgE levels and skin-test reactivity to allergens. *N Engl J Med* 1989; 320: 271–7.

20. Murray CS, Woodcock A, Custovic A. The role of indoor allergen exposure in the development of sensitisation and asthma. *Curr Opin Allergy Clin Immunol* 2001; 1: 407–12.

21. Sporik R, Holgate ST, Platts-Mills TAE, Coswell JJ. Exposure to house-dust mite allergen (*Der p 1*) and the development of asthma in childhood. *N Engl J Med* 1990; 323: 502–7.

22. Custovic A, Taggart S, Francis H, *et al*. Exposure to house dust mite allergens and the clinical activity of asthma. *J Allergy Clin Immunol* 1996; 98: 64–72.

23. Tunnicliffe WS, Fletcher TJ, Hammond K, Roberts K, Custovic A, Simpson A, Woodcock A, Ayres JG. Sensitivity and exposure to indoor allergens in adults with differing asthma severity. *Eur Respir J* 1999; 13: 645–9.

24. Hamid Q, Sprinall DR, Riveros-Moreno V, Chanez P, Howarth P, Redington A, Bousquet J, Godard P, Holgate S, Polak JM. Induction of nitric oxide in asthma. *Lancet* 1993; 342: 1510–13.

25. Kharitonov SA, Yates D, Robbins RA, Logan-Sinclair R, Shinebourne E, Barnes PJ. Increased nitric oxide in exhaled air of asthmatic patients. *Lancet* 1994; 343: 133–5.

26. Kharitonov SA, O'Connor BJ, Evans DJ, Barnes PJ. Allergen-induced late asthmatic reactions are associated with elevation of exhaled nitric oxide. *Am J Respir Crit Care Med* 1995; 151: 1894–99.

27. Jatakanon A, Lim S, Kharitonov SA, Chung KF, Barnes PJ. Correlation between exhaled nitric oxide, sputum eosinophils and methacholine responsiveness. *Thorax* 1998; 53: 91–5.

28. Kharitonov SA, Yates DH, Barnes PJ. Regular inhaled budesonide decreases nitric oxide concentration in the exhaled air of asthmatic patients. *Am J Respir Crit Care Med* 1996; 153: 454–7.

29. Peroni DG, Boner AL, Vallone G, Antolini I, Warner JO. Effective allergen avoidance at high altitude reduces allergen-induced bronchial hyperresponsiveness. *Am J Respir Crit Care* 1994; 149: 1442–6.

30. Peroni DG, Piacentini GL, Costella S, Pietrobelli A, Bodini A, Loiacono A, Aralla R, Boner AL. Mite avoidance can reduce air trapping and airway inflammation in allergic asthmatic children. *Clin Exp Allergy* 2002; 32: 850–5.

31. Rijssenbeek-Nouwens LHM, Oosting AJ, De Bruin-Weller MS, Bregman I, De Monchy JGR, Postma DS. Clinical evaluation of the effect of anti-allergic mattress covers in patients with moderate to severe asthma and house dust mite allergy: a randomised double blind placebo controlled study. *Thorax* 2002; 57: 784–90.

32. Woodcock A, Forster L, Matthews E, Martin J, Letley L, Vickers M, Britton J, Strachan D, Howarth P, Altmann D, Frost C, Custovic A and the Medical Research Council General Practice Research Framework. Control of exposure to mite allergen and allergen-impermeable bed covers for adults with asthma. *N Engl J Med* 2003; 349: 225–36.

33. Serra-Batlles J, Plaza V, Morejou E, Cornells A, Bruges J. Costs of asthma according to the degree of severity. *Eur Respir J* 1998; **12**: 1322–6.

34. Langley SJ, Goldthorpe S, Craven M, Morris J, Woodcock A, Custovic A. Exposure and sensitization to indoor allergens: association with lung function, bronchial reactivity, and exhaled nitric oxide measures in asthma. *J Allergy Clin Immunol* 2003; **112**: 362–8.

35. Szczeklik A, Stevenson DD. Aspirin-induced asthma: advances in pathogenesis, diagnosis and management. *J Allergy Clin Immunol* 2003; **111**: 913–21.

36. Caramago Jr CA, Weiss ST, Zhang S, *et al.* Prospective study of body mass index, weight change and risk of adult-onset asthma in women. *Arch Intern Med* 1999; **159**: 2582–8.

37. Beckett WS, Jacobs Jr DR, Yu X, Iribarren C, Williams OD. Asthma is associated with weight gain in females but not males, independent of physical activity. *Am J Respir Crit Care Med* 2001; **164**: 2045–50.

38. Castro-Rodriguez JA, Holberg JA, Morgan MJ, Wright AL, Martinez FD. Increased incidence of asthmalike symptoms in girls who become overweight or obese during the school years. *Am J Respir Crit Care Med* 2001; **163**: 1344–9.

39. Stenius-Aarniaia B, Poussa T, Kvarnstrom J, Gronlund EL, Ylikahri M, Mustajoki P. Immediate and long term effects of weight reduction in obese people with asthma: randomised controlled study. *BMJ* 2000; **320**: 827–32.

40. Tantisira KG, Weiss ST. Complex interactions in complex traits: obesity and asthma. *Thorax* 2001; **56**(Suppl II): ii64–74.

41. Carmichael J, Paterson IC, Diaz P, Crompton GK, Kay AB, Grant IWB. Corticosteroid resistance in chronic asthma. *BMJ* 1981; **282**: 1419–22.

42. Leckie MJ, Ten Brinke A, Khan J, Diamant Z, O'Connor BJ, Walls CM, Mathur AK, Cowley HC, Chung KF, Djukanovic R, Hansel TT, Holgate ST, Sterk PJ, Barnes PJ. Effects of an interleukin 5 blocking monoclonal antibody on eosinophils, airway hyperresponsiveness and the response to allergen in patients with asthma. *Lancet* 2000; **356**: 2144–8.

43. Bryan SA, O'Connor BJ, Matti S, Leckie KJ, Kanabar V, Khan J, Warrington SJ, Renzetti L, Rames A, Bock JA, Boyce JM, Hansel TT, Holgate ST, Barnes PJ. Effects of recombinant human interleukin-12 on eosinophils, airway hyper-responsiveness and the late asthmatic response. *Lancet* 2000; **356**: 2114–16.

44. Cox G. Glucocorticoid treatment inhibits apoptosis in human neutrophils. Separation of survival and activation outcomes. *J Immunol* 1995; **154**: 4719–25.

45. Strickland I, Kisich K, Hauk PJ, Vottero A, Chrousos GP, Klemm DJ, Leung DY. High constitutive glucocorticoid receptor β in human neutrophils enables them to reduce their spontaneous rate of cell death in response to corticosteroids. *J Exp Med* 2001; **193**: 585–94.

46. Sur S, Crotty TB, Kephart GM, Hyma BA, Colby TV, Reed CE, Hunt LW, Gleich GJ. Sudden onset fatal asthma: a distinct entity with few eosinophils and relatively more neutrophils in the airway submucosal. *Am Rev Respir Dis* 1993; **148**: 713–19.

47. Jatakanon A, Uasuf C, Maziak W, Lim S, Chung KF, Barnes PJ. Neutrophilic inflammation in severe persistent asthma. *Am J Respir Crit Care Med* 1999; **160**: 1001–8.

48. Ordonez CL, Shaughnessy TE, Matthay MA, Fahy JV. Increased neutrophil numbers and IL-8 levels in airway secretions in acute severe asthma—clinical and biological significance. *Am J Respir Crit Care Med* 2000; **161**: 1185–90.

49. Little SA, MacLeod KJ, Chalmers GW, Love JG, McSharry C, Thomson NC. Association of forced expiratory volume with disease duration and sputum neutrophils in chronic asthma. *Am J Med* 2002; **112**: 446–52.

50. Valley H, Taylor ML, Thompson PJ. The prevalence of aspirin intolerant asthma in Australian asthmatic patients. *Thorax* 2002; **57**: 569–74.

51. Szczeklik A, Stevenson DD. Aspirin-induced asthma: advances in pathogenesis, diagnosis, and management. *J Allergy Clin Immunol* 2003; **111**: 913–21.

52. O'Shaughnessy KM, Wellings R, Gilles B, Fuller RB. Differential effects of fluticasone propionate on allergen-evoked bronchoconstriction and increased urinary leukotriene E4 excretion. *Am Rev Respir Dis* 1993; **147**: 1472–6.

53. Dworski R, Fitzgerald GA, Oates JA, Sheller JR. Effect of oral prednisolone on airway inflammatory mediators in atopic asthma. *Am J Respir Crit Care Med* 1994; **149**: 953–9.

54. Robinson DS, Campbell D, Barnes PJ. Addition of leukotriene antagonists to therapy in chronic persistent asthma: a randomised double-blind placebo-controlled trial. *Lancet* 2001; **357**: 2007–11.

55. British Thoracic Society/Scottish Intercollegiate Guidelines Network. British guidelines on the management of asthma. *Thorax* 2003; **58**(Suppl 1): i1–94.

56. Ten Brinke A, Zwinderman AH, Sterk PJ, Rabe KF, Bel EH. Factors associated with persistent airflow limitation in severe asthma. *Am J Respir Crit Care Med* 2001; **164**: 744–8.

57. Rasmussen F, Taylor R, Flannery EM, Cowan JO, Greene JM, Herbison P, Sears MR. Risk factors for airway remodelling in asthma manifested by a low postbronchodilator FEV_1/vital capacity ratio. *Am J Respir Crit Care Med* 2002; **165**: 1480–8.

58. Bousquet J, Van Cauwenberge P. Allergic rhinitis and its impact on asthma (ARIA). *J Allergy Clin Immunol* 2001; **108**: S1–147.

3

The management of asthma

Introduction

The management of asthma is multifaceted and at its best involves a number of different healthcare professionals working together with the patient. It would be desirable to prevent the disease emerging in the first instance and some research has focused on the prevention of asthma emerging in high-risk individuals, so-called primary prevention. It is likely that any intervention would need to be applied during the pre- and perinatal periods and most research has tended to concentrate on manipulation of the maternal and neonatal diet and avoidance of allergens. At the time of writing there are currently no interventions that can be recommended.

Secondary prevention focuses on the period following sensitization, but preceding the clinical appearance of the disease, with the aim of reducing the burden of chronic persistent illness. Last year the Preventive Allergy Treatment Study reported that immunotherapy reduced the subsequent appearance of asthma in children with seasonal rhinoconjunctivitis |**1**|. Other studies have examined the potential of anti-histamines for modifying the anticipated progression from atopy to asthma and it is likely that other papers will be presented soon.

Tertiary prevention examines the role of reducing exposure to allergens with the aim of improving asthma control. The most popular attempt at tertiary prevention has been the examination of methods for reducing exposure to the house dust mite |**2–4**|. However, it has proven difficult to achieve significant and sustained reductions in the levels of exposure and definitive evidence of benefit is lacking |**5**|. Better studies are needed for providing good quality information on allergen avoidance.

The majority of patients presenting to their physician with symptoms of asthma will require pharmacological intervention. The recognition of the central role of inflammation in the pathogenesis of asthma has led to an emphasis on the administration of regular inhaled corticosteroids as anti-inflammatory therapy. Their pre-eminent position in the management of asthma is based on the recognition that regular administration is associated with reduced symptoms, improvements in lung function, a reduction in airway hyper-responsiveness, reduced hospitalizations and the prevention of death. Their use in patients with mild disease has not been fully established. Furthermore, an increasing body of evidence suggests that the maximum therapeutic effect may be attained for the majority of patients with low to moderate doses of these agents, with higher doses adding little and potentially contributing to unwanted systemic effects |**6,7**|. In recognition of this more information is becoming available on methods of stepping down therapy.

The role of short-acting β_2 agonists is directed towards the relief of symptoms (or the prevention of exercise-induced symptoms) and they should be prescribed on an as-required basis. Long-acting β_2 agonists have emerged as useful add-on therapy to inhaled corticosteroids and appear to confer additional benefit at all levels of asthma severity, including those with mild disease.

The leukotriene receptor antagonists have been launched relatively recently, but represent the first new therapy for asthma for many years. Their development was based on a series of *in vitro* observations showing that the cysteinyl leukotrienes replicate many of the pathophysiological features observed in the asthmatic lung. They are potent smooth muscle spasmogens, induce endothelial leakiness, reduce mucociliary clearance, enhance mucus secretion, contribute to the recruitment of eosinophils and increase airway hyper-responsiveness [8,9]. Elevated levels have been detected in the bronchoalveolar lavage fluid and urine of patients with asthma following allergen challenge or during an acute asthma attack. Over-expression of leukotriene C_4 synthase, the enzyme that directs the metabolism of leukotriene B_4 to leukotriene C_4, has been demonstrated in bronchial biopsy specimens from asthmatic patients.

Earlier studies in patients with allergic asthma and exercise-induced asthma have suggested that leukotriene receptor antagonists could produce modest improvements in lung function and reduce symptoms. In studies of patients on systemic corticosteroids the addition of leukotriene receptor antagonists could facilitate corticosteroid dose reduction [10]. Given their mode of action it has been suggested that they should be particularly beneficial in patients with aspirin-sensitive asthma [11]. They are well tolerated and may have advantages for some patients who prefer oral medication. However, debate continues as to their place in management and information has been lacking on their utility as an add-on therapy to inhaled corticosteroids. Currently they have been recommended at later stages of management protocols by most guidelines [12,13].

Although pharmacotherapy plays an important role in the management of asthma, we also need to recognize that there is considerable interest among patients in non-pharmacological options. Some have adopted the Buteyko technique and others yoga. Papers examining these as adjunct therapies have been limited. Furthermore, although considerable emphasis is placed on the development and delivery of new medications, it is generally acknowledged that a significant number of patients are poorly controlled because they have not enacted appropriate changes in their lifestyle or they cannot use or are poorly compliant with medications already prescribed. Improved control of asthma may therefore be achieved by encouraging patients to enter into a partnership of care with the healthcare team. Most guideline statements encourage practitioners to develop education and self-management programmes [14–16]. These programmes have developed with the aim of increasing patients' knowledge and supplying and reinforcing the skill base necessary for the patient (or their carers) to govern changes in their own therapy, the premise being that knowledge leads to improved day-to-day self-management behaviour. Such programmes are generally based on the delivery of an educational programme coupled with training in the principles of asthma therapeutics and the development of action plans that are based on the recognition of symptoms heralding deterioration in asthma.

Prevention strategies

Primary prevention

Eighteen-month outcomes of house dust mite avoidance and dietary fatty acid modification in the Childhood Asthma Prevention Study (CAPS)

Mihrshahi S, Peat JK, Marks GB, *et al.* for the Childhood Asthma Prevention Study Team. *J Allergy Clin Immunol* 2003; **111**: 162–8

BACKGROUND. A reduced intake of dietary fish and exposure and sensitization to house dust mites are recognized risk factors for the development of asthma in childhood. The Childhood Asthma Prevention Study (established in 1997 in Sydney, Australia) was designed for testing whether interventions promoting dietary supplementation with ω-3 fatty acids, the avoidance of house dust mite allergens or a combination of the two could decrease the incidence of allergy and asthma in high-risk children.

INTERPRETATION. Increasing dietary ω-3 fatty acids had no effect on serum immunoglobulin E (IgE), atopy or doctors' diagnosis of asthma, but reduced the prevalence of any wheeze and wheeze of >1 week. Avoidance of house dust mites was associated with a reduced requirement for oral steroids in the management of eczema, but had no effect on any of the other parameters.

Comment

In this study the authors attempted to target a population at high risk for the development of asthma by selecting families in which one parent or sibling had reported symptoms of asthma. They excluded cat owners, strict vegetarians, multiple births and those born before 36 weeks of gestation. They also excluded individuals with poor English, no telephone and who lived more than 30 km from the recruitment centre.

The study hypotheses were tested in a parallel-group, randomized, controlled trial in which the two interventions were tested separately and then together through the use of a factorial design. House dust mite avoidance included both physical (allergen-impermeable mattress covers) and chemical methods that were focused on the infants' beds and main play areas. The control group received standard advice on cleaning, vacuuming, dusting and maintaining adequate ventilation. Dietary intervention included the provision of a daily ω-3-rich tuna fish oil supplement from the age of 6 months onwards. Supplements were not required before 6 months unless the child was bottle-fed. Placebo supplements were provided to the control group. Outcomes were determined at 18 months and included information on symptoms and the diagnoses and treatment of asthma and eczema. Skin prick testing was used for testing for the development of allergy and collection of dust from the child's bed was used for quantifying house dust mite exposure. Plasma phospholipids were also measured.

Dietary intervention had no effect on the subjects' serum IgE, atopy or doctors' diagnosis of asthma, but did appear to influence the prevalence of wheeze. Compared to the control group wheeze-ever was 9.8% lower, the prevalence of wheeze for >1 week was 7.8% lower, the prevalence of wheeze for >1 week without a cold was 2.0% lower and the prevalence of doctor visits for wheeze was 6.3% lower in the active dietary intervention groups. Although this represents a positive outcome it remains unclear what the presence of wheeze means at this age as regards the later development of asthma [17,18]. The authors will be reporting outcomes again when the children are aged 3 and 5 years.

House dust mite allergen avoidance was actually associated with an 8.2% higher prevalence of reported eczema and a 6.9% higher prevalence of visible eczema in the active group than in the control house dust mite group. However, there was a lower prevalence of the use of oral steroids in the active house dust mite avoidance group that might indicate an effect of disease severity. There were no significant interactions between diet and house dust mite avoidance on any of the other outcome measures.

The authors suggested that they only achieved modest reductions in house dust mite levels and this may have been a factor in the outcome of the study and they alluded to three other important studies in this area [19–21]. The team in the Manchester Asthma and Allergy Study reduced house dust mite levels in bedding to five times lower than in this study [19]. This trial reported no difference in the prevalence of atopy, but did find a modest but significant reduction in wheeze. A study from Canada combined early dietary and environmental intervention and reported positive outcomes in terms of asthma and rhinitis at 1 year [20]. The Isle of Wight Study also combined house dust mite avoidance and dietary intervention and reported reductions in allergy, asthma and eczema at 1 year of age [21].

Tertiary prevention

Control of exposure to mite allergen and allergen-impermeable bed covers for adults with asthma

Woodcock A, Forster L, Matthews E, *et al.* and the Medical Research Council General Practice Research Framework. *N Engl J Med* 2003; **349**: 225–36

BACKGROUND. Exposure to high concentrations of house dust mite allergen (Der p1) in sensitized individuals is associated with greater severity of asthma, but the effectiveness of house dust mite avoidance in clinical practice has not been established. The aim of this study was to demonstrate that significant reductions in Der p 1 levels can be achieved and to determine whether this was associated with improvements in asthma control. The authors performed a randomized, parallel-group, double-blind, placebo-controlled trial of mite allergen avoidance with the use of allergen-impermeable covers for mattresses, pillows and quilts.

INTERPRETATION. The use of allergen-impermeable covers, as a single intervention, is unlikely to be effective in the management of patients with adult asthma.

Effect of mattress and pillow encasings on children with asthma and house dust mite allergy

Halken S, Høst A, Niklassen U, *et al. J Allergy Clin Immunol* 2003; **111**: 169–76

BACKGROUND. This prospective, double-blind, placebo-controlled study focused on a group of mite-allergic children and excluded those with other allergies that were likely to be clinically relevant. The primary effect measures were changes in exposure to house dust mite allergens and the need for asthma medication, particularly inhaled steroids.

INTERPRETATION. The use of mite-impermeable bed covers was associated with a significant long-term reduction in the mattresses' concentration of mite allergen and the need for inhaled corticosteroids in children with asthma and house dust allergy (Fig. 3.1).

Comment

Sensitization to a range of allergens followed by subsequent and continued exposure has been implicated in the initiation and perpetuation of the asthmatic response. The number of potential allergens is extensive and varies with climatic conditions. In the UK and other European countries house dust mites are a major source of allergens. Significant exposure in sensitized individuals is recognized in the development of asthma with those exposed to the highest levels reporting more severe disease |22–24|. The principal allergenic component is the protease Der p 1, which is found in their faeces.

The improvement of asthma in mite-free environments such as hospitals and the dry air of high altitude Alpine sanatoria suggest that avoidance of allergen may lead to a reduction in airway inflammation, airway hyper-reactivity and symptoms |25–28|. However, it has proven difficult to achieve significant and sustained reductions in levels of exposure. This was reflected by a recent Cochrane review on the topic including 23 studies and 686 subjects. However, most of the studies were small in number and no reported reduction in house dust mite allergen levels was observed in the majority (*n* = 17). The allergen levels were reduced in six studies, but only two of these were double blind |29|. In *Year in Respiratory Medicine 2003* (*YIRM 2003*) I included a paper by Rijssenbeek-Nouwens *et al.* Despite achieving significant

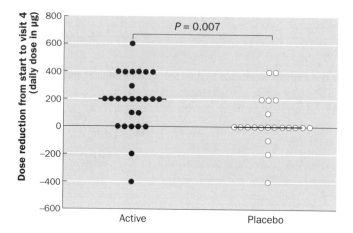

Fig. 3.1 Change in the need for inhaled steroids. The changes from baseline in the daily dose of inhaled steroid (in micrograms) by the end of the study in the active treatment (filled circles) and placebo (open circles) groups are shown. The results are expressed as individual data points and *P* values for the differences between medians are calculated by means of the Kruskal–Wallis test. Source: Halken *et al.* (2003).

reductions in Der p 1 with allergen-impermeable encasings on mattresses, pillows and bedcovers, it was not possible to demonstrate any clinically significant differences from the placebo group |30|.

The study this year by Woodcock *et al.* is impressive in size. Patients were recruited from 154 general practices in the Medical Research Council's General Practice Research Framework and 1122 patients aged between 18 and 50 years were enrolled. Sensitivity to Der p1 was determined by measurement of serum *Dermatophagoides pteronyssinus*-specific IgE. During a 4-week run-in period the patients kept a diary card of symptoms, peak flow and β agonist use and if they could perform this appropriately for 14 days were randomized to receive either Der p 1-impermeable mattress, pillow and quilt covers or non-impermeable polyester cotton (control) covers. The covers were fitted by a research nurse and left on the bedding for 1 year. No specific washing instructions for bed covers or any other information on the avoidance of mites were given to the patients in either group. A home visit was performed for all patients at the start of the study and for a 10% random sample further visits were performed at 6 and 12 months. An area of 1 m² of the mattress was vacuumed for 2 min through a filter device in order to collect dust samples.

The study was performed in two phases. In phase 1 (months 1–6) the patients were asked to maintain their inhaled corticosteroid therapy at the usual dose and in phase 2 (months 7–12) they were invited to participate in a programme of controlled reduction. The primary outcome measure for phase 1 was morning peak expiratory flow (PEF) and for phase II it was the proportion of patients who discontinued inhaled corticosteroid therapy.

At randomization 65% of the patients were mite sensitive (65.4% in the active intervention group and 65.1% in the control group), 55% had pets and 24% were current smokers. Follow-up was completed by 90% at 6 months and by 83% at 12 months. Although the authors were able to demonstrate significant reductions in recovering Der p 1 from mattress dust (geometric mean 0.58 μg/g compared to 1.71 μg/g in the control arm) they were unable to demonstrate an associated improvement in the clinical severity of asthma.

Following the end of phase 1 the authors reported that the morning PEF improved significantly in both groups, but there was no significant difference between the two groups. The difference in means between the active intervention group and the control group was −1.6 l/min (95% confidence interval [CI] = −5.9 to 2.7) among all patients and 1.5 l/min (95% CI = −6.9 to 3.9) among mite-sensitive patients. There was no significant difference between the groups in phase 2 with regard to the proportion who reduced or stopped inhaled corticosteroid therapy. This was true whether the authors considered the group as a whole or only those who were mite sensitive. They therefore concluded that, as a single intervention, the use of impermeable bedding was clinically ineffective in adult asthmatics.

The design and performance of such studies is formidable. The authors conducted a pragmatic and impressive study and their results are likely to be applicable to real-life day-to-day practice. Questions remain about the optimum method for expressing Der p 1 measurements and how best to quantify or estimate the actual exposure sustained by any individual patient. Whilst these issues may have influenced the results it is perhaps more reasonable to suggest that controlling one variable (in this case Der p 1 exposure) in a complex disease is overoptimistic [31]. For example, patients in this study owned cats and dogs and it is conceivable that sensitization and ongoing exposure to these allergens confounded the results.

Whilst the above study adds to a disappointing role of studies in this area the study by Halken et al. suggests that, in a carefully selected group of children, measures directed at the avoidance of house dust mites may have some utility. The study group was much smaller and the inclusion criteria more specific, requiring physician-diagnosed asthma, a positive skin prick test response to house dust mites, a positive bronchial provocation test with house dust mite allergen extract and a total house dust mite concentration of ≥2000 ng/g dust from the child's mattress. The authors excluded children with other allergies that might have been clinically relevant such as pollen and cats.

They reported that the mattress covers were highly effective in reducing house dust mite allergen exposure with 81–89% reductions that were maintained throughout the study. In the control group the reductions ranged from −1 to 70%. In this study the authors' primary outcome measure was medication requirement and they found that the daily dose of inhaled corticosteroids was reduced by at least 100 μg in most of the children in the active treatment group but not the placebo group. After 9 and 12 months the dose of inhaled corticosteroids was reduced by at least 50% in significantly more children in the active treatment group than in the placebo group. The median change from baseline was 200 μg/day in the active group and 0 μg/day in the placebo group, with the difference being significant ($P < 0.01$).

Pharmacological approaches in the management of asthma

Inhaled corticosteroids

Asthma is characterized by a persistent inflammatory response in the airways with the recruitment and activation of a variety of inflammatory cells and transformation of the structural airway cells into a pro-inflammatory phenotype. The optimal treatment for asthma therefore focuses on the delivery of anti-inflammatory medications. A number of agents available for asthma have anti-inflammatory effects, but inhaled corticosteroids remain pre-eminent. Regular administration of inhaled steroids in asthma produces a rapid improvement in symptoms, attenuates airway hyper-reactivity and reduces exacerbations |32–34|.

Early intervention with budesonide in mild asthma: a randomized, double-blind trial

Pauwels R, Pedersen S, Busse WW, *et al.* on behalf of the START Investigators Group. *Lancet* 2003; **61**: 1071–6

BACKGROUND. The benefits of inhaled corticosteroids have not been firmly established in patients with mild persistent asthma. The aim of this study was to determine the effectiveness of early intervention with budesonide in patients with mild persistent asthma of recent onset specifically examining the outcomes of severe asthma-related events and accelerated decline in lung function over a period of 3 years. The primary outcome was the time to first severe asthma exacerbation defined as admission, emergency treatment or death.

INTERPRETATION. Regular budesonide significantly reduced the hazard of and prolonged the time to the first severe asthma-related event. It was associated with improved lung function, significantly more symptom-free days and a reduced rescue requirement for systemic corticosteroids and other additional asthma therapies.

Comment

Inflammation is present in newly diagnosed patients with mild asthma and probably contributes to persistent symptoms and exacerbations |35|. There is also a reasonable concern that, if left unchecked, a persistent inflammatory process may lead to irreversible airflow limitation |36,37|. Inhaled corticosteroids are recognized as decreasing airway inflammation, improving symptoms, reducing exacerbations and improving lung function and may be associated with long-term gains in lung function |33,38|. It has been suggested that commencing inhaled corticosteroids early in the disease may be associated with a greater benefit than starting them later |39,40|.

The authors of this study enrolled 7241 patients who suffered from mild asthma as defined by wheeze, cough, dyspnoea or chest tightening at least once a week, but not as often as daily, whose disease had been present for less than 2 years and who had not received regular corticosteroid therapy. Patients were randomly allocated to receive 400 µg of once daily budesonide (200 µg for children <11 years) ($n = 3597$) or placebo ($n = 3568$). A total of 2607 patients completed the budesonide arm over the 3-year period of the study and 2548 patients completed the placebo arm.

Budesonide significantly reduced the risk of a first severe asthma-related event by 44% in all patients (hazard ratio = 0.56 and 95% CI = 0.45–0.71) ($P > 0.0001$) and by 47% for the 60% of patients who were not on any glucocorticoid at study entry when the trial began and whose pre-bronchodilator forced expiratory volume in 1 s (FEV_1) was >80%. Treatment with budesonide also prolonged the time to the first severe asthma-related event (Fig. 3.2). The budesonide group had 30 patients with two or more severe asthma-related events and nine patients with a life-threatening attack compared to 49 and 24 patients in the placebo group ($P = 0.003$ and $P = 0.009$), respectively. Despite a greater use of non-steroidal asthma therapies in the placebo group, patients taking budesonide had significantly more symptom-free days over the study period ($P < 0.0001$). Additional inhaled, oral or systemic steroids were required in 45% of the placebo group and 31% of the budesonide group and these were required earlier in the placebo group ($P < 0.0001$) (Fig. 3.3). Courses of oral

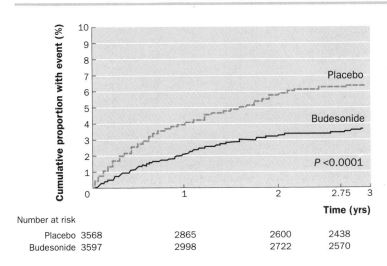

Fig. 3.2 Kaplan–Meier curve of the time to the first severe asthma-related event. Source: Pauwels *et al.* (2003).

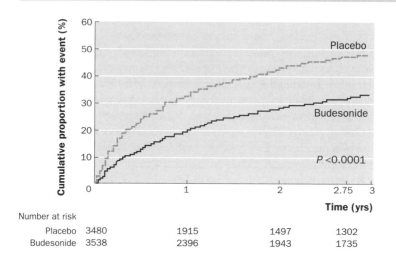

Fig. 3.3 Kaplan–Meier curve of the time to the first non-study glucocorticosteroid treatment. Source: Pauwels *et al.* (2003).

corticosteroids were administered in 23.1% of the placebo group and 15.2% of the budesonide group.

The patients entered the study with a mean pre-bronchodilator FEV_1 of 86.45% and a mean post-bronchodilator FEV_1 of 96.31%. Treatment with budesonide significantly improved both the patients' pre- and post-bronchodilator FEV_1 after 1 year (2.24 and 1.48%, respectively) (P <0.0001 for both) and after 3 years (1.71 and 0.88%) (P <0.0001 and P = 0.0005, respectively). The between-group difference in the post-bronchodilator FEV_1 diminished over time, although it remained significant throughout, but this may have been an artefact of the intention to treat analysis. The design of this study allowed patients in the placebo arm to commence inhaled corticosteroids during the study and, as more of the placebo group commenced regular inhaled corticosteroids, an analysis such as this began to underestimate the benefit in the active arm of the study. Indeed, the authors contended that their design resulted in a comparison of early versus delayed introduction of inhaled corticosteroids. A further possibility could be decreased adherence to therapy in the budesonide group.

The study suggests that, even in mild asthma, some loss of lung function occurs over time. The mean changes from baseline for the post-bronchodilator FEV_1 at 1 and 3 years were 0.62% and −1.79% for budesonide and −2.11% and −2.68% for placebo (P <0.001). The mean difference in the subjects' post-bronchodilator FEV_1 between the budesonide and placebo groups at 3 years was 0.88% (P <0.0005). The decline in post-bronchodilator FEV_1 in both treatment groups was more marked for males, active smokers and patients >18 years (P <0.001 for all) and the smallest treatment effect of budesonide was seen in adolescents when compared to children or adults. The effect of budesonide was independent of the baseline pre-bronchodilator FEV_1 and other asthma medication used.

The authors were unable to identify characteristics in patients who might benefit most from regular inhaled steroid therapy. The effectiveness of budesonide was independent of lung function or the medications being used at baseline and none of the baseline characteristics were associated with a high risk of severe or life-threatening exacerbations. This study therefore recommends that inhaled corticosteroids should be commenced early in the management of all patients with mild asthma.

It is reasonable to explore concerns that such a recommendation may be associated with a risk of treatment-related adverse events. The authors examined the impact of regular budesonide therapy on height and reported that children in the budesonide group aged 5–15 years at randomization grew less than those in the placebo group. However, the authors pointed out that studies reporting regular treatment with budesonide for 10 years have reported attainment of normal adult height |**41**|.

In summary, this study shows that the regular administration of inhaled corticosteroids in patients with mild asthma decreases severe asthma-related events, the requirement for corticosteroids and other therapies and is effective in a broad age range of patients.

Stepping down inhaled corticosteroids in asthma: randomized controlled trial

Hawkins G, McMahon AD, Twaddle S, Wood SF, Ford I, Thomson NC. *BMJ* 2003; **326**: 1115–18

BACKGROUND. High doses of inhaled corticosteroids are associated with a diminished therapeutic ratio and once asthma control has been achieved it is important to employ the lowest dose of corticosteroids that continues to provide acceptable control. As little information is available on how to reduce the dose of inhaled corticosteroids the authors undertook a study in a Scottish general practice population who were currently being prescribed 800 μg of beclomethasone dipropionate (or equivalent) per day and either reduced or sham reduced the dose of inhaled corticosteroid over a period of 1 year.

INTERPRETATION. A reduction in the dose of inhaled corticosteroids was achieved in 83% of the step-down group. Despite receiving less beclomethasone dipropionate than the control group no significant differences were observed between the step-down and the control group in relation to the number of asthma exacerbations, asthma-related events and health status. Thus, advocating step down is safe in patients receiving high doses of inhaled corticosteroids daily.

Steroid-sparing effects of fluticasone propionate 100 μg and salmeterol 50 μg administered twice daily in a single product in patients previously controlled with fluticasone propionate 250 μg administered twice daily

Busse W, Koenig SM, Oppenheimer J, *et al. J Allergy Clin Immunol* 2003;
111: 57–65

BACKGROUND. The aim of this study was to determine whether the use of the long-acting β_2 agonists salmeterol combined with fluticasone could be used for reducing the dose of inhaled corticosteroid whilst maintaining asthma control in patients currently stable on medium doses of inhaled steroid.

INTERPRETATION. In patients requiring 250 μg of twice daily fluticasone propionate, the use of salmeterol facilitated a 60% reduction in the dose of inhaled corticosteroid while effectively maintaining asthma control.

Comment

Inhaled corticosteroids remain the most effective therapy for asthma, controlling symptoms, reducing inflammation, minimizing morbidity and preventing death. However, concern exists regarding a number of potential side effects, including skin bruising, the formation of cataracts, glaucoma, reduced bone density and adrenal suppression |42,43|. Thus, most guidelines on the management of asthma advocate that the dose of inhaled corticosteroids is reduced once control of asthma has been achieved and maintained for an acceptable period. The Global Initiative for Asthma recommended that the dose of inhaled corticosteroids be reduced by approximately 25% every 3 months with close monitoring of patients' symptoms, clinical signs and lung function, but assigned a grade D to the level of evidence of this statement |44|.

The authors of this study attempted to provide information on this important topic. They designed a multicentre, randomized, double-blind, parallel-group trial and recruited 259 patients from a general practice population who were currently being prescribed at least 800 μg of beclomethasone dipropionate (or equivalent) per day. The mean dose of the patients recruited was 1430 μg/day. Starting doses were allocated from beclomethasone dipropionate (1000, 1500 or 2000 μg/day) or fluticasone propionate (500, 1000, 1500 or 2000 μg/day) according to prior use of inhaled corticosteroids. Two packs of inhaled corticosteroid were formulated for each patient and labelled either 'usual dose' or 'reduced dose'. For those patients randomized to the step-down arm the usual dose pack contained the patient's starting dose of corticosteroid and the reduced dose pack contained 50% of the starting dose. For those patients randomized to the control arm both the usual dose and reduced dose packs contained the starting dose of inhaled corticosteroid. Patients were followed up for 1 year. The primary objective was to compare the proportion of patients who experienced an asthma exacerbation. Secondary objectives were to determine the proportion of patients achieving a 50% reduction in their daily dose of inhaled corticosteroid without compromising asthma control in the step-down group and to compare the number of asthma-related events, the total dose of inhaled and oral corticosteroid administered and any changes in health status between the two groups.

Overall 84% of the step-down group and 81% of the control group from the original group of 259 participants met and maintained the criteria for good control and were issued with a reduced dose pack. On average the authors reported that the step-down group received 348 µg (95% CI = 202–494 µg) of beclomethasone dipropionate less per day than the controls (a difference of 25%), yet they did not find any significant difference in the rate of asthma exacerbations or asthma events between the two groups. Neither was there any difference between health status measures and the asthma morbidity. Thus, the authors suggested that advocating a step down in the dose of inhaled corticosteroids is safe in patients receiving high doses of inhaled corticosteroids daily.

The major strength of this study is that it took a pragmatic approach to a difficult and under-researched area. The patients, who included smokers and represented a broad socio-economic group, were typical of primary care and therefore the results are widely applicable. Previous studies have demonstrated that it is possible to reduce the dose of inhaled corticosteroids safely in patients with asthma of mild and moderate severity, but this paper provided information on patients receiving high doses of inhaled corticosteroids |45,46|. In YIRM 2003 I included a paper suggesting that the dose of inhaled corticosteroid could be safely reduced in the presence of a reduced sputum eosinophil count, but this study employed outcome measures that are applicable in general practice |47|.

It is possible that the authors' finding may have been explained by a trial effect. It is widely held that patients with asthma are less compliant than their doctor would like to believe. Recruitment into the study may have prompted previously non-compliant patients to improve adherence to a treatment regime. It is also possible that prior to the study patients had a suboptimal inhaler technique and this would have been addressed during recruitment.

In YIRM 2003 I reviewed a paper from the Asthma Clinical Research Network (ACRN) demonstrating that long-acting β_2 agonists could reduce asthma exacerbations and facilitate a reduction in inhaled corticosteroids |48|. The combined use of inhaled steroids with a long-acting β_2 agonist has been shown to improve asthma control and reduce exacerbations and both bronchoalveolar lavage and bronchial biopsy have shown equivalent anti-inflammatory effects |49,50|. In the study by Hawkins et al., 37% of the step-down group and 30% of the control group were using long-acting β_2 agonists, but a further subgroup analysis following removal of these patients from the study population did not alter the finding.

The study by Busse et al. explored the use of long-acting agents for facilitating corticosteroid step down. In this study a moderate dose of inhaled corticosteroids was defined as any of the following: 504–840 µg/day beclomethasone dipropionate, 400–800 µg/day budesonide, 440–660 µg/day fluticasone, 1000–1500 µg/day flunisolide or 1200–1600 µg/day triamcinolone acetonide.

A particularly commendable component of the study design was that the minimum steroid dose required for maintaining asthma control was verified during the run-in period. Thus, they only included those patients who they then knew had clinically unstable asthma when maintained on a lower dose of study steroid, in this case 100 µg of fluticasone propionate twice daily. Loss of control prompted the authors to step up therapy to 250 µg of fluticasone propionate twice daily and the patient then entered the study and was randomized to receive either fluticasone propionate 100/salmeterol Diskus combination product or 250 µg of fluticasone propionate Diskus twice daily. The primary efficacy end-point was the proportion of patients who remained in the study after 12 weeks of double-blind treatment with no evidence of worsening asthma control.

The authors found that the combination of salmeterol and fluticasone propionate facilitated a 60% reduction in the dose of inhaled corticosteroid while effectively maintaining asthma control. This study complements the study by the ACRN and a further study performed in general practice in the UK demonstrated that eformoterol allowed the dose of inhaled corticosteroid to be reduced whilst decreasing the rate of mild exacerbations |48,51|.

The mechanism behind the apparent synergy of long-acting β_2 agonists and inhaled corticosteroids remains unclear. A number of different complementary and synergistic actions have been suggested and these may be maximized by delivering the two agents simultaneously |52,53|. However, it is not clear whether the apparent molecular and cellular synergy of these agents for anti-inflammatory activity is also associated with a synergy in the side-effect profile.

Leukotriene receptor antagonists

Leukotrienes are lipid mediators derived from arachidonic acid, which following activation is released from the cell wall by phospholipase A_2 and is then metabolized either by a cyclooxygenase pathway, generating prostaglandins and thromboxanes or by a 5-lipoxygenase pathway, which, in association with 5-lipoxygenase-activating protein, produces the cysteinyl leukotrienes. The 5-lipoxygenase pathway is expressed in myeloid cells including mast cells, basophils, neutrophils, eosinophils and alveolar macrophages. Leukotriene C_4 is metabolized to leukotriene D_4 and leukotriene E_4 and these are rapidly degraded in the body. Leukotriene E_4 can be measured in the urine.

Inhaled glucocorticoids versus leukotriene receptor antagonists as single-agent asthma treatment: systematic review of current evidence

FM Ducharme. *BMJ* 2003; **326**: 621–3

BACKGROUND. The aim of this study was to update the previously published Cochrane review with a systematic review of randomized, controlled trials comparing antileukotrienes with inhaled glucocorticoids for 28 days or more in children and adults with asthma. This paper aimed to compare the safety and efficacy of antileukotrienes and inhaled glucocorticoids as monotherapy in people with asthma. Five additional trials were identified that had not been included in the original review.

INTERPRETATION. Inhaled glucocorticoids in doses equivalent to 400 μg/day beclomethasone are more effective than leukotriene receptor antagonists in the treatment of adults with mild to moderate asthma. There is insufficient evidence on which to draw conclusions on the efficacy of antileukotrienes in children. Inhaled corticosteroids remain the drug of first choice for the control of asthma.

Effect of montelukast added to inhaled budesonide on control of mild to moderate asthma

Vaqueriza MJ, Casan P, Castillo J, *et al.* for the Capacidad de Singular Oral en la Prevncion de Exacerbaiones Asmaticas Study Group. *Thorax* 2003; **58**: 204–11

BACKGROUND. In this study the authors performed a placebo-controlled, randomized, parallel-group study conducted at 80 secondary care centres in Spain in order to evaluate the efficacy of adding oral montelukast to a constant dose of inhaled budesonide for treating adult patients with mild to moderate asthma.

INTERPRETATION. For patients with mild to moderate airway obstruction and persistent asthma symptoms despite budesonide treatment, concomitant treatment with montelukast is associated with modest but significant improvements in asthma control.

Randomized, controlled trial of montelukast plus inhaled budesonide versus double-dose inhaled budesonide in adult patients with asthma

Price DB, Hernandez D, Magyar P, *et al.* for the Clinical Outcomes with Montelukast as a Partner Agent to Corticosteroid Therapy International Study Group. *Thorax* 2003; **58**: 211–16

BACKGROUND. In this study the investigators examined the potential of leukotriene receptor antagonist therapy as an add-on treatment to patients whose asthma was poorly controlled despite what might be considered high doses of inhaled corticosteroid therapy. Patients inadequately controlled on 800 μg/day budesonide were entered into a double-blind, randomized, parallel-group, non-inferiority, multicentre, 16-week study comparing the clinical benefit of adding montelukast to doubling the dose of inhaled budesonide.

INTERPRETATION. The study reported that the addition of montelukast to 800 μg/day inhaled budesonide was as effective as increasing the dose of inhaled budesonide to 1600 μg/day.

Montelukast and fluticasone compared with salmeterol and fluticasone in protecting against asthma exacerbation in adults: 1-year, double-blind, randomized, comparative trial

Bjermer L, Bisgaard H, Bousquet J, *et al. BMJ* 2003; **327**: 891–5

BACKGROUND. The aim of this study was to assess the effect of montelukast versus salmeterol added to inhaled fluticasone propionate on asthma exacerbation in patients whose asthma was inadequately controlled with fluticasone alone.

INTERPRETATION. Adding montelukast to the treatment of patients whose symptoms remain uncontrolled with inhaled flucticasone alone could provide equivalent clinical control compared with adding salmeterol.

Comment

Inhaled corticosteroids remain the most effective anti-inflammatory agent for the treatment of asthma |**32–34**|. The systematic review by Ducharme reinforced this point and demonstrated that they remain the controller therapy of first choice. Ducharme included all randomized, controlled trials that compared antileukotrienes with a stable dose of inhaled glucocorticoid for at least 28 days in adults and children aged ≥2 years. The *a priori* specified outcome was the number of exacerbations requiring systemic glucocorticoids. Patients treated with a leukotriene receptor antagonist were 60% more likely to experience an exacerbation requiring systemic glucocorticoids than those treated with inhaled glucocorticoids. (relative risk = 1.6 and 95% CI = 1.2–2.2). Inhaled corticosteroids also proved superior on reported secondary outcomes including lung function, nocturnal awakenings, the use of β_2 agonists and days with symptoms. Antileukotriene treatment was also associated with an increased risk of withdrawal because of poor asthma control.

Although meta-analyses are considered to provide high-quality scientific results, the conclusions reached depend on the quality of the original studies, how appropriately their findings were reported and how they have been identified by the meta-analyst.

Studies may be included yet differ in study populations, experimental design and quality control. There may be issues of publication bias and issues regarding the operational definitions employed by different investigators. However, it is unlikely that this result will be tested and most practising respiratory physicians will feel comfortable with the advice to prescribe inhaled corticosteroids rather than leukotriene receptor antagonists as first-line controller therapy.

Last year I included a meta-analysis by the same author examining the potential of leukotriene receptor antagonists as add-on therapy to inhaled glucocorticoids. The addition of leukotrienes to inhaled corticosteroids appeared to be associated with modest improvements in asthma control, but is not as effective as increasing the dose of inhaled corticosteroids. A significant reduction in exacerbations was observed, but only when higher than licensed doses |**54**|. It was concluded that it would be more appropriate to await appropriately powered, randomized, controlled trials. Three such papers have been published this year.

When patients remain symptomatic despite adequate doses of inhaled corticosteroids guideline statements currently favour the addition of long-acting β_2 agonists. This recommendation is backed up by a wealth of published data |**52**|. However, it is recognized that corticosteroids may not completely inhibit the synthesis and release of cysteinyl leukotrienes in the lungs, thereby suggesting that leukotriene receptor antagonists may have a role as add-on therapy |**55,56**|. Vaquerio et al. reported the results from a 16-week, randomized, controlled trial in 639 patients with uncontrolled asthma despite taking inhaled corticosteroids. In terms of lung function (the mean FEV_1 at baseline was 81% predicted) their asthma was mild in severity, but their inhaled corticosteroid doses ranged between 400 and 1600 µg/day. These patients were then randomized to receive either 10 mg/day montelukast or to maintain a constant dose of inhaled budesonide. The group receiving montelukast reported a 35% reduction in the median percentage of asthma exacerbation days and a 56% higher median percentage of asthma-free days. Patients receiving montelukast had significantly fewer nocturnal awakenings and significantly greater improvement in their β_2 agonist use and morning PEF. The number needed to treat to avoid one exacerbation day was 13 and the number needed to treat to gain one asthma-free day was ten. The authors were able to divide their patients into three groups on the basis of the prescribed corticosteroid dose and reported that the efficacy of montelukast was evident at both low and high doses of budesonide.

The study by Vaquerio et al. is important, as it is the first published study with montelukast to use exacerbation days as a primary end-point. However, one of the problems inherent with such studies is a lack of clarity as to what constitutes an exacerbation of asthma and definitions of exacerbations used in papers do vary. This study defined an exacerbation on the basis of symptoms, rescue medication use and unscheduled medical care. The authors also performed a post hoc analysis in which they applied two further definitions of asthma exacerbation and found that their results were broadly similar.

It is an interesting ethical point that Vaquerio et al. felt it was appropriate to leave poorly controlled patients on the same dose of inhaled corticosteroid! Price et al. reported the results of a 16-week, randomized, controlled trial in 889 adults with asthma that was inadequately controlled despite 800 µg/day budesonide. The patients in this study received either 800 µg/day budesonide plus 10 mg of montelukast or 1600 µg/day budesonide. The results suggest that adding montelukast is at least as good as doubling the dose of inhaled budesonide in terms of the primary outcome of PEF and the secondary outcomes of symptom control, exacerbations and asthma-specific quality of life.

The study may be criticized because of the absence of a placebo group. This means that it is not possible to judge the magnitude of effect against the 'trial effect'. It is usual that all patients who are entered into a clinical trial tend to improve and so we are unclear whether this explains the improvements reported by the investigators. This is particularly pertinent as we might reasonably expect the clinical effectiveness of inhaled budesonide to plateau at doses of 800 µg/day |**57,58**|. However, the authors answered this criticism by highlighting that, in the last 2 weeks of the run-in period, the patients were administered inhaled budesonide and a daily montelukast tablet in a single-blind fashion such that on day 1 of the study the patients were not aware that they had been switched to active drug or double-dose budesonide.

Although leukotriene receptor antagonists are not an alternative to inhaled corticosteroids it is possible that they may represent an alternative to long-acting β_2 agonists in patients whose asthma is inadequately controlled on appropriate doses of inhaled corticosteroids. Previous studies have reported that the efficacy of leukotriene receptor antagonists is less that that of inhaled long-acting β_2 agonists as an add-on treatment to inhaled corticosteroids, as assessed by changes in lung function and symptoms |**59,60**|. However, their anti-inflammatory potential suggests that they may provide additional benefit when assessing other end-points such as exacerbations |**61**|.

Bjermer *et al.* reported a randomized, double-blind, double-dummy, parallel-group, multicentre study assessing the effect of montelukast versus salmeterol added to inhaled fluticasone propionate on asthma exacerbations in patients whose asthma was inadequately controlled with fluticasone alone. The investigators recruited 2144 patients from 148 sites and 37 countries. They entered 1490 patients and randomized 747 patients to the montelukast–fluticasone arm of the study and 743 patients to the salmeterol–fluticasone arm.

The main finding from this study was that montelukast was not inferior to salmeterol in terms of the exacerbations experienced by the patients. Overall 20.1% patients in the montelukast–fluticasone arm experienced at least one asthma exacerbation compared with 19.1% for the salmeterol–fluticasone group, the difference being 1% (95% CI = –3.1 to 5.0%). A Kaplan–Meier plot that accounted for censored observations did not change this conclusion and there was no difference in the time to first exacerbation between the two groups. An analysis of the distribution of patients according to the number of exacerbations showed no difference between the two groups (Fig. 3.4).

Exacerbations represent an important clinical end-point, as they are associated with decreased quality of life, substantial morbidity, unscheduled healthcare visits, expense and even death. The role of long-acting β_2 agonists used in combination with inhaled corticosteroids for reducing exacerbations has been demonstrated by numerous studies, but this paper suggested that the combination of an inhaled corticosteroid with the leukotriene receptor antagonist montelukast represents an alternative strategy for some patients. The paper also reported that both treatment groups demonstrated improvements in lung function, reduced episodes of nocturnal awakenings and significantly improved PEF over baseline values.

The montelukast–fluticasone treatment reduced the patients' peripheral blood eosinophil counts compared with baseline (least-squares mean ± SE change –0.04 ± 0.01) ($P \leq 0.001$), whereas salmeterol–fluticasone did not. Whilst the

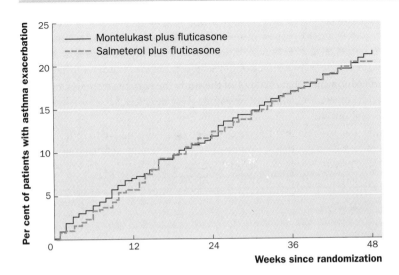

Fig. 3.4 Cumulative percentage of patients with asthma exacerbations ($P = 0.599$ by a log-rank test). Source: Bjermer *et al.* (2003).

authors chose to highlight this finding most respiratory physicians are unlikely to be impressed by a minor reduction in peripheral blood eosinophilia. Of potentially greater interest is the subset of patients who underwent induced sputum analysis and demonstrated that montelukast may produce a decline in sputum eosinophil counts. The exact role of eosinophils in the sputum is unclear, but this is a potentially important finding as it begins to substantiate the claims that these agents may have anti-inflammatory properties of real importance. Last year I included a study by Green *et al.* suggesting that therapy directed towards maintaining sputum eosinophils within a defined target provides superior asthma control than more traditional methods recommended in the British Thoracic Society guidelines |**62**|.

Aspirin desensitization in aspirin-sensitive asthma

Aspirin and other non-steroidal anti-inflammatory agents can aggravate asthma in between 3 and 15% of asthmatic individuals. Aspirin-sensitive asthma characteristically appears in the thirties and is heralded by the appearance of persistent rhinitis that is then followed by asthma, aspirin sensitivity and nasal polyposis. It is typically more common and severe in women and has been reported as a factor in life-threatening asthma |**63**|. Definitive confirmation of the diagnosis is made by provocation tests with increasing doses of aspirin.

A number of observations have been forwarded to explain why some individuals develop aspirin-sensitive asthma. These include the overproduction of leukotrienes by mast cells and eosinophils, which may in part be due to increased expression of leukotriene C_4 synthase. Aspirin-sensitive asthma is characterized by the over-production of prostaglandin D_2, a potentially critical prostanoid for inducing vasodilatation and bronchospasm and the up-regulation or synthesis of the critical leukotriene receptors that mediate inflammation and the aspirin-sensitive asthma-induced reactions, coupled with reduced synthesis of the inhibitory prostaglandin E_2. Diminished synthesis of the 5-lipoxygenase and 15-lipoxygenase products lipoxin and 15-epimer lipoxin, which are anti-inflammatory antagonists of leukotrienes, has recently been reported [63].

Long-term treatment with aspirin desensitization in asthmatic patients with aspirin-exacerbated respiratory disease

Berges-Gimeno MP, Simon RA, Stevenson DD. *J Allergy Clin Immunol* 2003; **111**: 180–6

BACKGROUND. The desensitization of patients with aspirin-sensitive asthma with the use of daily aspirin treatment has been validated by several studies. The aim of this study was to determine whether beneficial effects could be demonstrated within 6 months and to determine the duration of response. The authors also planned to determine how many patients experienced improvement, how many did not and what the side-effect profile was.

INTERPRETATION. Aspirin desensitization followed by daily aspirin is efficacious by at least the first 6 months of treatment and continues to be effective for up to 5 years of follow-up.

Comment

The use of aspirin for desensitization was first described in 1922 [64]. The most extensive experience with this treatment has been at the Scripps Clinic and Research Institute [65,66]. In this paper the authors reported their experience with 172 patients with aspirin-sensitive asthma who had been identified by a standard, single-blind, oral aspirin challenge. These patients then underwent aspirin desensitization, following which they were maintained on 650 mg of aspirin twice daily. The aspirin doses were gradually reduced after 1 year unless the patient experienced gastritis or bruising, when they were reduced earlier. Follow-up at 6 months and then 6-monthly intervals was obtained by the use of questionnaires and telephone interviews by nursing staff.

Data were collected on a range of outcome measures including the number of sinus infections, the number of surgical procedures, hospital admissions for asthma, symptom scores for sense of smell, topical corticosteroids for nasal insufflation, topical corticosteroids for bronchial inhalation, the use of systemic corticosteroids and leukotriene-modifier drugs and a global assessment of asthma activity and nasal sinus symptoms.

The authors reported that 24 (13%) of the 172 patients discontinued aspirin in the first year due to side effects. Of the remaining 148 patients 17 (11%) probably failed to respond and discontinued treatment during the first year. Therapy was discontinued for other reasons in five patients who had probably responded to therapy.

Sixteen (11%) of the 126 patients who took treatment for at least 1 year were deemed not to have responded. The clinical course was improved in 110 (87%) and deemed an excellent response in 60 and a good response in 50. There were highly significant reductions in the numbers of sinus infections, improvements in sense of smell and global assessments of nasosinus and asthma symptoms (Tables 3.1 and 3.2).

Table 3.1 Analysis of changes in markers of clinical disease after greater than 1 year of treatment with aspirin densensitization ($n = 126$)

	Baseline		≥1 y after therapy		P value
	Median	Range	Median	Range	
No. of sinus infections/y	5.0	0–12	2.0	0–12	<0.0001
Smell scores	0.0	0–5	3.0	0–5	<0.0001
Nasal symptom scores	2.0	0–4	4.0	0–4	<0.0001
Asthma symptom scores	3.0	0–4	4.0	0–4	<0.0001
Sinus operations/y	0.22	0–3	0.0	0–2	<0.0001
Hospitalizations for asthma/y	0.0	0–5	0.0	0–3	<0.0001
Emergency department visits for asthma/y	0.15	0–15	0.0	0–5	<0.0001

Values were determined with the Wilcoxon signed-rank statistic. Two-sided P values were reported.
Source: Berges-Gimeno et al. (2003).

Table 3.2 Analysis of the treatment with corticosteroids before, at 6 months after and greater than 1 year after starting aspirin desensitization therapy

	Baseline		Aspirin treatment at 6 mo			Aspirin treatment at >1 y		
	Mean	SEM	Mean	SEM	P value*	Mean	SEM	P value*
Nasal corticosteroids (μg/d)	271.4	10.3	252.2	10.5	0.004	216.3	15.0	<0.0001
Inhaled corticosteroids (μg/d)	867.3	52.1	829.9	49.2	0.06	656.7	35.4	<0.0001
Daily corticosteroids (mg/d)	10.8	1.8	8.1	1.6	0.01	3.6	0.8	<0.0001
Short courses of corticosteroids/y	2.7	0.7	0.8	0.9	<0.0001	0.5	1.3	<0.0001

Values were determined with the paired t test.
* Comparisons were made between baseline and 6 months and baseline and greater than 1 year.
Source: Berges-Gimeno et al. (2003).

A potential confounder in this study was that, during the study period, many patients were started on leukotriene-modifying agents. However, in the discussion of the paper the authors analysed their data in several different manners in order to overcome this and were able to suggest that desensitization therapy is effective.

Non-pharmacological strategies in the management of asthma

Adjuvant treatment for asthma

 Effect of two breathing exercises (Buteyko and pranayama) in asthma: a randomized controlled trial
Cooper S, Osborne J, Newton S, *et al. Thorax* 2003; **59**: 674–9

BACKGROUND. Breathing exercises practised in both yoga and Buteyko have been advocated for the management of asthma, but it remains unclear as to whether these techniques can improve asthma outcomes. The authors conducted a study using a parallel group design and randomized participants to follow the Eucapnic Buteyko technique or to use the Pink City Lung Exerciser, which is a device that mimics the breathing patterns employed in Pranayama Yoga. A third group received a Pink City Lung Exerciser placebo. The participants performed the exercises at home for 6 months and were also invited to participate in an optional steroid reduction phase. The primary

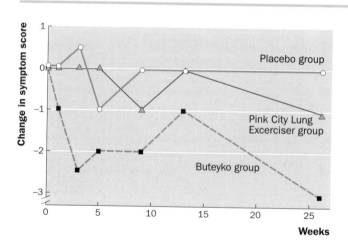

Fig. 3.5 Median change in symptom scores during the 6-month study. Source: Cooper *et al.* (2003).

outcome measures were symptom scores and a change in airway hyper-reactivity to methacholine.

INTERPRETATION. In adult patients with asthma the Eucapnic Buteyko breathing technique was associated with symptomatic improvement and a reduced requirement for rescue bronchodilator therapy (Fig. 3.5). The use of the Pink City Lung Exerciser was not associated with benefit in any of the outcome measures.

Breathing retraining for dysfunctional breathing in asthma: a randomized controlled trial

Thomas M, McKinley RK, Freeman E, Foy C, Prodger P, Price D. *Thorax* 2003; **58**: 110–15

BACKGROUND. The authors of this study had previously reported that one-third of women and one-fifth of men treated for asthma in a single general practice had symptoms suggestive of dysfunctional breathing. As a follow-up to this study they designed a randomized, controlled trial comparing breathing retraining led by a physiotherapist with an educational programme led by an asthma nurse specialist in order to determine whether breathing retraining could produce symptomatic improvements in this group. The outcome measures were asthma-specific health status and Nijmegen Questionnaire scores.

INTERPRETATION. Over half of the patients treated for asthma who had symptoms of dysfunctional breathing obtained benefit from breathing retraining and in over one-quarter this benefit was still apparent 6 months later. The number needed to treat at 1 month was 1.96 and at 6 months 3.57 (Table 3.3).

Comment

There is considerable interest amongst patients in the use of techniques designed for modifying the pattern of breathing |**67**|. Amongst the most popular of these are the

Table 3.3 Numbers (proportions) of patients showing clinically relevant changes in health status (overall AQLQ score change of >0.5) in breathing retraining and asthma education groups and the number needed to treat (NNT) for one patient to benefit

	Improved	Unchanged	Deteriorated	*n*	NNT
1 month					
Breathing retraining	9/16 (0.56)	7/16 (0.44)	0/16 (0)	16	
Asthma education	2/15 (0.13)	10/15 (0.67)	3/15 (0.20)	15	1.96
6 months					
Breathing retraining	9/16 (0.56)	5/16 (0.31)	2/16 (0.20)	16	
Asthma education	3/12 (0.25)	7/12 (0.58)	2/12 (0.17)	12	3.57

Source: Thomas *et al.* (2003).

use of yoga and the controversial Butyeko method. The two papers detailed above were designed for developing our knowledge of the use of breathing techniques further.

The study by Cooper *et al.* focused attention on the potential of the Buteyko method and yoga. The Butyeko technique is founded on the scientifically dubious principle that hyperventilation causes asthma and therefore proposes that adopting techniques for reducing hyperventilation should lead to a cure from asthma [68]. The Butyeko Breathing Centre has reported that over 90% of the 100 000 participants who have completed their course require no further asthma medication [69]. The only randomized, controlled trial of the method failed to show that the Buteyko method had any effect on the subjects' end-tidal carbon dioxide, but demonstrated reductions in the use of β_2 agonist use [70]. However, it should be noted that a central component to Buteyko is discouraging the use of reliever medications. The Eucapnic Buteyko technique is a Western modification of the Russian Buteyko technique. Exercises are designed for reducing the frequency and depth of breathing and patients are only encouraged to use bronchodilator therapy if this fails.

The practice of yoga has been established for centuries and a variety of disciplines exist. The use of techniques of meditation in Sahaja yoga has been explored in patients with asthma requiring treatment with moderate to high doses of inhaled corticosteroids, but only limited benefits were observed [71]. The term Pranayama refers to the study of the control of breathing and in yoga is usually designed for promoting a slow relaxed breathing pattern. In a trial of 18 patients it was possible to show that the use of a device for promoting a pattern of breathing similar to that observed in yoga was associated with decreased airway hyper-responsiveness [72]. The Pink City Lung Exerciser is a cylinder with an expiratory resistance valve that reduces the respiratory rate and increases the duration of expiration, similar to that encouraged in certain forms of yoga. The control group had an identical device without resistance.

In this study the authors recruited symptomatic adult patients treated with inhaled corticosteroids who had reversible airflow obstruction and hyper-responsiveness to methacholine from an asthma volunteer database and by advertisement. They made significant attempts to control for non-specific intervention effects by comparing a variety of asthma outcome measures. Randomization produced appropriately balanced groups except that the patients receiving Buteyko were younger, took slightly more inhaled corticosteroids and had slightly greater airway hyper-reactivity. The primary outcome measures were symptoms and airway hyper-reactivity (as assessed by PD_{20} methacholine).

The authors reported significant improvements in asthma symptom scores in the patients following Buteyko. The median change in the daily symptoms scores was 0 (interquartile range [IQR] = −1 to 1) in the placebo group, −1 (IQR = −2 to 0.75) in the Pink City Lung Exerciser group and −3 (IQR = −4 to 0) in the Buteyko group. There was no significant change in airway hyper-reactivity. As regards secondary outcome measures, patients in the Buteyko group had significantly less requirement for β_2 agonists, but there were no differences in lung function, the number of asthma exacerbations, days requiring an increase in inhaled corticosteroid dose or courses of prednisolone in any of the groups. There were no significant differences in steroid reduction between the three groups.

The authors suggested that these results indicate that the Buteyko method may help patients to feel more in control. Nevertheless, the magnitude and clinical relevance of the improvements were not clear and, as the Butekyo group received five sessions of 2 h compared to a single session of training on the Pink City Lung Exerciser, it is possible that the results reflect confounding by professional attention. Although the subjects in the Butyeko arm were able to reduce their β_2 agonist use, this was probably to be expected, as it is a fundamental part of the teaching. There was no change in quality of life as measured by the SF36 Questionnaire, save for one dimension (role limitation due to physical problems), which improved more in the Buteyko group. There were no changes in the Asthma Quality of Life Questionnaire (AQLQ) domains.

The study by Thomas et al. suggested that physiotherapy-led breathing retraining improves the quality of life of patients with asthma whose illness may be complicated by dysfunctional breathing. They identified patients aged 17–65 years who were registered as suffering asthma on the basis that they had been prescribed at least one bronchodilator or prophylactic anti-asthma medication in the previous year. The team examined the medical records for the presence of variable or reversible air-flow obstruction as a validation of the diagnosis of asthma. This was not possible in five patients. The presence of clinically relevant hyperventilation was identified by a Nijmegen Questionnaire score ≥23. The Nijmegen Questionnaire consists of a series of questions scored 0–4 covering respiratory, cardiac, neurological and psychiatric domains |73|. A score of ≥23 has been suggested to be highly specific for hyperventilation syndrome (HVS). However, the use of the Nijmegen Questionnaire score is controversial. It should be noted that it was designed and validated in normal individuals and remains to be properly examined in patients with asthma. Furthermore, a high score can be associated with the symptoms of poorly controlled asthma or other pulmonary or cardiac pathologies.

Patients were then randomized to either a physiotherapy-led breathing retraining programme or a nurse-led asthma education programme. The physiotherapist saw patients in groups of four to five patients for sessions of 45 min and then individual sessions of 15 min on the second and third weeks. Patients received instruction on breathing techniques emphasizing slow regular breathing and the use of diaphragmatic respiratory effort |74| and were encouraged to practice this for 10-minute periods each day. The control group underwent 60 min of nurse-led asthma education and, although they were then invited to attend for an individual asthma review, only six out of 16 patients took up this offer. The main outcome measures were health status as assessed by the AQLQ and the Nijmegen Questionnaire score.

After 1 month the intervention group demonstrated significant changes in the activities, symptoms and environment domains of the AQLQ. However, only the improvement in the activities domain persisted at 6 months. The Nijmegen Questionnaire score fell in the intervention group after 1 month and this persisted and

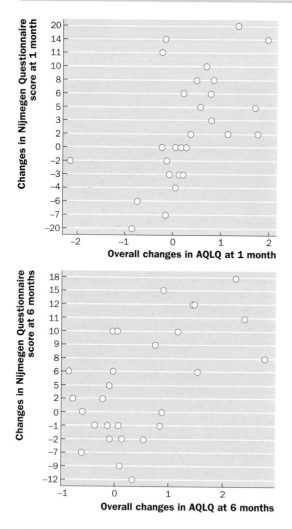

Fig. 3.6 Scatter plots of the changes in the AQLQ score and Nijmegen Questionnaire score at 1 and 6 months following intervention and control. Source: Thomas *et al.* (2003).

achieved significance at 6 months. In order to achieve an improvement at 1 and 6 months the numbers needed to treat were 2 and 3.65, respectively.

The authors were able to demonstrate a correlation between the changes in the overall AQLQ scores and Nijmegen Questionnaire scores at 6 months (Fig. 3.6). This observation provides some indication that the Nijmegen Questionnaire score may be clinically valid and alludes to the fact that uncontrolled hyperventilation may contribute to a lower health status in patients with asthma.

The authors acknowledged limitations inherent in their study, namely that they were a single centre with one physiotherapist and these observations need to be extended to other practices. Nevertheless, this is an important piece of work that should herald the beginnings of further research into this difficult area.

An alternative strategy for follow-up

Accessibility, acceptability and effectiveness in primary care of routine telephone review of asthma: pragmatic, randomized, controlled trial

Pinnock H, Bawden R, Proctor S, *et al.* BMJ 2003; **326**: 477–9

BACKGROUND. It has been suggested that telephone care has the potential for reducing morbidity, drug use and the use of health services in patients with a range of chronic disorders. The aim of this study was to determine whether nurse-led review by telephone improved access to care for asthmatic patients and could be substituted as an acceptable alternative to consultation in family practice units. The primary outcome measures included the proportion of patients reviewed within 3 months of randomization and change in their asthma-specific quality of life.

INTERPRETATION. Compared to consultations at the surgery the use of the telephone increased the number of individuals it was possible to review by 26% compared to surgery consultations. These reviews were shorter than surgery consultations, but did not amount to loss of satisfaction or clinical disadvantage.

Comment

The authors suggested that the culture of consultation is changing and acknowledged that the use of the telephone for assessing and delivering care may become more acceptable. Previous studies have suggested that consultation by telephone has the potential for reducing morbidity, drug use and the use of health services in patients with a range of chronic disorders |**75**|. Certainly important information can be relayed by telephone and the medium offers the potential for enhanced flexibility in consultation. The aim of this study was to examine the utility of telephone consultation for the management of asthma in primary care.

The authors enrolled patients with asthma from four general practices in England. The patients were included in the study if the computerized asthma register identified that they had requested a prescription for a bronchodilator inhaler in the previous 6 months, but had not had a regular review in 11 months. The patients were then centrally randomized in blocks of ten to either telephone review or face-to-face consultation with an asthma nurse. A letter was sent to patients who were randomized to telephone care to inform them that they should expect a telephone call from a nurse. No specific instructions were given to the nurses as to the structure or content of the call other than that it should reflect their normal practice. Follow-up consultations (either by telephone or in the practice) were arranged as deemed appropriate. The patients were also free to arrange any consultation they wished.

Applying an intention to treat analysis, the authors reported that 74% of those allocated to the telephone arm were reviewed compared to 48% of those allocated to a face-to-face consultation (risk difference = 26% with 95% CI = 14–37% and number needed to treat = 3.8 with 95% CI = 2.7–7.1) (P <0.001). The telephone interviews were shorter, even allowing for 141 abortive phone calls and five missed appointments. Although the authors suggested that they were able to address similar aspects of asthma care over the telephone as compared with a face-to-face consultation it would not have been possible to perform chest auscultation, measure peak flow or assess and identify deficiencies in inhaler technique.

This is an interesting study in a topical area, but it may be limited in application. Only 278 of 932 eligible patients agreed to participate and it should be acknowledged that the population studied by the authors failed to represent the greater population of asthma patients in primary care, perhaps excluding many patients who dislike telephone consultations |76|. This is important as the authors used patient satisfaction as one of their end-points. The authors also acknowledged that the practices were 'asthma interested' and this may have biased the findings. Furthermore, as it was not possible to blind the study it is impossible to determine whether the bias was introduced. The nurses were allowed to telephone patients up to four times, but if the patients did not attend a clinic only one further written invitation was given, thus it is possible that the higher follow-up rates reflected the reward of persistence. It should also be noted that the study was of relatively short duration (only 3 months) and, thus, does not provide any information on the utility of this method for longer term follow-up and does not provide a reliable assessment of more important outcome measures such as asthma exacerbations.

Thus, in conclusion, the authors reported an interesting and timely study exploring an alternative method of assessing asthma control and providing advice on asthma management. Further studies will be needed in order to determine the utility of the telephone consultation, but this study at least provided some reassuring data that may be applicable to patients who dislike attending surgery.

Conclusion

An important goal in the management of asthma will be to prevent its appearance in high-risk individuals. Epidemiological research such as that summarized in Chapter 1 continues to identify targets that appear to be implicated in this process and some of these may be modifiable. The paper from Mihrshahi *et al.* provides the beginnings of such studies and the longer term results of these are eagerly awaited. The work of Langley *et al.* (Chapter 2) suggesting that ongoing exposure to allergens appears to be important in determining asthma persistence and severity suggests that avoiding or minimizing exposure to allergens should be helpful in disease management. The study by Halken *et al.* does suggest that in specific subgroups of children avoidance of minimizing exposure to house dust mites may be beneficial, but the study by Woodcock *et al.* reminds us that extrapolating these findings to a greater number of adult asthmatics may not produce the same sort of beneficial outcomes.

Inhaled corticosteroids remain the controller therapy of first choice for asthma and the study by Pauwels *et al.* suggests that this should be the case even in patients with mild asthma. They offer tentative information that starting therapy early may prevent the loss of lung function seen in some patients with asthma. Nevertheless, it is important to prescribe both judiciously and prudently. New knowledge that, for many patients, the maximum effects of inhaled corticosteroids are achieved at modest doses should remind us to explore the possibility of stepping down therapy once asthma control has been achieved. The papers by Hawkins *et al.* and by Busse *et al.* increase our understanding of this neglected area.

Several worthwhile studies have been published on the use of leukotriene receptor antagonists as adjunctive treatments to inhaled corticosteroids. The best of these is probably that of Bjermer *et al.* suggesting that these agents may positively influence asthma exacerbations. More information on the potential anti-inflammatory potential of these drugs is awaited. Leukotriene receptor antagonists make a logical choice in patients with aspirin-sensitive asthma. However, the paper by Berges-Gimeno *et al.* provides important data on the utility and long-term outcome from aspirin desensitization.

Adjuvant therapy for asthma is likely to gain increasingly widespread acceptance. Concern remains over the scientific basis for the Buteyko method and a gap remains between the claims from the Buteyko organization and the outcomes of carefully conducted randomized, controlled trials. Nevertheless, the use of breathing training techniques is likely to be useful to many patients, particularly if they have a evidence of dysfunctional breathing.

Finally, more work needs to be performed on the optimum methods of educating patients and providing them with the confidence and skill base necessary for enacting the lifestyle and treatment choices necessary for improving the day-to-day control of their disease.

References

1. Moller C, Dreborg S, Ferdousi HA, Halken S, Host A, Jacobsen L, Koivikko A, Koller DY, Niggemann B, Norberg LA, Urbanek R, Valovirta E, Whan U. Pollen immunotherapy reduces the development of asthma in children with seasonal rhinoconjunctivitis (The PAT Study). *J Allergy Clin Immunol* 2002; **109**: 251–6.

2. Platts-Mills TA, Tovey ER, Mitchell EB, Moszoro H, Nock P, Wilkins SR. Reduction of bronchial hyperreactivity during prolonged allergen avoidance. *Lancet* 1982; **2**: 675–8.

3. Ehnert B, Lau-Schadendorf S, Weber A, Buettner P, Schou C, Wahn U. Reducing domestic exposure to dust mite allergen reduces bronchial hyperreactivity in sensitive children with asthma. *J Allergy Clin Immunol* 1992; **90**: 135–8.

4. Peroni DG, Boner AL, Vallone G, Antolini I, Warner JO. Effective allergen avoidance at high altitude reduces allergen-induced bronchial hyperresponsiveness. *Am J Respir Crit Care* 1994; **149**: 1442–6.

5. Gøtzsche PC, Johansen HK, Burr ML, Hammarquist C. House dust mite control measures for asthma (Cochrane Review). In: *The Cochrane Library*, Issue 4. Oxford: Update Software, 2002.

6. Szefler SJ, Martin RJ, Sharp King T, Boushey HA, Cherniak RM, Chinchilli VM, Craig TJ, Dolovich M, Drazen JM, Fagan JK, Fahy JV, Fish JE, Ford JK, Israel E, Kiley J, Kraft M, Lazarus SC, Lemanske RF, Mauger E, Peters SP, Sorkness CA, Pharm D for the Asthma Clinical Research Network of the National Heart, Lung and Blood Institute. Significant variability in response to inhaled corticosteroids for persistent asthma. *J Allergy Clin Immunol* 2002; **109**: 410–18.

7. Holt S, Suder A, Weatherall M, Cheng S, Shirtcliffe P, Beasley R. Dose–response relation of inhaled fluticasone propionate in adolescents and adults with asthma: meta-analysis. *BMJ* 2001; **323**: 1–8.

8. Lipworth BJ. Leukotriene receptor antagonists. *Lancet* 1999; **353**: 57–62.

9. O'Hickey SP, Hawsworth RJ, Fong CY, Arm JP, Spur BW, Lee TH. Leukotrienes C_4, D_4, and E_4 enhance histamine responsiveness in asthmatic airways. *Am Rev Respir Dis* 1991; **144**: 1053–7.

10. Lipworth BJ. Leukotriene receptor antagonists. *Lancet* 1999; **353**: 57–62.

11. Dahlén SE, Malmström K, Nizankowska E, Dahlén B, Kuna P, Kowalski M, Lumry WR, Picade C, Stevenson DD, Bousquet J, Pauwels R, Holgate ST, Shahane A, Reiss TF, Szczeklik A. Improvement of aspirin-intolerant asthma by montelukast, a leukotriene receptor antagonist. *Am J Respir Crit Care Med* 2002; **165**: 9–14.

12. British Thoracic Society. Scottish Intercollegiate Guidelines Network. *Thorax* 2003; **58**(Suppl 1): 1–94.

13. GINA Workshop Report. Global Initiative for Asthma Management and Prevention. Available on-line at http://www.ginasthma.com

14. UK National Asthma Campaign. Available on-line at http://www.asthma.org.uk

15. International Asthma Management Plan 'Zone System'. Available on-line at http://www.nhlbisupport.com/asthma/index.html

16. New Zealand 'Credit Card' System. Available on-line at http://www.asthmanz.co.nz

17. Sherriff A, Peters TJ, Henderson J, Strachan D. Risk factor associations with wheezing patterns in children followed longitudinally from birth to 3 years. *Int J Epidemiol* 2001; **30**: 1473–84.

18. Martinez FD, Wright AL, Taussig LM, Holberg CJ, Halonen M, Morgan WJ. Asthma and wheezing in the first six years of life. *N Engl J Med* 1995; **332**: 133–8.

19. Custovic A, Simpson BM, Simpson A, Kissen P, Woodcock A. Effect of environmental manipulation in pregnancy and early life on respiratory symptoms and atopy during the first year of life. *Lancet* 2001; **358**: 188–93.

20. Chan-Yeung M, Manfreda J, Dimich-Ward H, Ferguson A, Watson W, Becker A. A randomised controlled study on the effectiveness of a multifaceted intevention program

in primary prevention in the primary prevention of asthma in high-risk infants. *Arch Pediatr Adolesc Med* 2000; **154**: 657–63.

21. Hide DW, Matthews S, Tariq S, Arshad SH. Allergen avoidance in infancy and allergy at 4 years of age. *Allergy* 1996; **1**: 89–93.

22. Sporik R, Holgate ST, Platts-Mills TAE, Coswell JJ. Exposure to house-dust mite allergen (*Der p 1*) and the development of asthma in childhood. *N Engl J Med* 1990; **323**: 502–7.

23. Custovic A, Taggart S, Francis H, Chapman MD, Woodcock A. Exposure to house dust mite allergens and the clinical activity of asthma. *J Allergy Clin Immunol* 1996; **98**: 64–72.

24. Tunnicliffe WS, Fletcher TJ, Hammond K, Roberts K, Custovic A, Simpson A, Woodcock A, Ayres JG. Sensitivity and exposure to indoor allergens in adults with differing asthma severity. *Eur Respir J* 1999; **13**: 645–9.

25. Peroni DG, Boner AL, Vallone G, Antolini I, Warner JO. Effective allergen avoidance at high altitude reduces allergen-induced bronchial hyperresponsiveness. *Am J Respir Crit Care* 1994; **149**: 1442–6.

26. Peroni DG, Piacentini GL, Costella S, Pietrobelli A, Bodini A, Loiacono A, Aralla R, Boner AL. Mite avoidance can reduce air trapping and airway inflammation in allergic asthmatic children. *Clin Exp Allergy* 2002; **32**: 850–5.

27. Platts-Mills TA, Tovey ER, Mitchell EB, Moszoro H, Nock P, Wilkins SR. Reduction of bronchial hyperreactivity during prolonged allergen avoidance. *Lancet* 1982; **2**: 675–8.

28. Ehnert B, Lau-Schadendorf S, Weber A, Buettner P, Schou C, Wahn U. Reducing domestic exposure to dust mite allergen reduces bronchial hyperreactivity in sensitive children with asthma. *J Allergy Clin Immunol* 1992; **90**: 135–8.

29. Gøtzsche PC, Johansen HK, Burr ML, Hammarquist C. House dust mite control measures for asthma (Cochrane Review). In: *The Cochrane Library*, Issue 4. Oxford: Update Software, 2002.

30. Rijssenbeek-Nouwens LHM, Oosting AJ, De Bruin-Weller MS, Bregman I, De Monchy JGR, Postma DS. Clinical evaluation of the effect of anti-allergic mattress covers in patients with moderate to severe asthma and house dust mite allergy: a randomised double blind placebo controlled study. *Thorax* 2002; **57**: 784–90.

31. Boggs PB. Bed covers and dust mites. *N Engl J Med* 2003; **349**: 1668.

32. Djukanovic R, Wilson JW, Britten KM, Wilson SJ, Walls AF, Roche WR, Howarth PH, Holgate ST. Effect of an inhaled corticosteroid on airway inflammation and symptoms in asthma. *Am Rev Respir Dis* 1992; **145**: 669–74.

33. Haahtela T, Jarvinen M, Kava T, Kiviranta K, Koskinen S, Lethonen K, Nikander K, Persson T, Reinikainen K, Selroos O, Sovijärvi A, Stenius-Aarniala B, Svahn T, Tammivaara R, Laitinen LA. Comparison of a beta 2-agonist, terbutaline, with an inhaled corticosteroid, budesonide, in newly detected asthma. *N Engl J Med* 1991; **325**: 388–92.

34. Pauwels R, Pedersen S, Busse WW, Tan WC, Chen Y-Z, Ohlsson SV, Ullman A, Lamm CJ, O'Byrne PM on behalf of the START Investigators Group. Early intervention with budesonide in mild asthma: a randomised, double-blind trial. *Lancet* 2003; **361**: 1071–6.

35. Laitinen LA, Laitenan A, Haahtela T. Airway mucosal inflammation even in patients with newly diagnosed asthma. *Am Rev Respir Dis* 1993; **147**: 697–704.

36. Chetta A, Foresi A, Beertorelli G, Pesci A, Oliveieri D. Airways remodelling is a distinctive feature of asthma and is related to the severity of the disease. *Chest* 1997; **111**: 852–7.

37. Elias J. Airway remodelling in asthma. Unanswered questions. *Am J Respir Crit Care Med* 2000; **161**: S168–71.

38. Juniper EF, Kline PA, Vanzieleghem MA, Ramsdale EH, O'Bryne PM, Hargreave FE. Effect of long-term treatment with an inhaled corticosteroid (budesonide) on airway hyperresponsiveness and clinical asthma in nonsteroid dependent asthmatics. *Am Rev Respir Dis* 1990; **142**: 832–6.

39. Agertoft L, Pedersen S. Effects of long-term treatment with an inhaled corticosteroid on growth and pulmonary function in asthmatic children. *Respir Med* 1994; **88**: 373–81.

40. Selroos O, Pientinalho A, Lofroos A-B, Riska H. Effect of early vs late intervention with inhaled corticosteroids in asthma. *Chest* 1995; **108**: 1228–34.

41. Agertoft L, Pederson S. Effect of long-term treatment with inhaled budesonide on adult height in children with asthma. *N Engl J Med* 2000; **343**: 1064–9.

42. Barnes PJ, Pedersen S, Busse WW. Efficacy and safety of inhaled corticosteroids; new developments. *Am J Respir Crit Care Med* 1998; **157** (Suppl): S1–53.

43. Lipworth BJ. Systemic adverse effects of inhaled corticosteroid therapy. *Arch Intern Med* 1999; **159**: 941–55.

44. Global Initiative for Asthma (GINA). *Global Strategy for Asthma Management and Prevention.* Bethesda, MD: National Institutes of Health; National Heart, Blood and Lung Institute, 2002 (publication no. NIH-NHLI 02-3659).

45. Haahtela T, Jarvinen M, Kava T, Kiviranta K, Sirkka K, Lehtonon K, Nikander K, Persson T, Selroos O, Sovijärvi A, Stenius-Aarniala B, Svahn T, Tammivaara R, Laitinen LA. Effects of reducing or discontinuing inhaled budesonide in patients with mild asthma. *N Engl J Med* 1994; **331**: 700–5.

46. Leuppi J, Salome CM, Jenkins CR, Anderson SD, Xuan W, Marks GB, Koskela H, Brannan JD, Freed R, Anderson M, Chan HK, Woolcock AJ. Predictive markers of asthma exacerbation during stepwise dose reduction of inhaled corticosteroids. *Am J Respir Crit Care Med* 2001; **163**: 406–12.

47. Green RH, Brightling CE, McKenna S, Hargadon B, Parker D, Bradding P, Wardlaw AJ, Pavord ID. Asthma exacerbations and sputum eosinophil counts: a randomised controlled trial. *Lancet* 2002; **360**: 1715–21.

48. Lemanske RF, Sorkness CA, Mauger EA, Lazarus SC, Boushey HA, Fahy JV, Drazen JM, Chinchilli VM, Craig T, Fish JE, Ford JG, Israel E, Kraft M, Martin RJ, Nachman SA, Peters SP, Spahn JD, Szefler SJ for the Asthma Clinical Research Network for the National Heart, Lung, and Blood Institute. Inhaled corticosteroid reduction and elimination in patients with persistent asthma receiving salmeterol. *J Am Med Assoc* 2001; **285**: 2594–603.

49. Kips JC, O'Connor BJ, Inman MD, Svensson K, Pauwels RA, O'Byrne PM. A long-term study of the anti-inflammatory effect of low dose budesonide plus formoterol versus high dose budesonide in asthma. *Am J Respir Crit Care Med* 2000; **161**: 996–1001.

50. Sue-Chu M, Wallin A, Wilson S, Ward J, Sandstrom T, Djukanovic R, *et al.* Bronchial biopsy study in asthmatics treated with low- and high-dose fluticasone propionate (FP) compared to low dose FP combined with salmeterol. *Eur Respir J* 1999; **14**: 124s.

51. Price D, Dutchman D, Mawson A, Bodalia B, Duggan S, Todd P. Early asthma control and maintenance with eformoterol following reduction of inhaled corticosteroid dose. *Thorax* 2002; **57**: 791–8.

52. Barnes PJ. Scientific rationale for inhaled combination therapy with long-acting β_2-agonists and corticosteroids. *Eur Respir J* 2001; **19**: 182–91.

53. Nelson HS, Chapman KR, Pyke SD, Johnson M, Pritchard JN. Enhanced synergy between fluticasone propionate and salmeterol inhaled from a single inhaler versus separate inhalers. *J Allergy Clin Immunol* 2003; **112**: 29–36.

54. Ducharme FM. Anti-leukotrienes as add-on therapy to inhaled glucocorticoids in patients with asthma: systematic review of current evidence. *BMJ* 2002; **324**: 1545–52.

55. O'Shaughnessy KM, Wellings R, Gilles B, Fuller RB. Differential effects of fluticasone propionate on allergen-evoked bronchoconstriction and increased urinary leukotriene E_4 excretion. *Am Rev Respir Dis* 1993; **147**: 1472–6.

56. Dworski R, Fitzgerald GA, Oates JA, Sheller JR. Effect of oral prednisolone on airway inflammatory mediators in atopic asthma. *Am J Respir Crit Care Med* 1994; **149**: 953–9.

57. Busse WW, Chervinsky P, Condemi J, Lumry WR, Petty TL, Rennard S, Townley RG. Budesonide delivered by turbohaler is effective in a dose-dependent fashion when used in the treatment of adult patients with chronic asthma. *J Allergy Clin Immunol* 1998; **101**: 457–63 (erratum: *J Allergy Clin Immunol* 1998; **102**: 511).

58. Busse WW, Brazinsky S, Jacobson K, Stricker W, Schmitt K, Vanden Burgt J, Donnell D, Hannon S, Colice GL. Efficacy of inhaled beclomethasone dipropionate in asthma is proportional to dose and is improved by formulation with a new propellant. *J Allergy Clin Immunol* 1999; **104**: 1215–22.

59. Nelson HS, Busse WW, Kerwin E, Church N, Emmett A, Rickard K, Knobil K. Fluticasone propionate/Salmeterol combination provides more effective asthma control than low dose inhaled corticosteroid plus montelukast. *J Allergy Clin Immunol* 2000; **106**: 1088–95.

60. Fish JE, Israel E, Murray JJ, Emmett A, Boone R, Yancey SW, Rickard KA. Salmeterol powder provides significantly better benefit than montelukast in asthmatic patients receiving concomitant inhaled corticosteroid therapy. *Chest* 2001; **120**: 423–30.

61. Pizzichini E, Leff JA, Reiss TF, Hendeles L, Boulet LP, Wei LX, Efthimiadis AE, Zhang J, Hargreave FE. Montelukast reduces airway inflammation in asthma: a randomised, controlled trial. *Eur Respir J* 1999; **14**: 12–18.

62. Green RH, Brightling CE, McKenna S, Hargadon B, Parker D, Bradding P, Wardlaw AJ, Pavord ID. Asthma exacerbations and sputum eosinophil counts: a randomised controlled trial. *Lancet* 2002; **360**: 1715–21.

63. Szczeklik A, Stevenson DD. Aspirin-induced asthma: advances in pathogenesis, diagnosis and management. *J Allergy Clin Immunol* 2003; **111**: 913–21.

64. Widal MF, Abrami P, Lermeyaz J. Anaphylaxie et idiosynctasie. *Presse Med* 1922; **30**: 189–92.

65. Stevenson DD, Pleskow WW, Simon RA, Mathison DA, Lumry WR, Schatz M, Zeiger RS. Aspirin sensitive rhinosinusitis: a double-blind cross-over study of treatment with aspirin. *J Allergy Clin Immunol* 1984; **73**: 500–7.

66. Stevenson DD, Hankammer MA, Mathison DA, Christensen SC, Simon RA. Long term ASA desensitisation-treatment of aspirin sensitive asthmatic patients: clinical outcome studies. *J Allergy Clin Immunol* 1996; **98**: 751–8.

67. Ernst E. Breathing techniques: adjunctive treatment modalities for asthma. A systematic review. *Eur Respir J* 2000; **15**: 969–72.

68. Stalmatski A. *Freedom from Asthma: Buteyko's Revolutionary Treatment*. London: Kyle-Cathie Ltd, 1997.

69. Buteyko Breathing Centre. See http://www.buteyko.co.uk/trials.html

70. Bowler SD, Green A, Mitchell CA. Buteyko breathing techniques in asthma: a blinded randomised controlled trial. *Med J Aust* 1998; **169**: 575–8.

71. Manocha R, Marks GB, Kenchington P, Peters D, Salome CM. Sahaja yoga in the management of moderate to severe asthma: a randomised controlled trial. *Thorax* 2002; **57**: 110–15.

72. Singh V, Wisniewski A, Britton J, Tattersfield A. Effect of yoga breathing exercise (pranayama) on airways reactivity in subjects with asthma. *Lancet* 1990; **335**: 1381–3.

73. Van Dixhorn J, Duivenvoorden HJ. Efficacy of Nijmegen Questionnaire in recognition of the hyperventilation syndrome. *J Psychosom Res* 1985; **29**: 199–206.

74. Innocenti DM. Hyperventilation. In: Pryor JA, Prasad SA (eds). *Physiotherapy for Cardiac and Respiratory Problems*, 3rd edn. London: Churchill Livingstone, 2002: 563–79.

75. Wasson J, Gaudette C, Whaley F, Sauvigne A, Baribeau P, Welch HG. Telephone care as a substitute for routine clinic follow-up. *J Am Med Assoc* 1992; **267**: 1788–93.

76. Huynh T, Lavars C. Measurement of quality dimensions causes concern. *BMJ* 2003; **326**: 1267.

4

Acute asthma and asthma death

Introduction

Acute asthma is a common medical emergency and in recent years the total number of hospital admissions attributed to asthma has risen. These encounters are not only distressing and life threatening for the patient, but have a significant economic impact in terms of healthcare expenditure |1|. The goals of therapy are therefore to allay anxiety, remove hypoxaemia, improve airflow limitation and prevent death. In the recovery period it is important to identify factors that may have contributed to the attack and whenever possible to remove or modify them.

During an acute attack high concentrations of oxygen should be administered in order to maintain the oxygen saturation above 92% (95% in children). A β_2 agonist such as salbutamol is usually the bronchodilator of first choice. The dose administered depends on the severity of the exacerbation. In hospital it is most conveniently administered through a nebulizer driven by oxygen, but in primary care the delivery of salbutamol via a metered dose inhaler through a volumatic provides equivalent bronchodilation |2,3|. Up to 30% of acute asthma patients fail to respond adequately to short-acting β_2 agonists |4|. Additional bronchodilator therapy may be provided by the addition of ipratropium bromide |5|. Systemic corticosteroids reduce the inflammatory response and hasten the resolution of exacerbations |6|. They can usually be administered orally, but will not be effective for at least 4 h |7|.

In patients who fail to improve following these treatments a number of options exist with varying degrees of evidence base. The use of intravenous magnesium has been supported by several trials and has been suggested to confer additional benefit in those who fail to respond to initial therapy, particularly in those whose presenting peak expiratory flow (PEF) is <30% predicted |8|. Intravenous methylxanthines may represent an alternative and are favoured by many on an anecdotal basis. Evidence of benefit is lacking and concern has been raised over the potential for side effects |9,10|. Some physicians recommend the administration of intravenous β_2 agonists. Again clear evidence of benefit is lacking, but they may be useful in patients in whom inhaled therapy is not feasible |11|. More esoteric therapies such as the delivery of heliox have been suggested, but are not widely available |12|. Continued deterioration despite aggressive medical therapy or presentation in coma or with an impending respiratory arrest should signal admission to the intensive care unit and consideration of mechanical ventilation. Several papers have been published this year in an attempt to clarify the evidence base for treatment and evaluate potential new therapies.

Important advances in the medical management of asthma mean that death from asthma is fortunately rare, with an incidence of less than one up to eight per 100 000 per year |13,14|. However, whilst this figure is relatively low, particularly when one considers other causes of pulmonary death, it represents a continuing tragedy as a considerable number of these deaths occur in young people and many are preventable.

Most attacks of asthma are characterized by a gradual deterioration over several hours to days |15|, but some appear to occur with little or no warning: so-called brittle asthma |16–18|. Studies focusing on asthma death have identified several areas in which factors attributable to the death may be observed, including the underlying disease severity, the delivery of medical care and the pattern of health behaviour by the patient including the influence of psychological factors |19–23|.

Certain features may identify patients at risk of asthma death. Asthma death appears more common in patients with severe persistent asthma, but severe asthma attacks can occur in patients with mild asthma and a previous history of mechanical ventilation should be regarded as an important factor in any assessment |24–26|. Certain trigger factors may be important including the ingestion of aspirin, high levels of outdoor allergens or food allergy |27–29|. Despite the advances in the understanding and delivery of therapy for asthma some patients continue to demonstrate poor adherence and, particularly when this relates to inhaled corticosteroids, may represent an important risk factor |30|. A subset of patients may have a blunted perception of bronchospasm and fail to recognize the severity of their attack |31|. Other studies have suggested that psychological factors may be important in determining health behaviour.

Randomized pragmatic comparison of UK and US treatment of acute asthma presenting to hospital

Innes NJ, Stocking JA, Daynes TJ, Harrison BDW. *Thorax* 2002; **12**: 1040–4

BACKGROUND. The British Thoracic Society (BTS) and American Thoracic Society (ATS) guideline statements on the management of acute asthma differ with respect to β_2 agonists and corticosteroids. The ATS guidelines recommend lower doses of salbutamol at a higher frequency of dosing than the UK with continuous nebulization being recommended in the ATS guidelines. As regards corticosteroid dosages, American authors recommend up to 60 mg of prednisolone at intervals of 4 h for up to 72 h and then 60 mg/day thereafter, while the UK guidelines recommend 30–60 mg once daily.

INTERPRETATION. Treatment with higher doses of continuous, nebulized salbutamol leads to a greater immediate improvement in PEF, but the degree of recovery at 24 h and speed of recovery thereafter is achieved as effectively with lower corticosteroid doses, as recommended in the BTS guidelines.

Comment

Patients with acute asthma are less likely to be admitted in the USA than in the UK |**32**|. Whilst this may reflect differences in the structure and provision of healthcare, it is possible that differences in treatment protocols with respect to the administration of inhaled β_2 agonists and systemic corticosteroids influence the recovery from acute asthma attacks |**33,34**|. This study was aimed at examining whether these differences were associated with different outcomes.

The authors considered all patients presenting to the Norfolk and Norwich Hospital, UK, with an acute asthma attack for entry into a prospective, pragmatic, randomized, parallel-group study. Patients were considered eligible for the study if their PEF on presentation was ≤75% of their personal (or predicted) best, but they excluded patients who were *in extremis* as defined by collapse, respiratory arrest, hypercapnia or the need for immediate intubation. They enrolled 170 patients.

Patients randomized to the BTS arm of the study received 40 mg of prednisolone orally on presentation and then 40 mg once daily until asthma was controlled. Nebulized salbutamol was administered by a bolus of 5 mg at times 0 and 30 min and then, if admitted, at intervals of 4 h for at least 24 h. This was reduced to intervals of 6 h and as the patient improved the nebulizer was discontinued and the patient changed to a metered dose inhaler. Patients randomized to follow the ATS guidelines received 60 mg of prednisolone orally on presentation and then 60 mg at intervals of 6 h for 14 h and subsequently 60 mg once daily until asthma was controlled. Salbutamol was administered as a dose of 10 mg continuously nebulized over 1 h. This was repeated over the second hour if the PEF remained below 75% of best and was followed by 2.5 mg of salbutamol nebulized at intervals of 4 h for the first 24 h in those admitted, reducing in frequency and dose as per the BTS arm. Indications for the administration of ipratropium bromide and intravenous bronchodilators were the same for each group and as recommended in the BTS guidelines |**19**|. Patients discharged following initial treatment were prescribed prednisolone at a dose of 40 mg/day in the BTS group and 60 mg/day in the ATS group. In both arms prednisolone was given for a minimum course of 5 days and until PEF was ≥80% best on two consecutive days with ≤20% variability. No attempt was made to control for treatment received prior to presentation, but the discharge criteria were standardized.

The authors reported that the more intensive ATS protocol was associated with a significantly greater ΔPEF at 2 h (BTS = 49 l/min, ATS = 101 l/min and confidence interval [CI] = 28–77) ($P <0.0001$), although this did not result in any significant difference in the rate of discharge. The authors suggested that this was because they followed BTS guidance on admitting all patients whose presenting PEF was <50% best regardless of whether their PEF improved or not. Were it not for this, significantly more patients in the ATS arm could have been discharged with a 78% rate of achieving discharge PEF (>60%) in the ATS group as compared to 64% in the BTS group. After 24 h there was no difference in outcomes between the treatment arms.

As corticosteroids are unlikely to be effective within 2 h the authors suggested that the observed outcomes are more likely to reflect differences in the use of β_2 agonists

|7|. Indeed, there is evidence that the administration of inhaled bronchodilators as a single bolus provides less effective bronchodilation than sequential delivery |35–37| and other clinical studies have suggested that continuous nebulizations offer greater benefit than intermittent delivery |38–40|. This may reflect greater drug delivery to the peripheral airways once the central airways have bronchodilated.

The optimal dose of corticosteroids remains debated. It has been suggested that 60–80 mg of methyprednisolone is adequate in hospitalized patients with acute asthma |6|. A dose–response effect has been suggested, with doses below 0.6 mg/kg being less effective |41|. This study suggested there is little to choose between the different doses of systemic corticosteroids and proposed that 40 mg/day is acceptable. They did acknowledge that this could represent a type II error (concluding that treatment is not effective when it is), but felt this was unlikely as there was no significant difference between the time to discharge between the groups and the time for regaining control of asthma was in favour of the BTS arm.

Use of isotonic nebulized magnesium sulphate as an adjuvant to salbutamol in treatment of severe asthma in adults: randomized, placebo-controlled trial

Hughes R, Goldkorn A, Masoli M, Weatherall M, Burgess C, Beasley R. *Lancet* 2003; **361**: 2114–17

BACKGROUND. Magnesium may be administered intravenously during an acute asthma attack, but previous studies on the role of nebulized magnesium have provided conflicting results. The authors of this study conducted a randomized, placebo-controlled trial for investigating the effectiveness of nebulized isotonic magnesium sulphate as an adjuvant to salbutamol administered by nebulizer according to a standard emergency protocol for the treatment of severe asthma.

INTERPRETATION. Administration of isotonic magnesium sulphate as an adjuvant to salbutamol nebulizer solution results in an enhanced bronchodilator response in severe asthma.

Comment

The role of magnesium in the management of asthma has recently been recognized by the incorporation of intravenous magnesium into several guideline statements on the management of acute asthma. It acts as a powerful smooth muscle relaxant and causes bronchodilation, but is also known to modulate inflammatory processes believed to be important in asthma |42,43|. Depletion has been reported in chronic asthma |44|.

Intravenous administration of magnesium may be associated with hypotension and can cause flushing, nausea and phlebitis. Delivery by the nebulized route may avoid some of the potential side effects, but previous reports have failed to provide conclusive evidence of benefit |45–47|. Thus, the authors of this study conducted a randomized, placebo-controlled trial in order to investigate the effectiveness of nebulized isotonic magnesium sulphate as an adjuvant to salbutamol administered by nebulizer according to a standard emergency protocol for the treatment of severe asthma.

Fifty-two patients were enrolled following presentation with acute asthma at two university hospitals in New Zealand. Inclusion required a known history of asthma and presentation with a severe exacerbation with a recorded forced expiratory volume in 1 s (FEV_1) of less than 50% predicted normal values. Patients were excluded if they required immediate intubation or had evidence of pneumonia, hypotension, previously documented chronic airflow limitation with fixed airways obstruction, cardiac or renal disease or were pregnant. Patients were enrolled 30 min post-2.5 mg of nebulized salbutamol if their FEV_1 remained <50% of predicted normal values. The primary outcome measure was FEV_1 at 90 min (30 min after the third administration of the study drug).

In this study administration of the salbutamol nebulizer solution with the magnesium adjuvant resulted in approximately twice the increase in FEV_1 than the same dose of salbutamol administered with an isotonic saline nebulizer solution. The FEV_1 at 90 min in the magnesium group was 1.96 l (95% CI = 1.68–2.24) and in the saline group was 1.55 l (95% CI = 1.24–1.87) (Fig. 4.1). The difference in the mean FEV_1 between the magnesium and saline groups was 0.37 l (95% CI = 0.13–0.61)

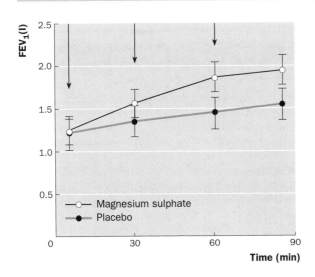

Fig. 4.1 FEV_1 after administration of 2.5 mg of nebulized salbutamol with either magnesium sulphate or saline adjuvant. Arrows indicate the start of study drug administration. The data are mean and 95% CIs (bars). Source: Hughes *et al.* (2003).

Table 4.1 Change in FEV$_1$ in the subgroups defined by baseline FEV$_1$ measurements*

	Baseline FEV$_1$ <30% predicted		Baseline FEV$_1$ >30% predicted	
	Magnesium (n = 12)	Saline (n = 12)	Magnesium (n = 16)	Saline (n = 12)
FEV$_1$ at baseline (l)	0.90 (0.35)	0.82 (0.17)	1.50 (0.30)	1.58 (0.30)
FEV$_1$ at 90 min (l)	1.73 (0.70)	1.01 (0.22)	2.14 (0.71)	2.09 (0.68)

The values are mean (standard deviations).
*Baseline FEV$_1$ at the time of randomization.
Source: Hughes *et al.* (2003).

($P = 0.003$). Expressed as a change from the baseline, the FEV$_1$ in the magnesium group improved by 0.72 l (95% CI = 0.50–0.94) and in the saline group by 0.35 l (95% CI = 0.18–0.52) after three administrations of salbutamol. Twelve patients were admitted in the magnesium group compared with 17 in the placebo group (relative risk = 0.61 and 95% CI = 0.37–0.99) ($P = 0.04$). Five patients in the magnesium group and one in the placebo group were discharged despite an FEV$_1$ below 50% predicted. Guidelines are not always followed, even under the spotlight of a study!

A *post hoc* subgroup analysis of 24 patients with life-threatening asthma (baseline FEV$_1$ <30% at the time of randomization) demonstrated that nebulized magnesium provided a greater additional benefit (difference = 0.64 l and 95% CI = 0.34–0.93) (P <0.0001) (Table 4.1). The authors considered that this could be regression to the mean, but felt that the observation was consistent with other studies where magnesium appeared to be effective in severe exacerbations, but not clearly so in less severe exacerbations.

The authors pointed out that appropriate care must be taken regarding the constitution of magnesium for nebulized purposes as both hypotonic and hypertonic nebulizer solutions cause bronchoconstriction. In this study the use of nebulized magnesium appeared safe with no clinically significant adverse events reported.

A randomized, controlled trial of intravenous montelukast in acute asthma

Camargo Jr CA, Smithline HA, Malice M-P, Green SA, Reiss TF. *Am J Respir Crit Care Med* 2003; **167**: 528–33

BACKGROUND. Intravenous montelukast has been shown to produce bronchodilatation in patients with chronic asthma. In this study the authors performed a multicentre, randomized, double-blind, placebo-controlled, pilot study designed for comparing the clinical efficacy, safety and tolerability of intravenous montelukast administered in addition to standard therapy with that of standard therapy alone in the management of acute exacerbations of asthma presenting to the emergency room. The primary outcome measure was an improvement in lung function as measured by the patients' FEV_1. Two doses of intravenous montelukast were evaluated: 7 mg and 14 mg.

INTERPRETATION. Compared with standard therapy and placebo, standard therapy and intravenous montelukast resulted in a rapid and significant improvement in patients' FEV_1 over the first 20 min following administration. This effect was still present at least 2 h later. Patients treated with montelukast tended to receive less β_2 agonists and have fewer treatment failures. The treatment was well tolerated.

Comment

As leukotriene pathways are activated in acute asthma |48,49| the investigators wished to explore the potential of a leukotriene receptor antagonist in the management of acute asthma attacks and report a pilot study in 16 US emergency departments. Montelukast, a leukotriene receptor antagonist, has been administered intravenously in chronic asthma and within 15 min provides an improvement in FEV_1 that is sustained for at least 24 h |50|.

The participants were aged between 15 and 54 years and reported a history of asthma for at least 1 year and less than ten pack years of tobacco use (one pack year = 20 cigarettes per day for one year). They had not been taking concomitant therapy with systemic corticosteroids, leukotriene modifiers, anticholinergics or long-acting β_2 agonists. Patients with pneumonia, congestive cardiac failure or other clinical explanations for dyspnoea were excluded, as were patients with significant co-morbid disorders requiring acute management. Following consent patients underwent initial spirometry followed by mandatory albuterol delivered by a nebulizer. They then performed a second spirometry. Most patients recruited had a moderate to severe asthma exacerbation. The initial FEV_1 was 39.2 ± 14.2% of the predicted value in the pooled montelukast groups and 46.4 ± 15.4% in the placebo group. The primary outcome measure was the average percentage change in FEV_1 from the pre-allocation baseline at 20 min after study medication infusion. Serial spirometry was performed at 10, 20, 40, 60 and 120 min and at 3 and 6 h after intravenous study drug administration.

Compared with the group receiving standard therapy plus placebo, a significant improvement in FEV_1 was observed among patients receiving standard therapy plus intravenous montelukast at the earliest time point measured (10 min). The mean percentage change from the pre-allocation baseline at 20 min was 14.8% versus 3.6% for the pooled montelukast and placebo groups, respectively, while the least-squares mean difference was 10% (95% CI = 2.8–17.3%) (P = 0.007) (Fig. 4.2). Benefit was maintained for at least 2 h. There was no difference in the treatment effect from either the doses of 7 mg or 14 mg of montelukast and the distribution of the response was unimodal, suggesting that there was no evidence of 'responders' and 'non-responders'. Whilst the use of intravenous magnesium has been associated with peripheral vasodilation, systolic hypotension, flushing, nausea and venous phlebitis the tolerability profile of intravenous montelukast was similar to that of placebo.

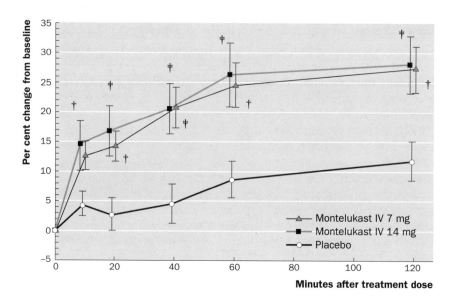

Fig. 4.2 Least-square mean ± standard error responses in FEV_1 for montelukast (doses of 7 and 14 mg) and placebo. The patients received standard therapy plus either intravenous montelukast or placebo and their FEV_1 responses were determined at individual times after the end of the 5-minute infusion. The results are expressed as the percentage changes from the pre-allocation baseline, which were 1.6, 1.6 and 1.7 l for the 7 mg of montelukast, 14 mg of montelukast and placebo groups, respectively. Montelukast at either dose caused a rapid improvement in the patients' FEV_1 compared with placebo. There were no differences between the montelukast treatment groups. † $P < 0.05$ for montelukast versus placebo; ‡ $P < 0.01$ for montelukast versus placebo. Source: Camargo *et al.* (2003).

A point for both this paper and the study by Hughes *et al.* is that it is pertinent to know how reliable spirometry is during an acute asthma attack. Hughes *et al.* did not discuss this, but in this study seven patients in Caramago *et al.*'s paper did not have valid FEV_1 data for the 10- and 20-minute time points and were not included in the primary end-point analysis. In addition, we also need to be reassured that there were no significant differences between the two groups. Camarago *et al.* examined the baseline characteristics of their groups, but could not identify any other factor for explaining the data. However, the montelukast group did have a lower FEV_1 so it is possible that some of the data is explained by regression to the mean. It is also interesting to note that, post-randomization, physicians prescribed less cortico-steroids to the montelukast group than those randomized to placebo (59.3 versus 75.8%, respectively) and fewer nebulized doses of β_2 agonist.

Standard therapy did not include the use of ipratropium bromide. The administration of nebulized ipratropium bromide to a nebulized β_2 agonist results in significantly greater bronchodilation than a nebulized β_2 agonist alone. The benefits include a faster recovery and shorter duration of admission [51–53]. As ipratropium bromide is frequently used by most practising physicians it would be interesting to know how the addition of montelukast compares to this.

The results from randomized, controlled trials on selected patients are often extrapolated to the greater body of unselected patients. The authors of this study excluded patients who were already taking leukotriene receptor antagonists and who had already received systemic corticosteroids so it remains unclear whether these patients would gain the same benefits seen in this study.

Psychological, social and health behaviour risk factors for deaths certified as asthma: a national case–control study

Sturdy PM, Victor CR, Anderson HR, *et al.* on behalf of the Mortality and Severe Morbidity Working Group of the National Asthma Task Force. *Thorax* 2002; **57**: 1034–9

BACKGROUND. Studies into asthma deaths have suggested that psychosocial and health behaviour factors may be important predictors of patients at risk of asthma death. Much of this information has been derived from studies of poor quality and the relationship between cause and effect remains unclear. In this study the authors conducted a large, community-based, case–control study in order to address some of these issues.

INTERPRETATION. Severe asthma *per se* appears to be associated with a high level of psychosocial factors. Associations between asthma death and either health behaviour or psychosocial factors appear to be complex. A limited number of factors show a positive relationship.

Comment

The authors performed a community-based, case–control study designed for examining how psychological, social and health behaviour factors may impact on the risk of death from asthma. Cases comprised deaths attributed to asthma as identified through the routine death certification system. This included any death in which asthma appeared anywhere in part I (but not part II), provided the underlying cause was a respiratory condition. Age-matched controls were identified as patients with severe asthma who had been admitted to the hospital relevant to the case within the same time frame.

The study examined 533 cases and 533 controls. The median age was 53 years and 60% of cases and 63% of controls were female. Cases had an earlier age of asthma onset, more chronic obstructive lung disease and were more obese. Health behaviour problems were found in 48% of cases and 42% of controls. Poor inhaler technique and repeated non-attendance for practice/hospital asthma appointments (including self-discharge) were associated with an increased risk of asthma death (odds ratio [OR] = 1.35 and 95% CI = 1.00–1.83 and OR = 1.47 and 95% CI = 1.03–2.09, respectively). Interestingly, non-compliance was not associated with asthma death.

Overall there was little difference in recorded psychosocial factors between the cases and the controls. Increased risk of asthma death was associated with any mention of psychosis (OR = 1.86 and 95% CI = 1.08–3.21) and when corroborated by the prescription of antipsychotic drugs in the previous 5 years (OR = 1.88 and 95% CI = 1.08–3.29). Learning difficulties were associated with a threefold increase in risk (OR = 3.07 and 95% CI = 1.31–7.20). A history of anxiety (including the prescription of antidepressant drugs) and sexual problems appeared to be associated with a reduced risk of death. Social factors were equally common in the cases and controls. An increased risk of asthma death was associated with a mention ever of financial problems (OR = 1.43 and 95% CI = 1.06–1.94), employment problems (OR = 1.60 and 95% CI = 1.19–2.17) and mention of alcohol abuse (OR = 1.49 and 95% CI = 1.08–2.07) or drug abuse (OR = 1.71 and 95% CI = 1.03–2.83). There was no significant association with mention of bereavement, separation, family problems, domestic abuse, isolation or housing problems.

This study is commendable as it was designed for avoiding many of the pitfalls associated with previous studies. The study was community based and enrolled a large number of cases, but 148 potential cases had to be excluded for legitimate reasons. The cases and controls were well balanced. By reviewing primary care records that had been made anonymous they ensured an unbiased method of ascertaining information, but accepted that this may have been at the expense of completeness of the data.

The authors' findings are broadly consistent with previous studies identifying repeated non-attendance, poor inhaler technique, psychosis (including the prescription of antipsychotic drugs), drug and alcohol abuse, and financial and employment problems as being associated with an increased risk of asthma death. They also reported an association with learning difficulties. However, association should not be regarded as synonymous with causation.

Conclusion

Acute asthma is a common cause of emergency call-outs and hospital admissions. Physicians and patients need to be educated on how to recognize, assess and manage these events. For the most part emergency treatment is straightforward and fortunately adverse outcomes remain rare. Nevertheless, there is no room for complacency and continued appraisal of this area remains an important component of asthma research. Innes *et al.* examined the differences between the UK and USA regimens and drew important conclusions on the delivery of β_2 agonists. The papers from Hughes *et al.* and Camargo *et al.* represent important evaluations of novel modes of bronchodilation by the nebulized and intravenous routes, respectively. The paper by Sturdy *et al.* provides us with further insight into the important psychological features in some of these patients and lastly Suissa and Ernst remind us that adherence to inhaled corticosteroids and also possibly montelukast may prevent untimely death.

References

1. Stroupe KTD, Gaskins D, Murray MD. Health-care costs of inner-city patients with asthma. *J Asthma* 1999; **36**: 645–55.

2. Cates CJ, Rowe BH. Holding chambers versus nebulisers for beta-agonist treatment of acute asthma. *Cochrane Database Syst Rev* 2000; **2**.

3. Turner MO, Patel A, Ginsburg S, Fitzgerald JM. Bronchodilator delivery in acute airflow obstruction. A meta-analysis. *Arch Intern Med* 1997; **157**: 1736–44.

4. Strauss L, Hejal R, Galan G, Dixon L, McFadden Jr ER. Observations on the effects of aerolized albuterol in acute asthma. *Am J Respir Crit Care Med* 1997; **155**: 454–8.

5. Rodrigo GJ, Rodrigo C. The role of anticholinergics in acute asthma treatment: an evidence-based evaluation. *Chest* 2002; **121**: 1977–87.

6. Manser R, Reid D, Abramson M. Corticosteroids for acute severe asthma in hospitalised patients (Cochrane review). In: *The Cochrane Library*, Issue 2. Oxford: Update Software, 2000.

7. Rowe BH, Spooner C, Ducharme FM, Bretzlaff JA, Bota GW. Early emergency department treatment of acute asthma with systemic corticosteroids (Cochrane review). In: Lasserson T, Picot J (eds). *The Cochrane Library*. Oxford: Update Software, 2001.

8. Rowe BH, Bretzlaff JA, Bourdon C, Bota GW, Camargo Jr CA. Magnesium sulfate for treating exacerbations of acute asthma in the emergency department. *Cochrane Database Syst Rev* 2000; **2**.

9. Parmeswaran K, Beida J, Rowe BH. Addition of intravenous aminophylline to beta-2 agonists in adults with acute asthma (Cochrane review). In: *Cochrane Library*, Issue 4. Oxford: Update Software, 2000.

10. Hart SP. Should aminophylline be abandoned in the treatment of acute asthma in adults? *Q J Med* 2000; **93**: 761–5.

11. Travers AH, Rowe BH, Barker S, Jones A, Camargo CA. The effectiveness of IV β-agonists in treating patients with acute asthma in the emergency department. *Chest* 2002; **122**: 1200–7.

12. Rodrigo G, Rodrigo C, Pollack C, Rowe B. Helium–oxygen mixture for nonintubated acute asthma patients (Cochrane review). In: Lasserson T, Picot J (eds). *The Cochrane Library*. Oxford: Update Software, 2001.

13. Sears MR. Descriptive epidemiology of asthma. *Lancet* 1997; **350**(Suppl 2): SII1–4.

14. McFadden ER, Warren EL. Observations on asthma mortality. *Ann Intern Med* 1997; **127**: 142–7.

15. Turner MO, Noertjojo K, Vedal S, Bai T, Crump S, Fitzgerald JM. Risk factors for near-fatal asthma: a case control study in hospitalised patients with asthma. *Am J Respir Crit Care Med* 1998; **157**: 1804–9.

16. Sur S, Crotty TB, Kephart GM, Hyma BA, Colby TV, Reed CE, Hunt LW, Gleich GJ. Sudden onset fatal asthma: a distinct entity with few eosinophils and relatively more neutrophils in the airway submucosal. *Am Rev Respir Dis* 1993; **148**: 713–19.

17. Kolbe J, Fergusson W, Vamos M, Garrett J. Case–control study of severe life threatening asthma (SLTA) in adults: psychological factors. *Thorax* 2002; **57**: 317–22.

18. Plaza V, Serrano J, Picado C, Sanchis J. Frequency and clinical characteristics of rapid-onset fatal and near-fatal asthma. *Eur Respir J* 2002; **19**: 846–52.

19. British Thoracic Society. Death from asthma in two regions of England. *BMJ* 1982; **285**: 1251–5.

20. Mohan G, Harrison BDW, Badminton RM, Mildenhall S, Wareham NJ. A confidential enquiry into deaths caused by asthma in an English health region: implications for general practice. *Br J Gen Pract* 1996; **46**: 529–32.

21. Bucknall CE, Slack R, Godley GC, Mackay T, Wright SC. Scottish confidential inquiry into asthma deaths (SCIAD), 1994–6. *Thorax* 1999; **54**: 978–84.

22. Burr ML, Davies BH, Hoare A, Jones A, Williamson IJ, Holgate SK, Arthurs R, Hodges IGC. A confidential inquiry into asthma deaths in Wales. *Thorax* 1999; **54**: 985–9.

23. Wright SC, Evans AE, Sinnamon DG, MacMahon J. Asthma mortality and death certification in Northern Ireland. *Thorax* 1994; **49**: 141–3.

24. Barnes PJ, Woolcock AJ. Difficult asthma. *Eur Respir J* 1998; **12**: 1209–18.

25. Roberston CF, Rubinfeld AR, Bowes G. Pediatric asthma deaths in Victoria: the mild are at-risk. *Pediatr Pulmonol* 1992; **13**: 95–100.

26. Fouchard T, Graff-Lonnevig V. Asthma mortality rate in Swedish children and young adults 1973–88. *Allergy* 1994; **49**: 616–19.

27. Matsuse H, Shimoda T, Matsuo N, Fukushima C, Takao A, Sakai H, Kohno S. Aspirin-induced asthma as a risk factor for asthma mortality. *J Asthma* 1997; **34**: 413–17.

28. O'Hollaren T, Yunginger JW, Offord KP, Sommers MJ, O'Connell EJ, Ballard DJ, Sachs MI. Exposure to an aeroallergen as a possible precipitating factor in respiratory arrest in young patients with asthma. *N Engl J Med* 1991; **324**: 359–63.

29. Roberts G, Patel N, Levi-Schaffer F, Habibi P, Lack G. Food allergy as a risk factor for life-threatening asthma in childhood: a case–control study. *J Allergy Clin Immunol* 2003; **112**: 168–74.

30. Suissa S, Ernst P, Benayoun S, Baltzan M, Cai B. Low-dose inhaled corticosteroids and the prevention of death from asthma. *N Engl J Med* 2000; **343**: 332–6.

31. Kikuchi Y, Okabe S, Tamura G, Hida W, Homma M, Shirato K, Takishima T. Chemo-sensitivity and perception of dyspnoea in patients with a history of near-fatal asthma. *N Engl J Med* 1994; **330**: 1329–34.

32. McFadden Jr ER, Elsanadi N, Dixon L, Takacs M, Deal EC, Boyd KK, Idemoto BK, Broseman LA, Panuska J, Hammons T, Smith B, Caruso F, McFadden CB, Shoemaker L, Warren EL, Hejal R, Strauss L, Gilbert IA. Protocol therapy for acute asthma: therapeutic benefits and cost savings. *Am J Med* 1995; **99**: 651–61.

33. British Thoracic Society. The British guidelines on asthma management. 1995 review and position statement. *Thorax* 1997; **52**(Suppl 1): S1–20.

34. National Heart, Lung and Blood Institute. *Guidelines for the Diagnosis and Treatment of Asthma*. Publication no. 97-4051. Bethesda, MD: National Institutes of Health, 1997.

35. Heimer D, Shim C, Williams MH. The effect of sequential inhalations of metaproterenol aerosol in asthma. *J Allergy Clin Immunol* 1980; **66**: 75–7.

36. Britton J, Tattersfield A. Comparison of cumulative and non-cumulative techniques to measure dose–response curves for beta-agonists in patients with asthma. *Thorax* 1984; **39**: 597–9.

37. Shrestha M, Bidadi K, Gourlay S, Hayes J. Continuous vs. intermittent albuterol, at high and low doses, in the treatment of acute severe asthma in adults. *Chest* 1996; **110**: 42–7.

38. Papa MC, Frank J, Thompson AE. A prospective randomised study of continuous versus intermittent nebulised albuterol for severe status asthmaticus in children. *Crit Care Med* 1993; **21**: 1479–86.

39. Rudnitsky GS, Eberlein RS, Schoffstall JM, Mazur JE, Spivey WH. Comparison of intermittent and continuously nebulised albuterol for treatment of asthma in an urban emergency department. *Ann Emerg Med* 1993; **22**: 1842–6.

40. Lin RY, Sauter D, Newman T, Sirleaf J, Walters J, Tavakol M. Continuous versus intermittent albuterol nebulisations in the treatment of acute asthma. *Ann Emerg Med* 1993; **22**: 1847–53.

41. Webb JR. Dose response of patients to oral corticosteroid treatment during exacerbations of asthma. *BMJ* 1986; **292**: 1045–7.

42. Spivey WH, Skobeloff EM, Levin RM. Effect of magnesium chloride on rabbit bronchial smooth muscle. *Ann Emerg Med* 1990; **19**: 1107–12.

43. Cairns CB, Kraft M. Magnesium attenuates the neutrophil respiratory burst in adult asthmatic patients. *Acad Emerg Med* 1996; **3**: 1093–7.

44. Emelyanov A, Fedoseev G, Barnes PJ. Reduced intracellular magnesium concentrations in asthmatic patients. *Eur Respir J* 1999; **13**: 38–40.

45. Rolla G, Bucca C, Arossa W, Bugiani M. Magnesium attenuates methacholine-induced bronchoconstriction in asthmatics. *Magnesium* 1987; **6940**: 201–4.

46. Rolla G, Bucca C, Caria E. Dose-related effect of inhaled magnesium sulphate on histamine bronchial challenge in asthmatics. *Drugs Exp Clin Res* 1988; **14**: 609–12.

47. Hill J, Lewis S, Britton J. Studies of inhaled magnesium on airway reactivity to histamine and adenosine monophosphate in asthmatic subjects. *Clin Exp Allergy* 1997; **27**: 546–51.

48. Drazen JM, O'Brien J, Sparrow D, Weiss ST, Martins MA, Israel E, Fanta CH. Recovery of leukotriene E_4 from the urine of patients with airway obstruction. *Am Rev Respir Dis* 1992; **146**: 104–8.

49. Sampson AP, Castling DP, Green CP, Price JF. Persistent increase in plasma and urinary leukotrienes after acute asthma. *Arch Dis Child* 1995; **73**: 221–5.

50. Dockhorn RJ, Baumgartner RA, Leff JA, Noonan M, Vandormael K, Stricker W, Weinland DE, Reiss TF. Comparison of the effects of intravenous and oral montelukast on airway function: a double blind placebo controlled, three period, crossover study in asthmatic patients. *Thorax* 2000; **55**: 260–5.

51. Lanes SF, Garrett JE, Wentworth III CE, Fitzgerald JM, Karpel JP. The effect of adding ipratropium bromide to salbutamol in the treatment of acute asthma: a pooled analysis of three trials. *Chest* 1998; **114**: 365–72.

52. Rodrigo G, Rodrigo C, Burschtin O. A meta-analysis of the effects of ipratropium bromide in adults with acute asthma. *Am J Med* 1999; **107**: 363–70.

53. Stoodley RG, Aaron SD, Dales RE. The role of ipratropium bromide in the emergency management of acute asthma exacerbation: a meta-analysis of randomised clinical trials. *Ann Emerg Med* 1999; **34**: 8–18.

Part II

Chronic obstructive pulmonary disease

Chronic obstructive pulmonary disease

A HILL

Introduction

Chronic obstructive pulmonary disease (COPD) is a major cause of chronic morbidity and mortality internationally and is currently the fourth leading cause of death in the world. Patients with COPD usually have progressive airflow obstruction that is not fully reversible, which leads to a history of progressive, worsening breathlessness that can impact on daily activities and health-related quality of life. In addition, patients with recurrent exacerbations can have further impairment of health status.

International guidelines have stratified the severity of COPD predominantly based on the measurement of the forced expired volume in 1 s (FEV_1) and forced vital capacity (FVC) and based on this severity there have been specific management recommendations. The classification of severity in the recent Global Initiative for Chronic Obstructive Lung Disease guidelines is shown in Table II.1 [**1**].

In view of the chronic morbidity and mortality with COPD there has been a flood of research trying to improve treatments. Twenty-five key papers from 1 October 2002 to 31 October 2003 have been selected for this section. The articles that have been selected have clinical relevance and address treatments for stable COPD, treatments

Table II.1 Disease severity for COPD based on FEV_1 (% predicted) and the ratio of FEV_1:FVC

	FEV_1	FEV_1/FVC
Mild	≥80% predicted	<70%
Moderate	50–79% predicted	<70%
Severe	30–49% predicted	<70%
Very severe	<30% predicted or <50% predicted and the presence of chronic respiratory failure or right heart failure	<70%

Respiratory failure is defined as a partial pressure of oxygen in arterial blood of <8 kPa (60 mmHg) with or without a partial pressure of carbon dioxide in arterial blood of >6.7 kPa (50 mmHg) whilst breathing air at sea level.
Source: Author's own.

for COPD exacerbations and treatments that may attenuate disease progression. The articles have an initial Background section, which is the scientific rationale for the study. Following this is an Interpretation section, which is the main message from the paper. The papers conclude with a final Comment section, which gives a more in-depth account of the papers and, in each paper, the scientific rationale is discussed, there is a summary of the study design/methodology, a summary of the main results and a final conclusion with comments on how this may impact on clinical practice.

The articles selected have been split into five chapters that deal with pharmacological treatments for stable COPD, oxygen treatment, pulmonary rehabilitation, surgical treatments and, finally, the treatment of exacerbations.

Reference

1. Global Initiative for Chronic Obstructive Lung Disease (GOLD). *Global Strategy for the Diagnosis, Management and Prevention of Chronic Obstructive Pulmonary Disease*. National Heart, Lung and Blood Institute (NHLBI)/World Health Organisation workshop report. Bethesda, NHLBI, April 2001; update of management sections, available on-line at www.goldcopd.com, accessed 1 July 2003.

5

Pharmacological treatments for stable COPD

Drug therapy for stable COPD

Inhaled corticosteroids

The recent Global Initiative for Chronic Obstructive Lung Disease (GOLD) guidelines recommend inhaled corticosteroids for patients with chronic obstructive pulmonary disease (COPD) with a forced expired volume in 1 s (FEV_1) <50% predicted and frequent exacerbations, for example three in the preceding 3 years, in order to reduce the frequency of exacerbations and improve health status [1].

In the GOLD guidelines an FEV_1 between 50 and 79% predicted represents moderate COPD, between 30 and 49% predicted represents severe COPD and <30% predicted represents very severe COPD. Mild COPD is defined as an FEV_1 ≥80% predicted with an FEV_1:FVC [forced vital capacity] ratio <70%.

Two papers are presented. The first paper was a meta-analysis of randomized, controlled trials of long-term inhaled corticosteroids in COPD from 1966 to 2002 examining whether inhaled corticosteroids can attenuate the relentless decline in FEV_1 in patients with different severities of COPD. The final paper was a randomized, controlled trial that evaluated the effect of discontinuing inhaled corticosteroids in patients with COPD.

Combination inhalers

In the GOLD guidelines long-acting bronchodilators are recommended in patients with moderate and severe COPD (FEV_1 <80% predicted), which can prolong the time to the next exacerbation and improve health status [1–3]. The two commonly used long-acting β_2 agonists used are salmeterol and formoterol fumarate, which are both administered twice daily and have the advantage over short-acting bronchodilators in being more effective and convenient than treatment with short-acting bronchodilators, but are more costly.

Inhaled corticosteroids, as previously discussed, are recommended in patients with severe COPD with an FEV_1 <50% predicted with recurrent exacerbations with the aim of reducing exacerbation frequency and attenuating the decline in health status.

Although these medications can be provided singly, the use of multiple inhalers can result in poor compliance. Combination inhalers are in vogue hopefully to improve compliance by simplifying the treatment regimen. Two 1-year randomized controlled studies were selected that compared the combination inhalers (a long-acting β_2 agonist and inhaled corticosteroid) with single agents and placebo.

Tiotropium

The recent GOLD guidelines recommend long-acting bronchodilators for patients with moderate and severe COPD, with an FEV_1 <80% predicted. The next random-ized controlled study compared 6 months of treatment with the new long-acting anticholinergic tiotropium with 6 months of the long-acting β_2 agonist salmeterol and placebo.

Effect of the phosphodiesterase inhibitor cilomilast

Inflammation is important in both the pathogenesis and progression of COPD. Cigarette smoking is a potent stimulus of the inflammatory process and smoking cessation is central to the management in patients with COPD. There is growing interest in anti-inflammatory agents in patients with COPD, with the aim of reduc-ing symptoms, reducing exacerbations and attenuating the decline in lung function parameters such as FEV_1. To date inhaled corticosteroids have remained the main anti-inflammatory agent in patients with COPD. The paper selected evaluated whether the phosphodiesterase inhibitor cilomilast influenced the inflammatory response in patients with COPD.

Long-term effects of inhaled corticosteroids on FEV_1 in patients with chronic obstructive pulmonary disease. A meta-analysis

Highland KB, Strange C, Heffner JE. *Ann Intern Med* 2003; **138**(12): 969–73

BACKGROUND. The aim of this meta-analysis was to evaluate the long-term (≥2 years) effects of inhaled corticosteroids on the rate of FEV_1 decline in patients with COPD.

INTERPRETATION. Independent of the severity of COPD, the use of inhaled corticosteroids had no impact on the rate of FEV_1 decline in 3571 patients followed for 24–54 months.

Comment

The role of inhaled corticosteroids in patients with COPD has been open to much debate. This meta-analysis evaluated the long-term effects of inhaled corticosteroids (≥2 years) on the rate of FEV_1 decline in patients with COPD.

The main data sources used included the MEDLINE, EMBASE, CISCOM and AMED databases and the Cochrane Library from 1966 to 2002. The inhaled cortico-steroid studies that were selected included randomized, placebo-controlled trials that examined the rate of FEV_1 decline as a primary outcome in patients with COPD.

Overall there were six studies with 3571 patients (1784 who were treated with inhaled corticosteroids and 1787 who received placebo) that were conducted over a period of 2–4.5 years. The mean baseline FEV_1 varied between the studies from approximately 40–87% predicted (39.6, 50.2, 63.8, 67.8, 76.8 and 86.6% predicted in the various studies). All studies had predominant fixed airflow obstruction with an FEV_1:FVC ratio <70%. The doses of inhaled corticosteroids used were moderate to high in all studies: 400 or 800 µg of budesonide twice daily, 750–1000 µg of beclomethasone diproprionate twice daily, 600 µg of triamcinolone twice daily and 500 µg of fluticasone propionate twice daily.

Analysing the six studies together, the summary estimate for the difference in FEV_1 decline between the placebo and inhaled corticosteroid treatment groups was -5.0 ± 3.2 ml/year (95% confidence interval [CI] $= -11.2$ to 1.2 ml/year) ($P = 0.11$).

When stratified by baseline FEV_1, the summary estimate for the difference in FEV_1 decline between the placebo and inhaled corticosteroid treatment groups in patients with more severe COPD with a mean FEV_1 <51% predicted ($n = 849$) was -11.0 ± 6.1 ml/year (95% CI $= -23.1$ to 1.0 ml/year) ($P = 0.10$).

In 2722 patients with less severe COPD with a baseline FEV_1 ≥51% predicted the summary estimate for the difference in FEV_1 decline between the placebo and inhaled corticosteroid treatment groups was -2.9 ml/year (95% CI $= -10.1$ to 4.3 ml/year) ($P = 0.17$).

In summary, this meta-analysis revealed that moderate- to high-dose inhaled corticosteroids offered no benefit over placebo on attenuating the decline in FEV_1 in patients with COPD, independent of the COPD severity.

However, the Inhaled Steroids in Obstructive Lung Disease in Europe (ISOLDE) Trial revealed that inhaled corticosteroids may affect other important end-points such as health status and exacerbation rates [4]. The ISOLDE Trial compared treatment with 500 µg of fluticasone propionate twice daily for 3 years with placebo in 751 patients with moderate to severe COPD (mean FEV_1 50.2% predicted). The exacerbation rates were reduced in patients treated with inhaled corticosteroids and there was a reduced rate of deterioration in health status.

Health status was assessed using the St George's Respiratory Questionnaire and a change of 4 units was a clinically significant difference. The placebo group's health status deteriorated by 3.2 units per year, while that of the inhaled corticosteroid group was less (2.0 units/year) ($P = 0.004$). Overall there was less deterioration in health status in the inhaled steroid group, but this was less than the difference of 4 units that signifies a clinically important difference.

Patients treated with inhaled corticosteroids had a 25% reduction in exacerbations (from a median of 1.32 to 0.99 exacerbations per year): an exacerbation was defined as worsening symptoms that required treatment with oral corticosteroids or antibiotics or both. A recent study [5] conducting a further analysis of the ISOLDE trial revealed that inhaled corticosteroids reduced the overall exacerbation rate in patients with a post-bronchodilator FEV_1 <50% predicted (median rate 1.47 exacerbations per year in the inhaled corticosteroid treated group and 1.75 exacerbations per year in the placebo group) ($P = 0.02$), but not in patients with an FEV_1 >50% predicted.

Effect of discontinuation of inhaled corticosteroids in patients with chronic obstructive pulmonary disease: the COPE study

Van der Valk P, Monninkhof E, Van der Palen J, Zielhuis G, Van Herwaarden C.
Am J Respir Crit Care Med 2002; **166**(10): 1358–63

BACKGROUND. The role of long-term inhaled corticosteroids in patients with COPD remains controversial. They do not attenuate the decline in FEV$_1$, but appear to reduce the number of exacerbations in patients with COPD with an FEV$_1$ <50% predicted and attenuate the decline in health status. The aim of this study was to examine the effect of discontinuing high-dose inhaled corticosteroids (1 mg/day fluticasone propionate) over a period of 6 months in a randomized, double-blind, placebo-controlled study.

INTERPRETATION. Discontinuation of high-dose inhaled fluticasone propionate (1 mg/day) was associated with a more rapid onset and higher recurrence rate of exacerbations and a significant deterioration in aspects of health-related quality of life over a period of 6 months.

Comment

The role of long-term inhaled corticosteroids remains controversial, but recent recommendations from the GOLD guidelines recommend inhaled corticosteroids for patients with COPD with an FEV$_1$ <50% predicted who have recurrent exacerbations. This study evaluated the effect of discontinuing inhaled corticosteroids over a period of 6 months.

The primary end-point was the time to first exacerbation and a rapid recurrence of well-defined exacerbations. An exacerbation was defined as worsening symptoms that required treatment with oral corticosteroids or antibiotics or both.

After 4 months of inhaled treatment with 1 mg/day fluticasone propionate 244 patients were randomized to either continue the inhaled corticosteroids (1 mg/day fluticasone propionate) for 6 months ($n = 123$; mean ± standard deviation [SD] age = 64.1 ± 6.8 years; mean ± SD FEV$_1$ = 57.5 ± 14.1% predicted and 86.2% had received inhaled corticosteroids at least 6 months before entering the study) or to receive placebo for 6 months ($n = 121$; mean ± SD age = 64.0 ± 7.7 years; mean ± SD FEV$_1$ = 56.1 ± 14.8% predicted and 80.2% had received inhaled corticosteroids at least 6 months before entering the study). These baseline measurements were not significantly different between the groups.

Over 6 months a greater percentage in the placebo group (57%) had at least one exacerbation compared with 47% in the inhaled corticosteroid group: the hazard ratio (HR) of a first exacerbation in the placebo group adjusted for smoking status was 1.5 (95% CI = 1.1–2.1) compared with the inhaled corticosteroid group.

Patients with placebo had a quicker exacerbation time (mean of 42.7 days in the placebo group and 75.2 days in the inhaled corticosteroid group) with a mean difference in the time to first exacerbation (34.6 days and 95% CI = 15.4–53.8 days) in favour of the inhaled corticosteroid group.

Overall, 21.5% in the placebo group experienced rapid recurrent exacerbations compared with 4.9% in the inhaled corticosteroid group (relative risk = 4.4 and 95% CI = 1.9–10.3). The time to first exacerbation was quicker in patients with an FEV_1 <50% predicted (HR = 2.1 and 95% CI = 1.1–3.6) compared with patients with an FEV_1 ≥50% predicted (HR = 1.2 and 95% CI = 0.8–2.0).

The placebo group had worse health status, assessed using the St George's Respiratory Questionnaire, compared with the inhaled corticosteroid group. A positive value indicates worsening health status, with a 4-unit change indicating a clinically significant difference. In comparison with the inhaled steroid group, the placebo group had a worsened health status (total score = 2.48 and 95% CI = 0.37–4.58), activity domain (total score = 4.64 and 95% CI = 1.6–7.68) and symptom domain (total score = 4.58 and 95% CI = 1.05–8.10) after adjustment of baseline scores and smoking status over 6 months (Fig. 5.1). There was no difference in the impact domain and overall there were no significant adverse effects with inhaled corticosteroids.

In summary, discontinuation of inhaled corticosteroids (after 4 months on high-dose inhaled corticosteroids) in patients with moderate COPD (mean FEV_1 57.5% predicted) led to a more rapid onset and higher recurrence risk of exacerbations and a significant deterioration in aspects of health-related quality of life.

This study highlighted that, although inhaled corticosteroids may not attenuate FEV_1 decline, they can influence other important parameters such as exacerbation frequency and health-related quality of life. The beneficial effect on health status with inhaled corticosteroids may be related to the reduced frequency of exacerbations, which is known to worsen health status.

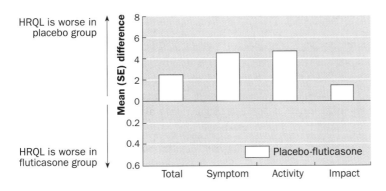

Fig. 5.1 Discontinuing inhaled corticosteroids led to worse health status as assessed by St George's Respiratory Questionnaire. A positive value indicates worse status, and a 4-unit change is clinically significant. HRQL, Health-Related Quality of Life.
Source: van der Valk *et al.* (2002).

This study supports the GOLD guidelines recommendation for the long-term use of inhaled corticosteroids in patients with COPD with an FEV_1 <50% predicted with frequent exacerbations as these patients are most likely to benefit |**1**|. The dose of inhaled corticosteroid required is not known and it may be that smaller doses of inhaled corticosteroids may be as effective, but further studies are needed.

Combined salmeterol and fluticasone in the treatment of chronic obstructive pulmonary disease: a randomized controlled trial

Calverley P, Pauwels R, Vestbo J, *et al*.; Trial of Inhaled Steroids and Long-acting Beta 2 Agonists Study Group. *Lancet* 2003; **361**(9356): 449–56

BACKGROUND. Patients with COPD normally have progressive deterioration in breathlessness associated with progressive decline in FEV_1, usually accompanied by intercurrent exacerbations and both have a major impact on health-related quality of life. Studies to date have revealed that inhaled long-acting β_2 agonists improve lung function and health status in symptomatic COPD and that inhaled corticosteroids can reduce the frequency of acute episodes of symptom exacerbation and delay deterioration in health status. The aim of this randomized, controlled study was to evaluate the efficacy of the combined inhaler with salmeterol (a long-acting β_2 agonist) and fluticasone propionate (a potent inhaled corticosteroid) with monotherapy with salmeterol or fluticasone propionate and placebo.

INTERPRETATION. Compared with placebo, combination therapy with salmeterol and fluticasone propionate in patients treated for 1 year improved their symptoms of breathlessness, improved their baseline FEV_1, reduced their exacerbation frequency and improved their health-related quality of life. In addition, combination therapy improved their FEV_1 and symptoms of breathlessness more than monotherapy with salmeterol or fluticasone propionate alone.

Comment

There has been much controversy regarding the therapeutic roles of both long-acting β_2 agonists and inhaled corticosteroids in patients with COPD. Some patients clearly benefit with long-acting β_2 agonists, with improved health status and inhaled corticosteroids can reduce the number of exacerbations in patients with severe COPD (FEV_1 <50% predicted) and attenuate the decline in health status. Although each of these treatments can be prescribed singly, there is likely to be improved compliance with combination inhalers that simplify the treatment regimen. This study evaluated the efficacy of the combination inhaler with salmeterol and fluticasone propionate as compared to monotherapy with the individual components and placebo over a period of 1 year.

A total of 1465 patients with COPD were recruited from outpatient departments in 25 countries and were randomized to either 50 µg of salmeterol twice daily

($n = 372$), 500 µg of fluticasone propionate twice daily ($n = 374$), 50 µg of salmeterol and 500 µg of fluticasone propionate twice daily ($n = 358$) or placebo
($n = 361$) for 12 months. Inhaled corticosteroids and long-acting β_2 agonists were
withdrawn in the 2-week run-in period. Throughout the study the patients were
allowed to continue theophyllines, mucolytics and anticholinergic agents if they
were on these as maintenance therapy and were asked to use a β_2 agonist as relief
therapy throughout the study.

The patients selected had moderate to severe COPD (mean FEV_1 approximately
45% predicted) with less than 10% reversibility following a β_2 agonist and had a
mean age of approximately 63 years. The primary outcome was the pre-treatment
FEV_1 after 12 months' treatment after patients had abstained from all bronchodilators for at least 6 h and from study medication for at least 12 h.

The following information summarizes the results after 12 months' treatment
comparing combination therapy with placebo. Combined therapy improved the
symptoms of cough ($P <0.05$) and breathlessness ($P <0.001$) and required less daily
relief medication ($P <0.001$), although there was no impact on sputum production.
Combined therapy improved both the pre-treatment FEV_1 (mean treatment difference 133 ml) ($P <0.001$) and post-treatment FEV_1 with a mean treatment difference
of 76 ml ($P <0.001$) (Fig. 5.2). There were reduced exacerbation rates with combination therapy, defined as worsening symptoms that required antibiotics, oral corticosteroids or both (mean 0.97 per patient per year compared with 1.3 for those treated
with placebo) ($P <0.001$). The treatment effect of reduced exacerbations with combination therapy was more efficacious for patients with moderate to severe COPD.
There was a 30% reduction for patients with moderate to severe COPD with an FEV_1
<50% predicted and a 10% reduction in patients with less advanced COPD (FEV_1
$\geq$50% predicted). There was an improved St George's Respiratory Questionnaire
score with combination therapy with a mean reduction of 2.2 ($P <0.001$), a reduced
score of 4 indicating a significant clinical improvement. The combination therapy
was well tolerated, although oral candidiasis was more frequent at 8% compared with
2% for placebo, skin bruising was similar (8% with combination therapy and 6%
with placebo) and there was a mild reduction in serum cortisol, although this was not
thought to be clinically significant (3% fall with combination therapy).

The following results compare the combination therapy group with the groups
receiving monotherapy with salmeterol and fluticasone propionate. The patients
were less breathless at 12 months with combination therapy than with monotherapy
with either salmeterol ($P <0.01$) or fluticasone propionate ($P = 0.01$). Patients
with combination therapy required less relief medication than both salmeterol and
fluticasone propionate (both $P <0.001$) and had an improved pre-treatment FEV_1
with a mean difference of 73 ml for salmeterol ($P <0.001$) and 95 ml for fluticasone
propionate ($P <0.001$) (Fig. 5.2).

In summary, compared with placebo, 12 months' treatment with combination
salmeterol and fluticasone propionate improved the patients' symptoms and pre-
treatment FEV_1, had less exacerbation rates and a trend for improvement in health

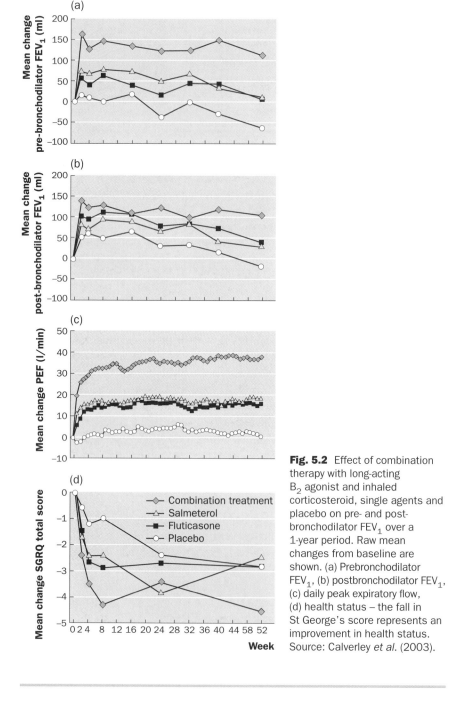

Fig. 5.2 Effect of combination therapy with long-acting B$_2$ agonist and inhaled corticosteroid, single agents and placebo on pre- and post-bronchodilator FEV$_1$ over a 1-year period. Raw mean changes from baseline are shown. (a) Prebronchodilator FEV$_1$, (b) postbronchodilator FEV$_1$, (c) daily peak expiratory flow, (d) health status – the fall in St George's score represents an improvement in health status. Source: Calverley *et al.* (2003).

status, although not quite reaching the 4-unit change that represents a clinically significant impact on health status.

Efficacy and safety of budesonide/formoterol in the management of chronic obstructive pulmonary disease
Szafranski W, Cukier A, Ramirez A, *et al. Eur Respir J* 2003; **21**(1): 74–81

BACKGROUND. A 1-year study was carried out in order to assess the efficacy and safety of the combination of budesonide and formoterol fumarate in a single inhaler compared with placebo, monotherapy with budesonide and monotherapy with formoterol fumarate in patients with moderate to severe COPD.

INTERPRETATION. Compared with placebo, combination therapy with budesonide and formoterol fumarate in patients treated for 1 year improved their symptoms of breathlessness, improved their baseline FEV_1, reduced their exacerbation frequency and improved their heath-related quality of life as assessed by the St George's Respiratory Questionnaire. In addition, combination therapy improved the patients' breathlessness and FEV_1 more than monotherapy with budesonide and had fewer severe exacerbations than monotherapy with formoterol fumarate.

Comment

As with the previous study combination treatments have been developed in order to simplify treatment regimens with the aim of improving compliance. This was a 12-month, randomized, double-blind, placebo-controlled, parallel-group study in 812 adults (mean age 64 years and mean FEV_1 36% predicted). Patients received two inhalations twice daily of either 160/4.5 μg (delivered dose) of budesonide/formoterol fumarate (Symbicort), 200 μg (metered dose) of budesonide, 4.5 μg of formoterol fumarate or placebo.

The primary end-points in this study were the number of severe exacerbations and FEV_1. Severe exacerbations were defined as exacerbations that required the use of oral corticosteroids and/or antibiotics and/or required hospitalization. In this study the FEV_1 end-point was the mean of available measurements during the treatment period.

A total of 812 patients with COPD were recruited. There were 208 patients in the combination budesonide and formoterol fumarate arm, 198 patients in the budesonide arm, 201 patients in the formoterol fumarate arm and 205 patients in the placebo arm. Only study medication was allowed throughout the study plus 500 μg of terbutaline as required as reliever medication.

The following information summarizes the results after 12 months' treatment comparing combination therapy with placebo. Combined therapy improved the symptoms of cough ($P <0.001$), breathlessness ($P <0.001$) and required less daily relief medication ($P <0.001$). Combined therapy improved the patients' FEV_1 by 15% ($P <0.001$) and the improvement in FEV_1 was maintained through the study period. There were reduced exacerbation rates with combination therapy, with a 24% reduction (P <0.001) in severe exacerbations (mean 1.42 exacerbations per patient per year for combination therapy and 1.87 for the placebo arm). There was also a 62% reduction in mild exacerbations with combination therapy (P <0.001). There was an improved St George's Respiratory Questionnaire score with combination therapy, with a mean reduction of 3.9 for combination therapy and –0.03 for the placebo arm (P <0.01), a reduction of 4 units, a clinically significant improvement. There were no significant adverse effects with combination therapy. There were more COPD events and greater discontinuation due to worsening COPD in the placebo arm of the study.

The patients were less breathless (P <0.001) and had an improved FEV_1 at 12 months with combination therapy compared with monotherapy with budesonide (P <0.001). There were less severe exacerbations with combination therapy compared with formoterol fumarate (P <0.05).

In summary, compared with placebo 12 months' treatment with combination budesonide and formoterol fumarate improved the patients' symptoms and FEV_1 and had less exacerbation rates and a trend for improvement in health status, very close to reaching the 4-unit change that represents a clinically significant impact on health status.

Further comment

Putting the latter two studies together, compared with placebo combination therapy with an inhaled corticosteroid and long-acting β_2 agonist for 1 year led to improved symptoms and FEV_1, lesser exacerbation rates (Table 5.1) and a trend for improvement in health status in patients with moderate to severe COPD. The improvement in health status was small and normally a four-point reduction in the St George's Respiratory Questionnaire is needed in order to determine clinical significance. There were some improvements over monotherapy with either of the individual components given singly.

Overall the treatment with combination inhalers should be reserved for patients with moderate to severe COPD and the patients most likely to benefit are probably

Table 5.1 Reduced mean numbers of exacerbations per patient per year in the inhaled steroid group (with or without long-acting β_2 agonists) compared with placebo

	Length of study	Exacerbations per patient per year in the inhaled steroid group	Exacerbations per patient per year in the placebo group	P-value
Burge et al. |4|	3 years	1.43	1.90	0.03
Calverley et al.	1 year	0.97	1.30	<0.001
Szafranski et al.	1 year	1.42	1.87	<0.001

Source: Author's own.

patients with COPD with frequent exacerbations. Although these studies indicated a significant group response, the same may not be true for the individual patient. A trial of 3–12 months is indicated for determining whether there are any subjective and/or objective improvements. If there is improvement then continuation may be indicated, but if there is no improvement the treatment should be reduced or stopped, but with careful monitoring to check there is no rebound worsening of symptoms after reduction or withdrawal of treatment. Finally, there may be additive effects with other bronchodilators, such as the long-acting anticholinergic tiotropium, but further studies are needed.

Health outcomes following treatment for 6 months with once daily tiotropium compared with twice daily salmeterol in patients with COPD

Brusasco V, Hodder R, Miravitlles M, Korducki L, Towse L, Kesten S. *Thorax* 2003; **58**(5): 399–404

BACKGROUND. Both short-acting β_2 agonists and anticholinergics have been long-established treatments that provide symptomatic benefit in patients with COPD. Tiotropium is a newer anticholinergic that has a long half-life, is prescribed once daily and is a more potent anticholinergic than the existing anticholinergics ipratropium bromide and oxitropium bromide. This study was undertaken in order to record exacerbations and health resource use in patients with COPD during 6 months of treatment with 18 μg of tiotropium once daily ($n = 402$), 50 μg of salmeterol twice daily ($n = 405$) or matching placebos ($n = 400$).

INTERPRETATION. Compared with placebo, 6 months of tiotropium led to an improved pre-dose FEV_1, reduced the time to first exacerbation, reduced the number of COPD exacerbations and led to a clinically significant improved health-related quality of life and dyspnoea. On the other hand, 6 months of salmeterol compared with placebo only improved the pre-dose FEV_1 and dyspnoea.

Comment

This trial used the newer anticholinergic tiotropium. It has a long half-life and lends itself to a once-daily prescription. Due to the slow disassociation of the M1 and M3 receptors it selectively inhibits the M1 and M3 receptors. It is also more potent than both ipratropium bromide and oxitropium bromide due to prolonged M3 receptor blockade and is delivered by a unique device, the HandiHaler.

This 6-month study compared 6 months of treatment with tiotropium with the long-acting β_2 agonist salmeterol, and placebo. It had useful end-points such as FEV_1, FVC, exacerbations, health-related quality of life, assessment of dyspnoea and adverse effects. The patients' health-related quality of life was assessed using the St George's Respiratory Questionnaire (a four-point reduction is a clinically significant improvement in health status) and dyspnoea assessed using the Transition Dyspnoea

Index (a one-point rise is a clinically significant improvement). An exacerbation was defined as worsening symptoms lasting at least 3 days and usually associated with a therapeutic intervention.

A total of 1207 patients participated in the study. Compared with placebo, tiotropium led to a delayed time to first exacerbation ($P \leq 0.01$) and fewer COPD exacerbations per patient-year (Table 5.2). However, tiotropium had no effect on the number that required hospital admission per patient-year for COPD exacerbations (0.10 patients treated with tiotropium and 0.15 for placebo) (P-value not significant).

Compared with placebo, patients treated with tiotropium had improved lung function (trough FEV_1), dyspnoea (a clinically significant improvement in their Transition Dyspnoea Index) and health-related quality of life (a clinically significant improvement in the St George's Respiratory Questionnaire) although a dry mouth was a common complication (Table 5.2).

Compared with placebo, patients treated with 6 months of salmeterol had an improved pre-treatment FEV_1 and breathlessness (there was an improvement in the Transition Dyspnoea Index although the improvement was just below the level that normally indicates a clinically significant improvement).

In summary, tiotropium was found to be a useful long-acting bronchodilator in patients with severe COPD (mean FEV_1 <40% predicted) with improved lung function, symptoms and health-related quality of life and a reduced number of COPD exacerbations. Its long half-life allows a once-daily prescription, which should improve compliance.

The study provides strong evidence that 6 months of tiotropium caused significant improvements in patients with severe COPD. For an individual patient the effects of any agent can be very variable. There certainly seems justification that

Table 5.2 The outcomes of the study at 6 months comparing tiotropium, salmeterol and placebo

Mean (SD) values expressed	Tiotropium	Salmeterol	Placebo
Number	402	405	400
Age (years)	63.8 (8.0)	64.1 (8.5)	64.6 (8.6)
FEV_1 (% predicted)	39.2 (11.6)	37.7 (11.7)	38.7 (12.1)
Unable to complete study (%)	7.2[**]	14.8	16.0
Number of COPD exacerbations per patient-year	1.1[*]	1.2	1.5
Improvement in the St George's Respiratory Questionnaire (units)	4.2 (0.7)[**]	2.8 (0.7)	1.5 (0.7)
Improvement of the Transition Dyspnoea Index compared with placebo	1.1[***]	0.7[*]	–
Improvement in trough FEV_1 compared with placebo (ml)	120 (100)[**]	90 (100)[**]	–
Dry mouth (%)	8.2[*]	1.7	2.3

*P <0.05, **P <0.01 and ***P <0.001 compared with placebo.

tiotropium should be tried in patients with severe COPD (FEV_1 <50% predicted) for a trial of 3–6 months. At the end of the trial period there should be a look at both subjective and objective improvements along with the side effects. If overall there is a positive effect, then long-term use of the agent can be considered.

There may be added efficacy in combining the long-acting anticholinergic with long-acting β_2 agonists or inhaled corticosteroids or combined long-acting β_2 agonists with inhaled corticosteroids, but further studies are needed in order to address this.

Anti-inflammatory effects of the phosphodiesterase-4 inhibitor cilomilast (Ariflo) in chronic obstructive pulmonary disease

Gamble E, Grootendorst DC, Brightling CE, *et al. Am J Respir Crit Care Med* 2003; **168**(8): 976–82

BACKGROUND. COPD is an inflammatory disease and the only established anti-inflammatory treatment remains inhaled corticosteroids. Cilomilast, a new oral phosphodiesterase-4 selective inhibitor, was evaluated to study its anti-inflammatory efficacy in patients with COPD.

INTERPRETATION. Cilomilast reduced the number of T lymphocytes and macrophages in bronchial biopsies following 12 weeks of therapy and represents a promising new anti-inflammatory treatment for patients with COPD.

Comment

The inflammatory process is thought to be important both in the pathogenesis and progression of COPD. There is a predominance of CD8+ T lymphocytes and macrophages in the airways and alveolar tissues of smokers with COPD, the CD8+ cells correlating inversely with FEV_1 (% predicted). In addition, the neutrophils are thought to be important in the inflammatory process, with increased neutrophils found from sputum and bronchoalveolar lavage fluid, and are associated with an accelerated decline in FEV_1.

The efficacy of inhaled corticosteroids in modulating this inflammatory process is controversial. Cilomilast, a new oral phosphodiesterase-4 selective inhibitor, was evaluated in order to study its anti-inflammatory efficacy in patients with COPD.

Fifty-nine patients with COPD were randomized to receive 15 mg of cilomilast twice daily ($n = 29$) or placebo ($n = 30$) for 12 weeks. Induced sputum differential cell counts were obtained at baseline and at five further visits at 1, 2, 4, 8, 10 and 12 weeks. Interleukin-8 (IL-8) (an important neutrophil chemoattractant) and neutrophil elastase (a protease released from the activated neutrophil) were measured in the induced sputum supernatant. Bronchial biopsies were obtained at baseline and at week 10 and were immunostained and counted for neutrophils, CD8+ (cytotoxic/suppressor) T lymphocytes and CD4+ (T helper) lymphocytes and

CD68+ monocytes/macrophages. Cells expressing the genes for IL-8 and tumour necrosis factor-α (TNF-α) were identified by *in situ* hybridization and quantified.

The mean age of the patients was approximately 61 years and patients had moderate COPD with an approximate mean FEV_1 of between 50 and 60% predicted. Only inhaled short-acting β_2 agonists and anticholinergics were used throughout the study. Inhaled corticosteroids were not permitted during the study and were stopped 4 weeks prior to the start of the study if they were on inhaled corticosteroids prior to this study (thus the patients were off inhaled corticosteroids for 6 weeks prior to the first bronchial biopsy).

Compared with placebo, analysis of variance of the change from baseline showed that cilomilast did not alter any sputum end-point (percentage of neutrophils, percentage of macrophages, total cell counts, IL-8 and neutrophil elastase), FEV_1 or Borg breathlessness score. However, the study was not powered for studying the effect of cilomilast on FEV_1. A larger study of 424 patients with COPD had shown an improvement of between 100 and 160 ml in their trough FEV_1 in patients treated with cilomilast compared with placebo [6].

However, at week 10 compared with baseline the bronchial biopsies demonstrated that cilomilast treatment compared with placebo was associated with reductions in subepithelial CD8+ T lymphocytes ($P = 0.001$) and CD68+ macrophages ($P < 0.05$).

In addition, the *post hoc* Poisson regression analysis confirmed the reductions in the cilomilast group compared with the placebo group in bronchial biopsy counts for CD8+ (48% reduction) ($P < 0.01$) and CD68+ (55% reduction) ($P < 0.001$) cells. In addition, there were reduced subepithelial neutrophils (37% reduction) ($P < 0.05$) and CD4+ (42% reduction) ($P < 0.05$) cells.

There were no side effects with cilomilast on haematology, biochemistry, vital signs or electrocardiogram findings. Diarrhoea occurred in 21 versus 13% in the placebo group (no statistical difference between the groups). Four patients taking cilomilast were withdrawn from the study due to serious adverse events, myocardial infarction, COPD exacerbation, dyspepsia, abdominal pain and/or nausea ($P < 0.05$). One patient in the placebo arm developed pancreatitis.

The extent of inflammation in COPD has been shown to correlate with the severity of COPD. Phosphodiesterase inhibitors promote the accumulation of intracellular cyclic adenosine monophosphate, a second messenger that suppresses the activity of immune cells and induces relaxation of airway smooth muscle. CD8+ cells have an important cytotoxic function, but if in excess are thought to promote tissue damage. Similarly alveolar macrophages can release proteinases that can promote both airway and alveolar damage. Cilomilast reduced the number of the CD8+ cells and tissue macrophages that may attenuate cell-mediated damage by these cells.

Another study by Profita *et al.* obtained bronchial epithelial cells from bronchial brushing and sputum cells from induced sputum in patients with moderate COPD (mean FEV_1 54% predicted) and cultured the cells *in vitro* for 24 h in the presence or absence of 1 μM of cilomilast [7]. Cilomilast reduced TNF-α release by bronchial epithelial and sputum cells (both $P < 0.01$) and granulocyte macrophage colony-stimulating factor release by sputum cells ($P < 0.01$), but had no effect on IL-8 release.

In addition, there was reduced neutrophil chemotaxis in the supernatants of bronchial epithelial and sputum cells treated with cilomilast (both P <0.01). Thus, cilomilast in this latter study has been shown to inhibit the production of some neutrophil chemoattractants by airway cells |7|.

In summary, phosphodiesterase-4 inhibitors represent a promising new class of substances for use as anti-inflammatory treatment in patients with COPD. Large, multicentred studies are needed for studying their clinical efficacy, such as exacerbation frequency, dyspnoea index, lung function parameters and health-related quality of life, and how they compare with inhaled corticosteroids. In addition, they may have greater effect in patients with severe COPD who have greater airways inflammation, but further studies are needed in order to clarify this.

References

1. Global Initiative for Chronic Obstructive Lung Disease. *Global Strategy for the Diagnosis, Management and Prevention of Chronic Obstructive Pulmonary Disease.* National Heart, Lung and Blood Institute (NHLBI)/World Health Organisation workshop report. Bethesda, NHLBI, April 2001; update of management sections, available on-line at www.goldcopd.com, accessed 1 July 2003.

2. Mahler DA, Donohue JF, Barbee RA, Goldman MD, Gross NJ, Wisniewski ME, Yancey SW, Zakes BA, Rickard KA, Anderson WH. Efficacy of salmeterol xinafoate in the treatment of COPD. *Chest* 1999; **115**: 957–65.

3. Jones PW, Bosh TK. Quality of life changes in COPD patients treated with salmeterol. *Am J Respir Crit Care Med* 1997; **155**: 1283–9.

4. Burge PS, Calverley PM, Jones PW, Spencer S, Anderson JA, Maslen TK. Randomised, double blind, placebo controlled study of the effect of inhaled fluticasone proprionate in patients with moderate to severe COPD: the ISOLDE Trial. *BMJ* 2000; **320**: 1297–303.

5. Jones PW, Willits LR, Burge PS, Calverley PM. Inhaled Steroids in Obstructive Lung Disease in Europe Study Investigators. Disease severity and the effect of fluticasone propionate on chronic obstructive pulmonary disease exacerbations. *Eur Respir J* 2003; **21**(1): 68–73.

6. Compton CH, Gubb J, Nieman R, Edelson J, Amit O, Bakst A, Ayres JG, Creemers JP, Schultze-Werninghaus G, Brambilla C, Barnes NC; International Study Group. Cilomilast, a selective phosphodiesterase 4 inhibitor for treatment of patients with chronic obstructive pulmonary disease: a randomised, dose-ranging study. *Lancet* 2001; **358**: 265–70.

7. Profita M, Chiappara G, Mirabella F, Di Giorgi R, Chimenti L, Costanzo G, Riccobono L, Bellia V, Bousquet J, Vignola AM. Effect of cilomilast (Ariflo) on TNF-alpha, IL-8, and GM-CSF release by airway cells of patients with COPD. *Thorax* 2003; **58**(7): 573–9.

6

Oxygen treatment

Introduction

Three papers have been selected for this chapter. The first paper addressed the important question of whether short-burst oxygen supplementation before or after submaximal exercise in patients with chronic obstructive pulmonary disease (COPD) is effective.

Long-term oxygen therapy for at least 15 h/day has been established as an effective treatment in patients with severe COPD with respiratory failure. Such treatment can improve exercise capacity, mental state and improve survival. It is however a cumbersome treatment that necessitates its usage for at least 15 h/day. The second paper evaluated the effectiveness of the respiratory stimulants acetazolamide and medroxyprogesterone acetate and whether they can delay the need for long-term oxygen therapy. The final paper evaluated patients on long-term oxygen therapy and evaluated whether there was added efficacy using adjunctive treatment with pulsed nitric oxide, a potent pulmonary vasodilator.

Oxygen supplementation before or after submaximal exercise in patients with chronic obstructive pulmonary disease
Nandi K, Smith AA, Crawford A, *et al. Thorax* 2003; **58**(8): 670–3

B ackground. In patients with severe COPD short-burst oxygen therapy is often used palliatively for relieving dyspnoea, usually post-exercise. This UK study was a randomized, placebo-controlled study and evaluated whether oxygen therapy both pre- and post-exercise could improve walking distances or either subjective or objective recovery times in patients with severe COPD (mean forced expiratory volume in 1 s [FEV_1] 29–34% predicted) with oxygen desaturation on exercise.

I nterpretation. This group of patients with severe COPD with oxygen desaturation on exercise derived no physiological or symptomatic benefit from 28% oxygen breathed for 10-minute periods before or 5 min post-exercise.

Comment

Oxygen is frequently prescribed in patients with severe COPD with an FEV_1 <40% predicted, in particular if there is oxygen desaturation on exercise. The reason for its prescription is that patients express marked symptoms with breathlessness and a long time for recovery. Oxygen is prescribed for palliative use that is believed to be of symptomatic benefit.

This was an important randomized, placebo-controlled study evaluating the evidence base for the use of short-burst oxygen therapy both pre- and post-exercise. The primary end-points were the 6-minute walking distance and the subjective and objective recovery times.

There were two studies. The first study evaluated 28% oxygen versus air being given for 10 min pre-exercise. The 34 patients selected had severe COPD with a mean FEV_1 34% predicted, a limited exercise tolerance (mean 6-minute walk distance on air 283 m) and >4% oxygen desaturation on submaximal exertion (corridor walking). Although with oxygen therapy the patients' oxygen saturations improved with pre-oxygenation, there was no improvement in their 6-minute walking distance, no change in their breathlessness assessed on the visualized analogue scale between the baseline and the end of the walk, and there was no improvement in either their subjective or objective recovery times post-exercise.

The second study evaluated 28% oxygen versus air given for 5 min post-exercise. As in the previous study the 18 patients selected had severe COPD with a mean FEV_1 29% predicted, a limited exercise tolerance (mean 6-minute walk distance on air 233 m) and >4% oxygen desaturation on submaximal exertion (corridor walking). Although with oxygen therapy their oxygen saturations improved quicker, there was no improvement in their breathlessness assessed on the visualized analogue scale at 5 min post-exercise and there was no improvement in either their subjective or objective recovery times post-exercise.

In summary, this study demonstrated that short-burst oxygen therapy either before or after exercise in patients with severe COPD with oxygen desaturation on exercise resulted in neither subjective nor objective benefits. A similar study by Lewis *et al.* obtained similar results revealing that short-burst oxygen therapy either immediately before or after exercise did not improve dyspnoea or exercise tolerance in patients with severe COPD (mean FEV_1 34% predicted) |1|. Short-burst oxygen therapy should therefore only be prescribed for patients if they have shown subjective or objective evidence of benefit on exercise testing.

Combined treatment with acetazolamide and medroxyprogesterone in chronic obstructive pulmonary disease patients

Wagenaar M, Vos PJ, Heijdra YF, Teppema LJ, Folgering HT. *Eur Respir J* 2002; **20**(5): 1130–7

BACKGROUND. Both hypoxia and hypercapnia can develop with advancing respiratory failure in patients with severe COPD. The authors evaluated the efficacy of the addition of the respiratory stimulants acetazolamide and medroxyprogesterone acetate, both singly and then in combination, in patients with advanced COPD with hypercapnia.

INTERPRETATION. The combination therapy with acetazolamide and medroxyprogesterone acetate improved the chemical drive, both daytime and overnight blood gases and the combination was superior to monotherapy. Longer term studies are needed in order to determine their tolerability and whether these agents can delay the requirements for long-term oxygen therapy.

Comment

Acetazolamide and medroxyprogesterone acetate are both respiratory stimulants and have the potential for improving blood gases in patients with advanced COPD. The carbonic anhydrase inhibitor acetazolamide has been successfully used in the treatment of hypoventilation in patients with COPD and is thought to work by inhibiting renal carbonic anhydrase causing a metabolic acidosis that induces an increase in respiratory drive. However, it may also work on the peripheral chemo-receptors and on the cerebral blood flow. Medroxyprogesterone acetate is thought to improve hypoxia and hypercapnia in patients with COPD, the ventilatory effect mediated by receptors in the hypothalamus, although action via the central and peripheral chemoreceptors has been described.

Patients with COPD with daytime hypercapnia (partial pressure of carbon dioxide in arterial blood [$PaCO_2$] $\geq$6 kPa) were selected. Patients that were excluded were patients on long-term oxygen therapy, patients with exacerbations within the pre-ceding 3 months, patients with abnormal baseline renal and liver function tests, patients already using respiratory stimulant drugs or patients known to have obstructive sleep apnoea or hypopnoea.

This randomized, controlled study determined to what extent combined treat-ment with acetazolamide and medroxyprogesterone acetate improved hypoxia and hypercapnia in patients with advanced stable COPD (Table 6.1) and compared the results with single-drug treatment in patients with hypercapnic COPD. Twenty-three patients were randomized. There was 2 weeks of placebo given and then the patients were randomly given 2 weeks' treatment of acetazolamide (250 mg twice daily) or medroxyprogesterone acetate (30 mg twice daily) and then both groups were given combined acetazolamide and medroxyprogesterone acetate for 2 weeks.

With combined treatment there was improvement in ventilation (tidal volume and minute ventilation), inspired mouth occlusion pressures, daytime arterial blood gases with improvement in both the partial pressure of oxygen in arterial blood (PaO_2) and hypercapnia and improvement in nocturnal gas measurements (Table 6.1).

In general the combined therapy gave superior results compared with monotherapy with either drug alone, although not all the differences reached statistical difference. Compared with acetazolamide, combined therapy had significantly improved ($P < 0.025$) minute ventilation, PaO_2, $PaCO_2$, mean nocturnal end tidal CO_2 and mean nocturnal oxygen saturation of arterial blood (SaO_2). Compared with medroxyprogesterone acetate, combined therapy had significantly improved ($P < 0.025$) PaO_2, mean nocturnal end tidal CO_2 and mean nocturnal SaO_2. The Medical Research Council (MRC) Dyspnoea Scale did not change significantly during therapy.

There were no serious adverse effects with the study medications and there were no withdrawals. However, four patients on medroxyprogesterone reported gastrointestinal discomfort and four reported fatigue, while two patients on acetazolamide reported gastrointestinal discomfort, one reported headache and three reported fatigue.

In summary, 2 weeks' combined treatment with acetazolamide and medroxyprogesterone acetate improved minute ventilation and both daytime blood gases and nocturnal oxygenation. Longer term studies are needed in order to determine their tolerability and whether such treatments can postpone the requirements for long-term oxygen therapy and improve long-term outcomes.

Table 6.1 Effect of combination therapy with acetazolamide and medroxyprogesterone acetate on ventilation, mouth pressures, arterial blood gases and nocturnal gas measurements

Mean ± standard error of the mean	Baseline	Combination therapy	P-value
Minute ventilation (l/min)	9.3 ± 0.5	11.2 ± 0.8	<0.025
Tidal volume (l)	0.6 ± 0.06	0.7 ± 0.1	<0.025
Inspiratory mouth occlusion pressure (kPa)	5.7 ± 0.5	6.7 ± 0.7	<0.025
Expiratory mouth occlusion pressure (kPa)	9.3 ± 0.7	9.6 ± 0.7	n.s.
pH	7.39 ± 0.01	7.36 ± 0.01	<0.025
PaO_2 (kPa)	7.9 ± 0.3	9.6 ± 0.4	<0.025
$PaCO_2$ (kPa)	6.5 ± 0.2	5.3 ± 0.2	<0.025
BE (mEq/ll)	4.5 ± 0.7	−2.4 ± 0.8	<0.025
SaO_2 (%)	89.0 ± 1.3	92.3 ± 1.0	<0.025
Nocturnal end tidal CO_2 (kPa)	5.5 ± 0.2	4.1 ± 0.2	<0.025
Mean nocturnal SaO_2 (%)	85.5 ± 1.6	90.2 ± 1.0	<0.025
Percentage time overnight SaO_2 <90%	61.8 ± 9.9	42.0 ± 10.4	<0.025

Combination therapy is compared with baseline measurements.
P-values are shown (n.s.= not significant).

Controlled prospective randomized trial on the effects on pulmonary haemodynamics of the ambulatory long-term use of nitric oxide and oxygen in patients with severe COPD

Vonbank K, Ziesche R, Higenbottam TW, *et al. Thorax* 2003; **58**(4): 289–93

BACKGROUND. Currently the only effective treatment for pulmonary hypertension related to severe COPD is long-term oxygen therapy for at least 15 h/day. In hypoxic lung disease there is evidence of impaired endothelin release of nitric oxide, a potent pulmonary vasodilator. This 3-month, randomized, controlled trial evaluated the safety and efficacy of the ambulatory use of adjunctive treatment with nitric oxide and oxygen in patients with severe COPD.

INTERPRETATION. This 3-month, prospective, randomized trial revealed that pulsed inhalation of nitric oxide with oxygen therapy was safe and improved the pulmonary haemodynamics. Longer term studies are needed in order to study its effect on mortality and heath-related quality of life.

Comment

Currently the recommended treatment for patients with severe COPD with hypoxia with a PaO_2 <7.3 kPa is long-term oxygen therapy for at least 15 h/day. Long-term oxygen therapy has been shown to improve the pulmonary haemodynamics, symptoms and mortality. This study evaluated the safety and efficacy of adjunctive treatment with nitric oxide. The rationale for the study is that, in hypoxic lung disease, there is impaired endothelial release of nitric oxide, a potent vasodilator. However, there are concerns about the use of nitric oxide in conjunction with oxygen therapy, as this can lead to the production of nitrogen dioxide. In order to limit this the authors devised a breathing circuit using pulsed nitric oxide so the contact time with nitric oxide and oxygen was <1 s. The amount of nitric oxide used was determined individually on the dose that led to the largest decrease in pulmonary vascular resistance without affecting the patients' PaO_2.

The patients selected were patients with severe COPD with pulmonary hypertension ($\geq$25 mmHg) that had been established on long-term oxygen therapy for over 6 months. The patients that were excluded were patients that had had an exacerbation within the preceding 3 months, significant coronary artery or left heart disease, atrial fibrillation or flutter, a previous myocardial infarct or a cerebrovascular accident within the preceding 6 months.

This was a 3-month study and 40 patients were randomized to continue long-term oxygen therapy ($n = 20$) or have combined treatment with nitric oxide and oxygen ($n = 20$) (mean nitric oxide used was 20 ppm). The primary end-point of the study was the pulmonary vascular resistance index.

The mean age was approximately 62 years and mean FEV_1 was 1.2 l (no predicted values given). Thirty-two completed the study and the reasons for dropout were

Table 6.2 Effects of 3 months' combination of pulsed nitric oxide and oxygen therapy

Mean ± standard deviation	Baseline	3 months	P-value
Mean pulmonary artery pressure (mmHg)	27.6 ± 4.4	20.6 ± 4.9	<0.001
Pulmonary vascular resistance (dyne/s/cm^5)	276.9 ± 96.6	173.1 ± 87.9	0.001
Pulmonary vascular resistance index (dyne/s/cm^5/m^2)	569.7 ± 208.1	351.3 ± 159.9	<0.001
Cardiac output (l/min)	5.6 ± 1.3	6.1 ± 1.0	<0.05
Cardiac index (l/min/m^2)	2.7 ± 0.6	3.0 ± 0.4	0.14
PaCO$_2$ (kPa)	7.4 ± 1.4	6.7 ± 1.1	<0.05

similar between the groups (exacerbations, non-compliance and coronary artery disease).

After 3 months' therapy long-term oxygen therapy had no impact on the patients' pulmonary artery pressure, pulmonary vascular resistance, pulmonary vascular resistance index, cardiac output, cardiac index or arterial blood pressure.

After 3 months of the group receiving the combination of pulsed nitric oxide and oxygen, there were improvements in their mean, systolic and diastolic pulmonary arterial pressure, pulmonary vascular resistance, pulmonary vascular resistance index and cardiac output (Table 6.2).

Patients in the group receiving a combination of pulsed nitric oxide and oxygen reported a 38.5% improvement in physical performance after 3 months compared with 12.5% in the long-term oxygen therapy group ($P <0.05$). It had no impact on the patients' heart rate, cardiac index, pulmonary capillary wedge pressure, arterial blood pressure, FEV$_1$, lung volumes or arterial blood gases with the exception of a reduced arterial CO$_2$ in the group receiving a combination of pulsed nitric oxide and oxygen (Table 6.2). The nitrogen dioxide production was <1 ppm in this study.

In summary, this is an important preliminary study that has shown that the addition of pulsed nitric oxide along with long-term oxygen therapy is safe and can improve the pulmonary haemodynamics. Longer term studies are needed in order to evaluate its long-term safety and efficacy in addition to its effect on health-related quality of life and mortality.

Reference

1. Lewis CA, Eaton TE, Young P, Kolbe J. Short-burst oxygen immediately before and after exercise is ineffective in nonhypoxic COPD patients. *Eur Respir J* 2003; 22(4): 584–8.

7

Pulmonary rehabilitation

Introduction

Pulmonary rehabilitation has been proven to be an effective treatment for chronic obstructive pulmonary disease (COPD), independent of its severity. It can reduce symptoms, improve exercise capacity, improve health-related quality of life and provide psychosocial benefits. A pulmonary rehabilitation programme ideally should be multidisciplinary, with components including exercise training, nutrition counselling and education and should run for at least 2 months. Longer programmes are likely to lead to more effective results. However, the benefits following rehabilitation tend to wane over a 2-year period.

Four papers were selected. The first was a meta-analysis of randomized, controlled trials that looked at the effectiveness of pulmonary rehabilitation and aimed to determine the optimal type and duration of rehabilitation. The next paper was a randomized, controlled trial that examined the benefits of maintenance following a pulmonary rehabilitation programme. The final two papers explored the adjunctive value of assisted ventilation and nutritional support for rehabilitation.

Rehabilitation for patients with chronic obstructive pulmonary disease: meta-analysis of randomized controlled trials
Salman GF, Mosier MC, Beasley BW, Calkins DR. *J Gen Intern Med* 2003; **18**(3): 213–21

BACKGROUND. Patients with moderate and severe COPD have progressive deterioration in exercise capacity and often enter a cycle of increasing disability. There has been increased interest in the role of pulmonary rehabilitation in such patients. This was a meta-analysis carried out to determine the effectiveness of pulmonary rehabilitation and to determine the optimal type and duration of rehabilitation.

INTERPRETATION. Pulmonary rehabilitation improved both the symptoms of breathlessness and exercise capacity in patients with COPD. The patients that benefited with rehabilitation used lower extremity training. Longer rehabilitation (at least 6 months) may be needed for patients with severe COPD ≤35% predicted, but further studies are needed to clarify this. However, shorter rehabilitation programmes may suffice for patients with less severe COPD.

Comment

Pulmonary rehabilitation has been shown to improve exercise capacity and health-related quality of life. The aim of the meta-analysis was to assess the impact of rehabilitation on exercise capacity and breathlessness and to determine the optimal type and duration of rehabilitation programmes.

There was a search in MEDLINE from 1966 to 2000, in CINHAL from 1990 to 2000 and the Cochrane database for randomized, controlled trials for rehabilitation (three times a week for at least 4 weeks) in patients with COPD. The effect of rehabilitation was calculated as the standardized effect size using random effects estimation techniques.

The primary outcome measures included exercise capacity and the effect on shortness of breath assessed by the Chronic Respiratory Disease Questionnaire (CRDQ) with rehabilitation.

Twenty trials were available for the final analysis (979 patients). There was improvement in the walking test following rehabilitation (effect size = 0.71 and 95% confidence interval [CI] = 0.43–0.99), equivalent to 50.57 m (CI = 30.3–70.8) and less breathlessness as assessed by 12 trials (723 patients) that measured the CRDQ (effect size = 0.62 and 95% CI = 0.35–0.89).

Further analysis found that rehabilitation using at least lower extremity training ($n = 820$) improved the walking test compared with controls. There were only two studies ($n = 159$) with respiratory muscle training only that had no significant effect on the walking test.

There was significant improvement in 126 patients with severe COPD (forced expiratory volume in 1 s [FEV_1] $\leq 35\%$ predicted) only when the rehabilitation programmes were ≥ 6 months. However, there was only one study ($n = 54$) receiving <6 months rehabilitation in this meta-analysis that showed no significant effect. Patients with less severe COPD improved with short- (≥ 4 weeks) and long-term rehabilitation.

In summary, this meta-analysis confirmed that pulmonary rehabilitation improved walking capacity and shortness of breath in patients with COPD. The patients that benefited with rehabilitation used lower extremity training. Longer rehabilitation (at least 6 months) may be needed for patients with severe COPD $\leq 35\%$ predicted, but further studies are needed to clarify this. Shorter rehabilitation programmes may suffice for patients with less severe COPD. Further larger trials are needed to evaluate the length of rehabilitation needed for the various severities of COPD and how to maintain the benefits with rehabilitation.

Maintenance after pulmonary rehabilitation in chronic lung disease: a randomized trial

Ries AL, Kaplan RM, Myers R, Prewitt LM. *Am J Respir Crit Care Med* 2003; **167**(6): 880–8

BACKGROUND. Pulmonary rehabilitation has been shown to improve exercise tolerance, symptoms and quality of life with a decrease in healthcare expenditure. There is increasing interest in how to maintain the benefits after pulmonary rehabilitation. This randomized, controlled trial evaluated the efficacy of a limited 1-year maintenance programme following pulmonary rehabilitation in patients with chronic lung disease.

INTERPRETATION. A 1-year intervention following pulmonary rehabilitation with once-weekly telephone calls and monthly supervised sessions produced only modest improvements in the maintenance of benefits after pulmonary rehabilitation.

Comment

Pulmonary rehabilitation has been shown to improve exercise tolerance, symptoms and the quality of life with a decrease in healthcare expenditure. There is increasing interest in how to maintain the benefits after pulmonary rehabilitation as the benefits with pulmonary rehabilitation normally gradually decline over a period of 1–2 years. This randomized, controlled trial evaluated the efficacy of a limited 1-year maintenance programme following pulmonary rehabilitation in patients with chronic lung disease.

A sample of 172 patients following 8 weeks' pulmonary rehabilitation were randomized to receive 1 year's weekly telephone calls with once-monthly supervised reinforcement sessions (1.5 h of supervised exercise, 1 h topic review and 30 min of social time) ($n = 87$) or standard care ($n = 85$) and followed for 2 years. The main outcomes were the assessment of physiological and psychosocial outcomes.

The mean age (standard deviation [SD]) was 67.1 (8.2) years and the mean FEV_1 was 45% predicted indicating moderate to severe impairment. The subjects were randomly assigned to the 12-month maintenance regimen described above ($n = 87$) or standard care ($n = 85$) and followed for 2 years. Except for a slight imbalance between the sexes (57% females in the control and 35% females in the maintenance group), the experimental and control groups were equivalent at baseline and showed similar improvements following 8 weeks of rehabilitation.

With 8 weeks' rehabilitation there was improvement in exercise performance (maximal treadmill workload and 6-minute walk), less symptoms of breathlessness and muscle fatigue with exercise, improved self-efficacy for walking, less depression, improved quality of life including both general (quality of well-being and Rand 36-Item Health Survey) and disease-specific (Chronic Respiratory Questionnaire [CRQ]) instruments and overall health status ($P < 0.01$).

Measures of exercise tolerance (maximal treadmill workload and 6-minute walk) and overall health status were better maintained over the 12-month intervention

Table 7.1 Comparisons of the maximum treadmill workload between the intervention and no intervention groups at baseline, post-8 weeks' rehabilitation and 1 and 2 years following rehabilitation

Maximum treadmill exercise workload (METS)	Baseline	Post-rehabilitation	12 months	24 months
Intervention group	4.4 (2.2)	5.6 (2.6)	5.7 (2.6)*	5.1 (2.5)
No intervention	4.4 (2.2)	5.6 (2.4)	5.0 (2.5)	4.8 (2.7)

The values are expressed as means (SD).
*$P \leq 0.05$.

programme in the experimental subjects together with a reduction in hospital days (Table 7.1 shows the results of the maximal treadmill workload). There were no group differences for other measures of pulmonary function (including FEV_1 and total lung capacity), dyspnoea, self-efficacy, generic and disease-specific quality of life and healthcare use.

In the post-intervention year there were 131 subjects who completed the 24-month follow-up. By 24 months there were no significant group differences. The patients returned to levels that were close to but above the pre-rehabilitation measures. There was no difference in survival at 2 years.

In summary, the maintenance programme was only modestly successful at maintaining health benefits and was not sufficient to prevent regression of beneficial health outcomes fully after successful pulmonary rehabilitation in patients with advanced chronic lung disease. Further work is needed to evaluate how to maintain the long-term benefits of rehabilitation.

Proportional assist ventilation as an aid to exercise training in severe chronic obstructive pulmonary disease
Hawkins P, Johnson LC, Nikoletou D, *et al. Thorax* 2002; **57**(10): 853–9

BACKGROUND. The use of pulmonary rehabilitation in patients with COPD has been shown to improve both exercise tolerance and health-related quality of life. The aim of this study was to assess the efficacy of proportional assisted ventilation as an aid to exercise training in patients with severe COPD.

INTERPRETATION. Proportional assisted ventilation in a 6-week rehabilitation programme enabled a higher level of training in patients with severe COPD that subsequently led to greater improvements in maximum exercise capacity.

Comment

Exercise training is an important part of pulmonary rehabilitation, but the optimal training strategy for patients with severe COPD is unknown. Patients with moderate

COPD can achieve a greater physiological benefit if the exercise is performed at a work rate exceeding their anaerobic threshold. However, this is not achievable in patients with severe COPD due to ventilatory limitation.

Inspiratory pressure support has been shown to increase endurance, improve breathlessness, unload the respiratory muscles and prolong exercise-induced lactataemia during exercise. Proportional assisted ventilation is a method that matches ventilator output to patient effort that is more tolerable and appears to be as effective as conventional inspiratory pressure support [1].

This randomized, controlled study evaluated the use of proportional assisted ventilation as an aid to exercise training in severe COPD. Nineteen patients participated in this 6-week randomized study. Patients received an exercise programme three times per week for 6 weeks and had a 30-minute session on a cycle ergometer aiming initially to achieve 70% of the peak work rate observed from the pre-training incremental exercise test and this was progressively increased by 5 W if the patient could achieve 30 min at that work rate.

The patients were randomized to receiving proportional assisted ventilation using a 'BIPAP Vision' (Respironics, USA), with a mean (SD) flow assistance of 3.6 (0.7) $cmH_2O/l/s$ and a first volume assist of 12.7 (1.5) cmH_2O/l. There was no educational component during the study and patients were encouraged to continue their normal activities at home, but not to perform extra exercise in between sessions. The primary outcome measure was the magnitude of the reduction in lactate concentration at an equivalent work rate after training.

Twenty-nine patients were recruited for the study, but only 19 completed it (withdrawal was due to exacerbations or non-compliance with the exercise programme, six of these in the unassisted group). Ten were randomized to the assisted ventilation and nine were unassisted. Pre-rehabilitation, the peak exercise capacity was markedly impaired in both groups with a mean of 26% predicted (95% CI = 20–31%) in the assisted group and 27% (95% CI = 21–34%) in the unassisted group.

Following 6 weeks' training, the mean training intensity was 15.5% (95% CI = 3.2–27.1%) higher in the assisted group ($P <0.05$). Both groups showed an improvement in exercise capacity ($P <0.001$) in the incremental test, but a greater improvement was found in the assisted group (Table 7.2).

However, there was no change in the patients' peak plasma lactate concentration with the 6 weeks' training. With identical workloads during the constant work rate test before and after training, the plasma lactate concentration reduced significantly in the assisted arm only ($P <0.01$). The reduction in plasma lactate concentration at an equivalent workload after training correlated with the increase in peak work rate ($r = –0.6; P <0.01$) and with the mean training intensity in the last week of training ($r = –0.7; P <0.001$).

In summary, patients with severe COPD who received ventilatory assistance during a 6-week exercise programme achieved greater training intensities and maximum exercise capacity. However, the primary outcome, the change of lactate concentration during the constant work rate test, did not achieve a significant difference between the groups, but this was only a small study.

Table 7.2 Comparison between the groups receiving assisted ventilation and the unassisted group

Mean (SD)	Assisted (n = 10)	Unassisted (n = 9)	P-value
Age (years)	68 (9.1)	66 (6.8)	n.s.
FEV$_1$ (% predicted)	26 (7)	28 (7)	n.s.
Pre-study peak exercise capacity (W)	45.6 (10.7)	43.5 (12)	n.s.
Mean (95% CI) increase in the peak exercise capacity (W) post-study (%)	32.9 (22–44)	14.5 (8–21)	0.005
Reduction in lactate concentration post study (%)	30 (16–44)	12 (–7 to 31)	0.09

N.s., not significant.

The pressure-assisted ventilation is thought to work by unloading the respiratory muscles enabling the patients to place a greater workload on the leg muscles during the training sessions. Further larger studies are needed.

Nutritional enhancement of exercise performance in chronic obstructive pulmonary disease: a randomized controlled trial

Steiner MC, Barton RL, Singh SJ, Morgan MD. *Thorax* 2003; **58**(9): 745–51

BACKGROUND. It is well established that pulmonary rehabilitation is effective in improving exercise performance and health status in patients with COPD. This UK study evaluated the role of nutritional support in the enhancement of the benefits of exercise training. A double-blind, randomized, controlled trial of carbohydrate supplementation was undertaken in patients attending outpatient pulmonary rehabilitation.

INTERPRETATION. In this small study carbohydrate supplementation when universally prescribed did not enhance the rehabilitation of patients with severe COPD. Larger studies are needed.

Comment

This study evaluated whether optimizing nutritional support would enhance the rehabilitation potential in patients with advanced COPD. Eighty-five patients with severe COPD were studied, with a mean FEV$_1$ of approximately 35% predicted, a mean body mass index (BMI) of approximately 24 kg/m^2, a mean incremental shuttle walk test of approximately 215 m and a mean endurance shuttle walk test of approximately 190 s. Patients with a BMI >30 kg/m^2 were excluded.

Patients were randomized to receive a 570 kcal carbohydrate-rich supplement or a non-nutritive placebo daily for the duration of a 7-week outpatient pulmonary rehabilitation programme. The primary outcome measures were peak (incremental shuttle walk test) and submaximal exercise performance (endurance shuttle walk test) using the shuttle walk tests.

Forty-two patients were randomized to the supplement arm and 43 patients to the placebo arm. The study unfortunately had a high dropout rate leaving 25 patients in the supplement arm and 35 in the placebo arm.

Patients receiving placebo lost weight (−0.58 kg) whereas supplemented patients gained weight (+0.63 kg) (P <0.01). With the 7-week rehabilitation programme, patients in both the supplement and placebo groups increased their incremental and endurance shuttle walking performance (P <0.01). The mean increase in the incremental shuttle walk test was 60 m in the supplement arm and 43 m in the placebo arm (no significant differences between these group results). The mean increase in the endurance shuttle walk test was 328 s in the supplement arm and 191 s in the placebo arm (no significant differences between these group results).

A subgroup analysis was carried out, but there were only small numbers (eight with a BMI <19 kg/m^2 and 52 with a BMI >19 kg/m^2). In patients with a normal BMI (>19 kg/m^2) the improvement in their incremental shuttle performance was significantly greater in the supplemented group (mean difference between groups 27 m and 95% CI = 1–53 m) (P <0.05). The increases in incremental shuttle performance correlated weakly with the increases in total carbohydrate intake ($r = 0.3$; $P = 0.01$).

In summary, when universally prescribed, carbohydrate supplementation did not enhance the rehabilitation of patients with COPD. However, this was a small study and an effect may have been found in a larger study. This study suggested that exercise training resulted in a negative energy balance that can be overcome by supplementation and that, in selected patients, this may improve the outcome of training. The finding of benefit in well-nourished patients may suggest a role for nutritional supplementation beyond the treatment of weight loss in COPD. Further larger studies are needed.

Reference

1. Dolmage TE, Goldstein RS. Proportional assist ventilation and exercise tolerance in subjects with COPD. *Chest* 1997; **111**: 948–54.

8

Surgical treatments

Introduction

There has been an increased interest in surgical options for patients with emphysema. Lung volume reduction surgery may improve the lung mechanics in patients with emphysema by reducing the dynamic hyperinflation. The aim with surgery would be to improve the patients' functional capacity and health-related quality of life without causing major morbidity or mortality. The first three papers that are presented explore the outcomes, cost-effectiveness and health-related quality of life from lung volume reduction surgery and help identify which patients should be referred for lung volume reduction surgery.

There have been international guidelines for lung transplantation available that identify which patients with chronic obstructive pulmonary disease (COPD) should be referred for lung transplantation |**1**|. Patients that are suitable for lung transplantation include patients (age <65 years) with no significant co-morbidities with a forced expiratory volume in 1 s (FEV$_1$) <25% predicted without reversibility and/or a raised partial pressure of carbon dioxide in arterial blood ($PaCO_2$) >7.3 kPa (55 mmHg) and/or raised pulmonary artery pressures with progressive deterioration such as corpulmonale. Preference is given for patients with a raised $PaCO_2$ with progressive deterioration who require long-term oxygen therapy as they have the poorest prognosis. The final paper selected for this chapter examined the 13-year outcome for lung transplantation in patients with COPD with and without α$_1$-antitrypsin deficiency.

A randomized trial comparing lung volume reduction surgery with medical therapy for severe emphysema
Fishman A, Martinez F, Naunheim K, *et al.*; National Emphysema Treatment Trial Research Group. *N Engl J Med* 2003; **348**(21): 2059–73

BACKGROUND. In advanced COPD lung hyperinflation accompanying advanced airflow obstruction is thought to contribute to respiratory disability. Lung volume reduction surgery has been proposed as a treatment for severe emphysema to allow the residual lung to function more effectively. This US, randomized, controlled study (**1218 patients**) compared lung volume reduction surgery with medical therapy, the primary end-points of which were maximal exercise capacity and mortality at 2 years.

INTERPRETATION. Exercise capacity at 2 years improved by >10 W in 15% in the lung volume surgery group compared with 3% in the medically treated group (P <0.001). On the other hand, lung volume reduction surgery conferred no survival advantage compared with medical therapy (0.11 deaths per person-year in both treatment groups).

Comment

In patients with severe emphysema, pulmonary function tests demonstrate significant airflow obstruction, gas trapping with a raised residual volume and a raised ratio of residual volume:total lung capacity and a reduced gas transfer. The lung hyperinflation component is thought to contribute to respiratory disability by impairing the normal lung mechanics.

Lung volume reduction surgery by a median sternotomy or video-assisted thoracoscopic surgery resects 20–35% of each lung, targeting the most diseased areas. This is thought to improve the pulmonary mechanics, which may ultimately improve lung function, exercise capacity and prognosis.

This US, randomized, controlled study randomized 1218 patients to lung volume reduction surgery ($n = 608$) or medical therapy ($n = 610$). Prior to randomization all patients underwent a 6–10-week period of pulmonary rehabilitation, which is now established as an important adjunct to treatment for COPD patients.

The inclusion criteria included patients with heterogeneous emphysema, lung function tests with an FEV_1 ≤45% predicted, total lung capacity ≥100% predicted, residual volume ≥150% predicted and arterial blood gases with a partial pressure of oxygen in arterial blood (PaO_2) ≥6 kPa (45 mmHg) and a $PaCO_2$ ≤8 kPa (55 mmHg). All patients had to have given up smoking for ≥4 months.

In the surgery group, the mean ± standard deviation (SD) age was 66.5 ± 5.3 years, post-bronchodilator FEV_1 26.8 ± 7.4% predicted, total lung capacity 128.0 ± 15.3% predicted, residual volume 220.5 ± 49.9% predicted, diffusing capacity for carbon monoxide (Dl_{co}) 28.3 ± 9.7% predicted, PaO_2 8.6 ± 1.4 kPa and $PaCO_2$ 5.8 ± 0.8 kPa. There were no significant differences with the medically treated group.

The primary end-points in the study were mortality and maximal exercise capacity after 2 years. The mortality rates at 90 days were significantly higher in the surgically treated group (7.9% in the surgically treated group compared with 1.3% in the medically treated group) (P <0.001). However, at 2 years there was no significant difference in mortality with 0.11 deaths per person-years in both groups. At 2 years there was however a greater improvement of >10 W exercise capacity in the surgically treated group (15% in the surgically treated group compared with 3% in the medically treated group) (P <0.001).

Table 8.1 looks at the outcomes at 2 years including mortality, the increase in exercise capacity (>10 W) and an eight-point improvement in the St George's Respiratory Questionnaire (a four-point improvement is clinically significant). Patients with predominant upper lobe emphysema fared better with lung volume reduction surgery and the greatest improvements were seen in patients with poor functional status.

Subgroup analysis was carried out to help determine the selection criteria for lung volume reduction surgery. Patients with an FEV_1 ≤20% predicted and either

Table 8.1 Comparison of the surgically treated group and medically treated group outcomes at 2 years

2 years	Upper lobe emphysema plus exercise capacity of ≤25 W for women and ≤40 W for men	Upper lobe emphysema plus exercise capacity of >25 W for women and >40 W for men	Non-upper lobe emphysema plus exercise capacity of ≤25 W for women and ≤40 W for men	Non-upper lobe emphysema plus exercise capacity >25 W for women and >40 W for men
Number	290	419	149	220
Mortality risk ratio for death				
Surgery versus medical treatment	0.47**	0.98	0.81	2.06*
Greater than 10 W increase in exercise capacity (%)				
Surgery treatment	30***	15**	12	3
Medical treatment	0	3	7	3
Greater than eight-point improvement in the St George's Respiratory Questionnaire (%)				
Surgery treatment	48***	41***	37**	15
Medical treatment	10	11	7	12

The distribution of emphysema was split into upper and non-upper lobe emphysema and exercise capacity into those who have either a low exercise capacity (≤25 W for women or ≤40 W for men) or a higher exercise capacity (>25 W for women or >40 W for men). Non-upper lobe emphysema is defined as emphysema predominantly in the lower lobes or diffuse emphysema. The outcomes include mortality, increase in exercise capacity (>10 W) and an eight-point improvement in the St George's Respiratory Questionnaire (a four-point improvement is clinically significant).
* P <0.05, ** P <0.01, *** P <0.001.

homogeneous emphysema on computed tomography (CT) scanning or a carbon monoxide gas transfer ≤20% predicted had a poor prognosis with lung volume reduction surgery with little chance for functional improvement (7% functional improvement in the surgical group compared with 2% in the medically treated group) (P-value not significant) and a high mortality rate (0.33 deaths per person-year in the surgical group compared with 0.18 deaths in the medically treated group) ($P = 0.06$).

In summary, lung volume reduction surgery overall at 2 years increased the chance of improved exercise capacity, but did not confer a survival advantage over medical therapy. However, subgroup analysis revealed a survival advantage for patients with both predominantly upper lobe emphysema and low baseline exercise capacity.

Poorer outcomes were identified in patients with either diffuse emphysema or predominant lower lobe emphysema, in particular in patients with very advanced airflow obstruction (FEV_1 ≤20% predicted) or a carbon monoxide gas transfer ≤20% predicted. In addition, there was an increased mortality rate with surgery in patients with an exercise capacity (>25 W for women or >40 W for men) in patients with diffuse or predominant lower lobe emphysema.

In summary, it would seem advisable to reserve lung volume reduction surgery for patients with predominant upper lobe emphysema, an FEV_1 21–45% predicted, total lung capacity ≥100% predicted, residual volume ≥150% predicted and patients with a poor exercise capacity (≤25W for women or ≤40 W for men), but without respiratory failure.

Cost-effectiveness of lung volume reduction surgery for patients with severe emphysema

Ramsey SD, Berry K, Etzioni R, Kaplan RM, Sullivan SD, Wood DE; National Emphysema Treatment Trial Research Group. *N Engl J Med* 2003; **348**(21): 2092–102

BACKGROUND. The latter National Emphysema Treatment Trial, a randomized, clinical trial comparing lung volume reduction surgery with medical therapy for severe emphysema, included a prospective economic analysis for evaluating whether lung volume reduction surgery was cost-effective.

INTERPRETATION. After exclusion of high-risk cases (FEV_1 ≤20% predicted and either homogeneous emphysema on CT scanning or a carbon monoxide gas transfer ≤20% predicted) the cost-effectiveness ratio for lung volume reduction surgery as compared with medical therapy was $190 000 per quality-adjusted life year (QALY) gained at 3 years and $53 000 per QALY gained at 10 years. Given its cost and benefits over 3 years of follow-up, lung volume reduction surgery is costly relative to medical therapy. Although the predictions are subject to substantial uncertainty, the lung volume reduction surgery may be cost-effective if the benefits from surgery can be maintained over time.

Comment

An economic analysis was carried out for the latter trial. Briefly, after pulmonary rehabilitation, 1218 patients were randomly assigned to lung volume reduction surgery or continued medical treatment. The costs for the use of medical care, medications, transportation and time spent receiving treatment were derived from Medicare claims and data from the trial. Cost-effectiveness was calculated over the duration of the trial and was estimated for 10 years of follow-up with the use of modelling based on observed trends in survival, cost and quality of life.

During the trial an interim analyses identified a group of patients with excess mortality and little chance of improved functional status after surgery (FEV_1 ≤20% predicted and either homogeneous emphysema on CT scanning or a carbon monoxide gas transfer ≤20% predicted) and these patients were excluded.

The mean total costs per person at 3 years were higher at $98 952 in the surgery group ($n = 531$) compared with $62 560 in the medical group ($n = 535$) ($P < 0.001$). The mean number of QALYs gained was higher in the surgery group (1.46) (95% confidence interval [CI] = 1.46–1.47) compared with the medically treated group (1.27) (95% CI = 1.27–1.28) ($P < 0.001$). The estimated cost-effectiveness ratio for lung volume reduction surgery as compared with medical therapy was $190 000 per QALY gained at 3 years and $53 000 per QALY gained at 10 years. This compares with $8300–64 000 per QALY gained for coronary artery bypass surgery or $130 000–220 000 for lung transplantation.

Subgroup analyses identified patients with predominantly upper lobe emphysema and low exercise capacity (≤25 W for women and ≤40 W for men) after pulmonary rehabilitation that had a lower mortality and better functional status than patients who received medical therapy. For this subgroup of patients the QALY gain was 1.54 (95% CI = 1.53–1.55) in the surgery group compared with 1.04 (95% CI = 1.03–1.05) in the medically treated group ($P < 0.001$). The cost-effectiveness ratio in this subgroup was $98 000 per QALY gained at 3 years and $21 000 at 10 years.

This cost-effectiveness ratio was less favourable at 3 years for patients with predominant upper lobe emphysema and exercise capacity (>25 W for women and >40 W for men) at $240 000 per QALY gained or those with non-upper lobe emphysema who had exercise capacity (≤25 W for women and ≤40 W for men) at $333 000 per QALY gained. Bootstrap analysis revealed substantial uncertainty for the 10-year estimates.

In summary, given the cost and benefits over 3 years of follow-up, lung volume reduction surgery is costly relative to medical therapy. Although the predictions are subject to substantial uncertainty, the procedure may be cost-effective if the benefits from lung volume reduction surgery can be maintained over a longer time such as 10 years, but this requires long-term prospective follow-up.

Influence of lung volume reduction surgery (LVRS) on health-related quality of life in patients with chronic obstructive pulmonary disease

Goldstein RS, Todd TR, Guyatt G, *et al. Thorax* 2003; **58**(5): 405–10

BACKGROUND. This randomized, controlled clinical trial examined the impact of lung volume reduction surgery on health-related quality of life.

INTERPRETATION. Lung volume reduction surgery in COPD patients with heterogeneous emphysema resulted in important benefits in disease-specific quality of life compared with medical management that were sustained at 12 months after treatment.

Comment

Disease-specific quality of life is a responsive interpretable outcome that enables health professionals to identify the magnitude of the effect of an intervention across several domains. The aim of this randomized, controlled study was to study the impact of lung volume reduction surgery on health-related quality of life over a period of 1 year.

Patients aged <75 years with severe COPD (FEV_1 <40% predicted and FEV_1:forced vital capacity <0.7), hyperinflation with a total lung capacity >120% predicted and evidence of heterogeneity of the emphysema from high resolution CT were randomized to surgical or control groups after 6 weeks of pulmonary rehabilitation. All patients had to have given up smoking for ≥6 months. Patients with hypercapnia >6.6 kPa or pulmonary hypertension (mean pressure >35 mmHg) were excluded.

Both groups were monitored at intervals of 3 months for 12 months with no cross-over between the groups. The primary outcome was disease-specific quality of life as measured by the Chronic Respiratory Questionnaire (CRQ). This focuses on four domains (dyspnoea, fatigue, emotional function and mastery). A minimal clinical important difference in CRQ score has been shown to be 0.5 units. Treatment failure was defined as death or functional decline (fall of 1 unit in any two domains of the CRQ). Secondary outcomes included the 6-minute walking distance, submaximal cycle endurance time and measures of pulmonary function including spirometry and lung volumes.

Following rehabilitation 28 patients received lung volume reduction surgery and 27 received medical therapy alone. Overall the mean ± standard error (SE) age was 64.9 ± 0.9 years, FEV_1 32.0 ± 1.4% predicted, total lung capacity 146.0 ± 2.6% predicted, residual volume 240 ± 7.9% predicted, DL_{co} 35.0 ± 1.6% predicted, PaO_2 9.3 ± 0.2 kPa and $PaCO_2$ 5.9 ± 0.1 kPa. There were no significant differences between the surgically and medically treated groups.

Lung volume reduction surgery was carried out by video-assisted thoracoscopic surgery or median sternotomy and aimed to remove 20–30% of the lung volume. Bilateral surgery was carried out in 19 and eight had unilateral surgery.

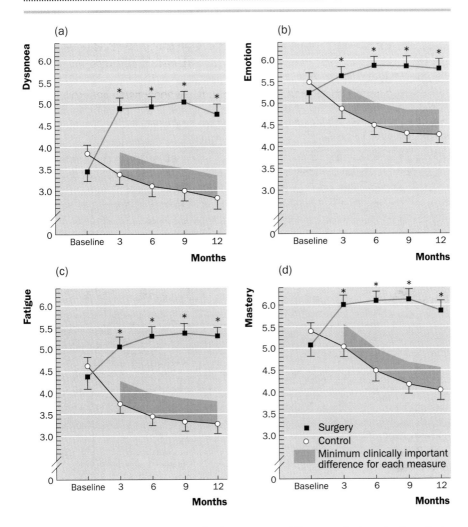

Fig. 8.1 The effect of lung volume reduction surgery and the group that received medical treatment alone on each of the 4 domains of the CRQ (dyspnoea, emotional function, fatigue and mastery) at baseline 3, 6, 9 and 12 months. The shaded area (0.5 units) shows the minimum clinically important difference. *$P < 0.0001$.
Source: Goldstein *et al.* (2003).

Overall by 1 year there were four deaths (14%) due to respiratory failure in the surgical group (two deaths within 30 days of surgery) and one death due to respiratory failure in the control group (4%).

There was significant morbidity with lung volume reduction surgery: four had serious complications including prolonged ventilation, non-fatal cardiac arrest, bleeding and sternal dehiscence. The other main side effects were prolonged air leak over 7 days in 36% and benign dysrhythmias, respiratory tract infections and transient confusion in 21%. Following discharge from hospital there were four admissions in the surgical group and three pulmonary complications, but none in the control group.

However, lung volume reduction surgery resulted in significant between-group differences in each domain of the CRQ at 3, 6, 9 and 12 months (a change of 0.5 represents a small but important difference): for dyspnoea a change of 1.9 (95% CI = 1.3–2.6) (P <0.0001), for emotional function a change of 1.5 (95% CI = 0.9–2.1) (P <0.0001), for fatigue a change of 2.0 (95% CI = 1.4–2.6) (P <0.0001) and for mastery a change of 1.8 (95% CI = 1.2–2.5) (P <0.0001) (Fig. 8.1).

Surgical treatment resulted in less treatment failure over 12 months (hazard ratio = 3.1 and 95% CI = 1.3–7.6) (P = 0.01). In the surgical group 25% had treatment failure (four out of 28 patients died and three experienced functional decline), whereas in the control group 63% had treatment failure (one out of 27 patients died and 16 experienced functional decline) over 12 months.

For secondary end-points the surgery group compared with the medical group led to improvements (P <0.05) in flow rates, lung volumes and exercise at 12 months. The surgical group in comparison with the medical group showed an improvement in FEV_1 of 0.3 l (95% CI = 0.1–0.5) (P = 0.0003), residual volume –47% predicted (95% CI = –71 to –23) (P = 0.0002), submaximal exercise 7.3 min (95% CI = 3.9–10.8) (P <0.0001) and 6-minute walk 66 m (95% CI = 32–101) (P = 0.0002).

In summary, COPD patients with heterogeneous emphysema, FEV_1 <40% predicted and lung hyperinflation can benefit with lung volume reduction surgery in terms of improvements in health-related quality of life and less treatment failures. Patients should be aware of the potential mortality with lung volume reduction surgery and the significant morbidity risk attached to the operation before being considered for surgical intervention.

Thirteen-year experience in lung transplantation for emphysema

Cassivi SD, Meyers BF, Battafarano RJ, *et al. Ann Thorac Surg* 2002; **74**(5): 1663–9

BACKGROUND. The aim of this retrospective study was to look at the results of a single-institution series of lung transplants for COPD with and without α_1-antitrypsin deficiency in order to identify outcome differences and the factors predicting mortality and morbidity in these two groups.

INTERPRETATION. As predicted patients with COPD with α_1-antitrypsin deficiency receive lung transplantation at an earlier age. The overall 5-year survival was approximately 59%, with no significant differences between patients with COPD with and without α_1-antitrypsin deficiency. The 5-year survival was superior with bilateral compared with single lung transplantation.

Comment

Patients with α_1-antitrypsin deficiency develop emphysema at a younger age and tend to require lung transplantation at a younger age. The aim of this retrospective study was to study the results of a single-institution series of lung transplants for COPD with and without α_1-antitrypsin deficiency in order to identify outcome differences and the factors predicting mortality and morbidity in these two groups.

This retrospective study included 306 lung transplants for COPD, including 86 patients with COPD and α_1-antitrypsin deficiency and 220 patients with COPD without α_1-antitrypsin deficiency.

The mean $\pm$ SD age of patients with α_1-antitrypsin deficiency was 48.9 $\pm$ 6.3 years, which was younger than patients without α_1-antitrypsin deficiency (55.2 $\pm$ 6.4 years) (P <0.001). The mean FEV_1 indicated advanced airflow obstruction in both groups (the FEV_1 in patients with α_1-antitrypsin deficiency was 17 $\pm$ 5% predicted and 16 $\pm$ 5% predicted in patients without α_1-antitrypsin deficiency) (P-value not significant).

The hospital mortality was 6.2%, with no difference between COPD patients with and without α_1-antitrypsin deficiency or between single lung transplants and bilateral lung transplants. The hospital mortality during the most recent 6 years of this 13-year study was significantly lower (3.9 versus 9.5%) ($P = 0.04$).

The 5-year survival was 58.6 $\pm$ 3.5%, with no significant difference between patients with α_1-antitrypsin deficiency (60.5 $\pm$ 5.8%) and without α_1-antitrypsin deficiency COPD (56.8 $\pm$ 4.4%). The 5-year survival was better with bilateral lung transplants (66.7 $\pm$ 4.0%) than with single lung transplants (44.9 $\pm$ 6.0%) (P <0.005) (Fig. 8.2) and this was also observed with the groups of COPD with and without α_1-antitrypsin deficiency. Independent predictors of mortality by Cox analysis were single lung transplantation (relative hazard = 1.98 and P <0.001) and need for cardiopulmonary bypass during the transplant (relative hazard = 1.84 and $P = 0.038$).

At 5 years post-transplantation there was an improved FEV_1 and 6-minute walk test. At 5 years in patients with α_1-antitrypsin deficiency the FEV_1 was 73 $\pm$ 3% predicted and the mean improvement from baseline in the 6-minute walk was 527 feet whilst for patients without α_1-antitrypsin deficiency the FEV_1 was 62 $\pm$ 3% predicted and the mean improvement from baseline in the 6-minute walk was 444 feet (135 metres).

Bronchiolitis obliterans syndrome occurred in 40.7% and post-transplant malignancy in 9.3% of patients with α_1-antitrypsin deficiency, which was not significantly different from patients without α_1-antitrypsin deficiency (36.8 and 7.7%, respectively).

In summary, this was a large cohort of patients with COPD with and without α_1-antitrypsin deficiency that had received lung transplantation. Despite patients with α_1-antitrypsin deficiency being younger they had a very similar prognosis post-transplantation to patients without α_1-antitrypsin deficiency. Bilateral lung transplantation was superior to single lung transplantation with improved 5-year survival figures.

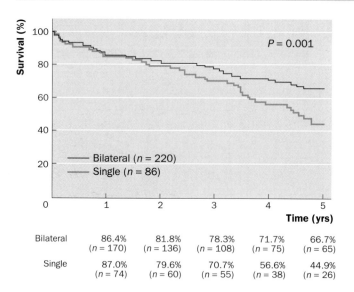

Bilateral	86.4%	81.8%	78.3%	71.7%	66.7%
	(n = 170)	(n = 136)	(n = 108)	(n = 75)	(n = 65)
Single	87.0%	79.6%	70.7%	56.6%	44.9%
	(n = 74)	(n = 60)	(n = 55)	(n = 38)	(n = 26)

Fig. 8.2 There was an improved actuarial survival for bilateral compared with single-lung transplants. Source: Cassivi *et al.* (2002).

Conclusion

The first three papers on lung volume reduction surgery will help guide the clinician as to who should be considered for lung volume reduction surgery. Prior to consideration for lung volume reduction surgery, patients should have optimization of their medical therapy, be non-smoking and have undergone pulmonary rehabilitation.

Lung volume reduction surgery is not without risk and there has been an increased mortality particularly in patients with an FEV_1 ≤20% predicted and either homogeneous emphysema on CT scanning or a carbon monoxide gas transfer ≤20% predicted (29% 90-day mortality). An increased mortality has also been found in patients who had an exercise capacity >25 W for women and >40 W for men that had emphysema predominantly in the lower lobes or that had diffuse emphysema.

The patients thought to benefit most are patients with heterogeneous predominant upper lobe emphysema, patients with an FEV_1 21–45% predicted, evidence of hyperinflated lung fields with an elevated total lung capacity ≥100% predicted and residual volume ≥150% predicted in patients without respiratory failure.

These selected patients can have long-term functional improvements in exercise tolerance, have improved health-related quality of life and less mortality. Along with the potential benefits with surgery, patients should be aware of the potential morbidity and mortality from lung volume reduction surgery (5–7% 90-day mortality).

Finally, lung volume reduction surgery is costly, at least over a 3-year period. However, the procedure may be cost-effective if the benefits with lung volume reduction surgery can be maintained over a longer time such as 5–10 years, but this requires long-term prospective follow-up.

Lung transplantation can improve both functional capacity and health-related quality of life, although its impact on survival is less clear [2]. In view of this, patients have to be selected very carefully. Patients should have severe irreversible airflow obstruction with preference given to patients that have respiratory failure that requires long-term oxygen therapy, as such patients have the poorest prognosis. Currently the age limits are <65 years for single lung transplantation and <60 years for bilateral lung transplantation.

Lung transplantation, although it can significantly improve exercise capacity and improve quality of life, is associated with significant morbidity and mortality. The morbidity associated with transplantation relates to lifelong immunosuppression, invasive investigations and the treatment of complications such as infection and lung rejection. There is an initial high mortality in the first 30 days (between 5 and 15%) and by 5 years it is approximately 40–50%.

Therefore, patients that are selected should have advanced COPD with an expected poor prognosis with an estimated life expectancy of <2 years. There continues to be a drive to improve both morbidity and mortality with lung transplantation, which will be helped by newer and more effective immunosuppressive agents and the prompt treatment of both infection and rejection. In light of the lack of donor organs there has been increased interest in single lung transplantation. However, the latter study in this chapter revealed that bilateral lung transplantation had a superior 5-year survival compared with single lung transplants without any increase in hospital stay, intensive care unit stay or mechanical ventilation. Bilateral lung transplantation would seem the preferred option, but the lack of donor organs is likely to hinder this.

References

1. Maurer JR, Frost AE, Estenne M, Higenbottam T, Glanville AR. International guidelines for the selection of lung transplant candidates. *J Heart Lung Tranplant* 1998; **17**: 703–9.
2. Hosenpud JD, Bennett LE, Keck BM, Edwards EB, Novick EJ. Effect of diagnosis on survival benefit of lung transplantation for end stage lung disease. *Lancet* 1998; **351**: 24–7.

9

Treatment of exacerbations

Introduction

Exacerbations of chronic obstructive pulmonary disease (COPD) are an important cause of both morbidity, which causes significant impairment of health status and mortality. Both infection of the tracheobronchial tree and air pollution are common causes of exacerbations, but a cause cannot always be identified. The presence of at least two of worsening symptoms, increased sputum purulence and increased sputum volume are usually due to a bacterial infection and in such patients antibiotic therapy is usually recommended.

The Global Initiative for Chronic Obstructive Lung Disease (GOLD) guidelines comment that inhaled bronchodilators, theophyllines, systemic glucocorticoids (preferably oral) and antibiotics (the latter if clinical signs of airway infection) are effective treatments for exacerbations of COPD |1|. The first three papers selected explored the use of methylxanthines and systemic steroids for exacerbations of COPD.

In severe exacerbations non-invasive positive pressure ventilation is a useful adjunct to other medical therapy and improves blood gases and pH, reduces in-hospital mortality, decreases the requirements for invasive mechanical ventilation and intubation and decreases the length of hospital stay. Three papers were selected including two systematic reviews of the use of non-invasive positive pressure ventilation in exacerbations of COPD and the other paper selected was a cost-effective analysis of the use of non-invasive positive pressure ventilation for severe exacerbations of COPD.

There has been increased interest in treating exacerbations of COPD at home that would normally be treated in hospital. After formal assessment in hospital a number of the less severe exacerbations of COPD, without co-morbidities and sufficient home support, can be treated at home with augmentation of medical therapy, for example with nebulized bronchodilators, oral corticosteroids and antibiotic therapy and nursing support. Two papers were selected. The first paper selected explored the usefulness of domiciliary community follow-up following hospital discharge with an exacerbation of COPD and the final paper explored home treatment, as described above, for exacerbations of COPD.

Methylxanthines for exacerbations of chronic obstructive pulmonary disease: meta-analysis of randomized trials

Barr RG, Rowe BH, Camargo Jr CA. *BMJ* 2003; **327**(7416): 643

BACKGROUND. Methylxanthines are considered as an adjunct to conventional treatment for exacerbations of COPD including bronchodilators, corticosteroids and antibiotic therapy. This meta-analysis reviewed four randomized, controlled trials (*n* = 169) comparing methylxanthines and placebo for exacerbations of COPD. This treatment occurred either in the emergency department or immediately on admission to hospital. The primary end-points were the patients' forced expiratory volume in 1 s (FEV$_1$) at 2 h and 3 days, clinical outcomes (admission to hospital, relapse and length of stay and symptom scores) and adverse events.

INTERPRETATION. The available data do not support the use of methylxanthines for the treatment of exacerbations of COPD. Overall there were no benefits with methylxanthines in FEV$_1$, clinical outcomes or symptom scores, but there was a greater likelihood of adverse events.

Comment

This study evaluated the evidence base behind the recommendations for the use of methylxanthines for acute exacerbations of COPD. Methylxanthines may be potentially advantageous during exacerbations by decreasing diaphragmatic muscle fatigue, increasing mucociliary clearance, blocking centrally mediated hypoventilation and decreasing capillary leakage. However, they have a significant side-effect profile and the potential side effects may outweigh the potential advantages.

There were four randomized, controlled studies from 1299 articles reviewed with only 169 patients collectively in these studies. The mean change in FEV$_1$ at 2 h was similar in the methylxanthines and placebo groups, but transiently increased with methylxanthines at 3 days. There was no significant benefit with methylxanthines in either clinical outcomes (admission to hospital, relapse and length of stay) or symptom scores, but there was a greater incidence of nausea and vomiting with methylxanthines compared with placebo (odds ratio = 4.6 and 95% confidence interval [CI] = 1.7–12.6).

In summary, there is a paucity of studies with a small number of patients evaluating the efficacy of methylxanthines for acute exacerbations of COPD. The data from these four randomized, controlled trials do not support the routine use of methylxanthines for the treatment of exacerbations of COPD as the side-effect profile seemed to outweigh the potential benefits. It may be that methylxanthines have a role in more severe exacerbations of COPD, but further randomized, controlled studies are needed to address this.

Out-patient oral prednisone after emergency treatment of chronic obstructive pulmonary disease

Aaron SD, Vandemheen KL, Hebert P, *et al. N Engl J Med* 2003; **348**(26): 2618–25

BACKGROUND. The mainstays of treatment for exacerbations of COPD are bronchodilator therapy, antibiotics and corticosteroids. The bronchodilators relieve the airflow obstruction and help the symptoms of dyspnoea. Antibiotics are recommended if there are at least two of the following symptoms: increased symptoms with increased sputum volume and purulence. This randomized, placebo-controlled study evaluated the efficacy of oral corticosteroids in exacerbations of COPD managed as outpatients.

INTERPRETATION. Compared with placebo, outpatient treatment with oral prednisone improved the symptoms of breathlessness over a 10-day period, improved FEV_1 over a 10-day period and reduced relapse rates at 30 days, but did not impact on disease-specific quality of life. The lack of effect on disease-specific quality of life was thought to be due to the increased side effects with corticosteroids, including insomnia and weight gain.

Comment

This randomized, placebo-controlled study evaluated the efficacy of oral cortico-steroids for exacerbations of COPD treated as outpatients.

A total of 147 patients admitted to an emergency department with an exacer-bation of COPD were enrolled. All patients had to have at least two of the following symptoms: worsening breathlessness, increased sputum volume and sputum puru-lence. Patients were randomly assigned to a 10-day course with 40 mg of oral pred-nisolone or placebo. All patients received regular bronchodilators for 30 days including both a β_2 agonist and an anticholinergic and all received a 10-day course of antibiotics (septrin or doxycycline).

The primary end-point of this study was the risk of relapse. This was defined as an unscheduled visit to a doctor or to the emergency department because of worsening breathlessness within 30 days after randomization.

The authors enrolled 147 patients who were being discharged from the emergency department after an exacerbation of COPD and randomly assigned to 10 days of treatment with 40 mg of oral prednisone ($n = 74$) once daily or identical appearing placebo ($n = 73$). All patients received oral antibiotics for 10 days, plus inhaled bronchodilators.

A criticism with this study was that, in approximately 11% of patients, the diag-nosis of COPD was made at the time of the acute exacerbation. There is a risk that there will not only be patients with COPD but also asthmatic patients and it would have been preferable if they had randomized only patients with known COPD that had been diagnosed according to international guidelines.

The mean age was around 69 years and the mean FEV_1 at the start of the

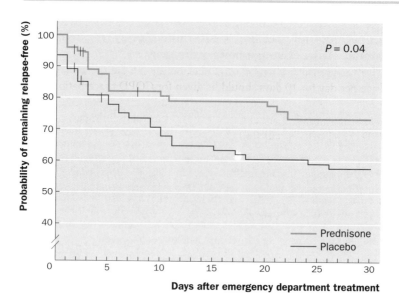

Fig. 9.1 Kaplan–Meier estimates of the probability of remaining relapse-free at 30 days in the prednisone and placebo-controlled groups. Tick marks represent censored data. $P = 0.04$ by the log-rank test. Source: Aaron *et al.* (2003).

exacerbation was 38% predicted. At 10 days there was a mean 34% improvement in FEV_1 in the group treated with oral corticosteroids compared with 15% in the placebo arm ($P < 0.01$). At day 10, the group treated with oral corticosteroids had a greater improvement in dyspnoea as part of the breathlessness domain from the Chronic Respiratory Disease Questionnaire (CRDQ) index ($P < 0.05$) and a higher Transitional Dyspnoea Index with a mean rise of 4.0 compared with 2.1 in the placebo arm ($P < 0.05$) (a 1-unit rise is a clinically significant improvement).

There was also a reduced relapse at 30 days of treatment with oral corticosteroids (27% compared with 43% in the placebo arm) ($P = 0.05$) and the time to relapse was prolonged in those taking prednisone ($P = 0.04$) (Fig. 9.1). There was no significant difference in the rate for hospitalization for COPD (11% in the corticosteroid arm and 21% in the placebo arm) ($P = 0.11$) although a larger study may have demonstrated a difference.

Despite the improvement in FEV_1 and breathlessness and a reduced relapse rate with corticosteroids, there was no improvement in the total score from the disease-specific quality of life questionnaire (the CRDQ index) at day 10, which may have been due to the increased adverse effects with corticosteroids, namely insomnia (48% in the steroid group compared with 21% in the placebo arm) ($P = 0.001$) and weight gain (13% in the steroid group compared with 1% in the placebo arm) ($P = 0.01$).

In summary, the addition of oral corticosteroids improved FEV_1 and breathlessness and had reduced relapsed rates. It is estimated that the number needed to treat is six in order to prevent one relapse in 30 days. Overall the advantages of oral corticosteroids outweigh the disadvantages for severe exacerbations of COPD treated as outpatients. This study supported the GOLD guidelines recommendation that 40 mg of oral prednisolone per day for 10 days should be given for COPD exacerbations that have a baseline FEV_1 <50% predicted |1|. Further studies are needed in order to determine whether there are similar benefits for acute exacerbations in patients with less severe COPD (FEV_1 >50% predicted).

Corticosteroid therapy for patients with acute exacerbations of chronic obstructive pulmonary disease: a systematic review

Singh JM, Palda VA, Stanbrook MB, Chapman KR. *Arch Intern Med* 2002; **162**(22): 2527–36

BACKGROUND. The aim of this systematic review was to evaluate the efficacy of the addition of oral corticosteroids in the management of exacerbations of COPD.

INTERPRETATION. Short courses of systemic corticosteroids up to 14 days in acute exacerbations of COPD improved both spirometric and clinical outcomes and are recommended as an adjunct to standard treatment for exacerbations of COPD.

Comment

This systematic review was carried out to determine whether systemic corticosteroids are of benefit to patients with acute exacerbations of COPD. Both MEDLINE (1966 to February 2002) and the Cochrane Library were reviewed in order to identify published clinical trials of systemic corticosteroid administration in acute exacerbations of COPD. All relevant English-language, randomized, placebo-controlled, clinical trials were considered.

Overall there were eight studies including 678 patients. There was an early improvement in FEV_1 within the first 5 days in patients treated with oral corticosteroids compared with placebo. However, the difference was small with a maximal rise up to 120 ml. However, this improvement in FEV_1 was not maintained after 2 weeks.

The largest study was by Niewoehner *et al.* ($n = 271$) in patients with severe COPD with mean FEV_1 values of 750, 772 and 785 ml in the placebo and in the 2- and 8-week steroid groups, respectively |2|. In this study patients with an exacerbation of COPD requiring hospital admission were randomized to placebo or 2 or 8 weeks of corticosteroid therapy. The 2-week corticosteroid group received 500 mg/day intravenous methylprednisolone for 3 days. Following this they received 60 mg/day oral prednisolone on days 4–7, 40 mg/day on days 8–11 and, finally,

20 mg/day on days 12–15. The 8-week corticosteroid group received 500 mg/day intravenous methylprednisolone for 3 days. Following this they received 60 mg/day oral prednisolone on days 4–7, 40 mg/day on days 8–11, 20 mg/day on days 12–43, 10 mg/day on days 44–50 and, finally, 5 mg/day on days 51–57. An important primary end-point in this study was treatment failure. They defined treatment failure as death, the requirement of intubation, augmentation of the therapeutic regimen or return for medical care after discharge.

At 30 days, there was less treatment failure in the steroid arm (23% treatment failure in the steroid arm compared with 33% in the placebo arm) (P <0.05). At 90 days, there was less treatment failure in the steroid arm (37% treatment failure in the steroid arm compared with 48% in the placebo arm) (P <0.05), but the treatment failure rates were similar at 6 months, independent of whether they received oral corticosteroids. There were no additional benefits with 8 weeks' compared with 2 weeks' corticosteroids. Although there was an initial benefit with oral corticosteroids (30 mg/day prednisolone for 14 days) in the smaller study by Davies *et al.* (n = 56) (mean FEV_1 27% predicted in the steroid-treated group and 21% in the placebo group), by 6 weeks there was no difference |3|.

These two latter studies revealed that, in the steroid-treated group, the length of hospitalization was reduced by 1–2 days (P <0.05).

The potential benefits have to be weighed up with the potential adverse effects with corticosteroids. Hyperglycaemia requiring treatment was found to be more frequent (P <0.005) in the glucocorticoid-treated group (15%) compared with placebo (4%) in the study by Niewoehner *et al.* |2|. There was some concern about the risk of infection with a prolonged 8 weeks' treatment, but this did not reach statistical significance. With prolonged use or use with frequent exacerbations there is particular concern about the development of osteoporosis.

In summary, there is evidence that oral corticosteroids as an adjunct to treatment in exacerbations of COPD that required hospital admission improved lung function parameters, reduced the length of hospital stay and reduced treatment failure. Oral corticosteroids are probably as effective as parenteral treatment as long as there is no malabsorption. The duration of treatment and optimal dose of oral corticosteroids has yet to be established, although the evidence suggests that ≤2 weeks will suffice. Recent recommendations from the GOLD guidelines recommend 30–40 mg/day oral prednisolone for 10–14 days in patients that require hospital management |1|. Further studies are needed to clarify the optimal dose, route, duration of treatment and long-term adverse effects.

Non-invasive positive pressure ventilation to treat respiratory failure resulting from exacerbations of chronic obstructive pulmonary disease: Cochrane systematic review and meta-analysis

Lightowler JV, Wedzicha JA, Elliott MW, Ram FS. *BMJ* 2003; **326**(7382): 185

BACKGROUND. The aim of this systematic review was to evaluate the effectiveness of non-invasive positive pressure ventilation in the management of respiratory failure resulting from an exacerbation of COPD.

INTERPRETATION. Non-invasive positive pressure ventilation is recommended in suitable patients as the first-line intervention in addition to usual medical care for managing respiratory failure secondary to an acute exacerbation of COPD. Non-invasive positive pressure ventilation should be tried early in the course of respiratory failure and before severe acidosis develops in order to reduce mortality, avoid endotracheal intubation and decrease treatment failure.

Comment

The aim of this systematic review was to evaluate the efficacy of non-invasive positive pressure ventilation in the management of respiratory failure resulting from exacerbations of COPD. This was a systematic review of the literature until 2002 of randomized, controlled trials with patients admitted with an exacerbation of COPD with respiratory failure with a baseline partial pressure of carbon dioxide in arterial blood ($PaCO_2$) >6 kPa. Treatment failure was defined as the combination of mortality, need for intubation and intolerance of the allocated treatment.

There were eight studies in this systematic review (546 patients). Non-invasive positive pressure ventilation was associated with a lower mortality rate (relative risk [RR] = 0.41 and 95% CI = 0.26–0.64), a lower need for intubation (RR = 0.42 and 95% CI = 0.31–0.59) and a lower likelihood of treatment failure (RR = 0.51 and 95% CI = 0.38–0.67).

In addition, there were greater improvements at 1 h in pH (weighted mean difference = 0.03, 95% CI = 0.02–0.04), $PaCO_2$ (weighted mean difference = –0.4 kPa, 95% CI = –0.78 to –0.03) and respiratory rate (weighted mean difference = –3.08, 95% CI = –4.26 to –1.89). Non-invasive positive pressure ventilation resulted in fewer complications associated with treatment (RR = 0.32 and 95% CI = 0.18–0.56) and shorter duration of stay in hospital (RR = –3.24 days and 95% CI = –4.42 to –2.06). Almost all the excess complications were due to the requirement for intubation, suggesting that avoidance of ventilation is the main benefit of non-invasive positive pressure ventilation.

The number needed to treat with non-invasive positive pressure ventilation in order to prevent one treatment failure was five (95% CI = 4–7). The number needed to treat in order to prevent one intubation was five (95% CI = 4–7) and that in order to prevent one death was eight (95% CI = 6–13).

In summary, in patients admitted with an exacerbation of COPD with respiratory failure (pH <7.35 and $PaCO_2$ >6 kPa or >45 mmHg) the use of non-invasive positive pressure ventilation significantly reduced mortality, endotracheal intubation, treatment failure, complications and length of hospital stay and improved blood gas tensions. Non-invasive positive pressure ventilation is often carried in high-dependency units or intensive care units (ICUs). However, it is sometimes used in medical wards and if such a set-up exists there should be training for staff and monitoring to be in place with 24-hour medical cover.

Which patients with acute exacerbation of chronic obstructive pulmonary disease benefit from non-invasive positive-pressure ventilation? A systematic review of the literature

Keenan SP, Sinuff T, Cook DJ, Hill NS. *Ann Intern Med* 2003; **138**(11): 861–70

BACKGROUND. The aim of this systematic review was to assess the impact of non-invasive positive pressure ventilation on the rate of endotracheal intubation, length of hospital stay and in-hospital mortality rate in patients admitted with an exacerbation of COPD as in the previous study, but in addition this study aimed to determine the effect of exacerbation severity on these outcomes.

INTERPRETATION. Non-invasive positive pressure ventilation benefited patients with severe exacerbations of COPD, but did not benefit hospitalized patients with milder exacerbations.

Comment

Non-invasive positive pressure ventilation is being increasingly used in severe exacerbations of COPD admitted to hospital. The aim of this systematic review was to assess the impact of non-invasive positive pressure ventilation on the rate of endotracheal intubation, length of hospital stay and in-hospital mortality rate in patients admitted to hospital with an exacerbation of COPD and aimed to determine the effect of exacerbation severity on these outcomes.

The main sources were MEDLINE (1966–2002), EMBASE (1990–2002) and the Cochrane Library. The studies selected were randomized, controlled trials that compared non-invasive positive pressure ventilation with standard therapy for acute exacerbations of COPD that required hospitalization and included the need for endotracheal intubation, length of hospital stay and hospital survival as outcomes. The main outcomes measured were the need for endotracheal intubation, length of hospital stay and hospital survival.

Overall there were 15 papers included in the meta-analysis. The addition of non-invasive positive pressure ventilation reduced the rate of endotracheal intubation (654 patients) (risk reduction 28% and 95% CI = 15–40%), length of hospital stay

(340 patients) (absolute reduction 4.57 days and 95% CI = 2.3–6.8 days) and in-hospital mortality rate (629 patients) (risk reduction 10% and 95% CI = 5–15%).

Subgroup analysis showed that these benefits with non-invasive positive pressure ventilation occurred only in patients with severe exacerbations (pH <7.3). With the use of non-invasive positive pressure ventilation in patients with severe exacerbations (pH <7.3 or hospital mortality rate >10% in the control group) there was a greater reduction in the hospital mortality rate (risk reduction 12% and 95% CI = 6–18%), rate of endotracheal intubation (risk reduction 34% and 95% CI = 22–46%) and length of hospital stay (absolute reduction 5.6 days and 95% CI = 3.7–7.5 days). There were only two trials enrolling 72 patients who did not have severe exacer-bations (pH >7.3) and non-invasive positive pressure ventilation demonstrated no benefit in hospital survival (risk reduction 2% and 95% CI = –8 to 12%), intubation (risk reduction 0% and 95% CI = –11 to 11%) or hospital stay (absolute reduction 0.8 days and 95% CI = –0.1 to 1.8 days).

In summary, this systematic review confirmed that non-invasive positive pressure ventilation confers advantages in patients with severe exacerbations of COPD that have respiratory failure with acidosis (pH <7.3), with reduced intubation rates, length of hospital stay and mortality rates. The beneficial effect with non-invasive positive pressure ventilation in severe exacerbations was not found with less severe COPD exacerbations (pH >7.3). Smaller numbers were studied in this latter group and further studies are needed. The GOLD recommendations for non-invasive positive pressure ventilation include an exacerbation of COPD with respiratory failure (pH <7.35 and $PaCO_2$ >6 kPa or >45 mmHg) and a respiratory rate >25 breaths/min |**1**|.

Cost-effectiveness of ward-based non-invasive ventilation for acute exacerbations of chronic obstructive pulmonary disease: economic analysis of randomized controlled trial

Plant PK, Owen JL, Parrott S, Elliott MW. *BMJ* 2003; **326**(7396): 956

BACKGROUND. Non-invasive positive pressure ventilation has been established as a clinically effective treatment for severe exacerbations of COPD with respiratory acidosis. This study evaluated the cost-effectiveness of ward-based non-invasive positive pressure ventilation for acute exacerbations of COPD.

INTERPRETATION. Non-invasive positive pressure ventilation was found to be cost-effective and improved the hospital mortality rate for patients admitted with an exacerbation of COPD with respiratory acidosis.

Comment

Non-invasive positive pressure ventilation is now a well-established treatment for exacerbations of COPD requiring hospital admission with respiratory acidosis. The aim of this study was to evaluate whether this was cost-effective, as expected from the improvements in reduced intubation rates, hospital days and mortality from previous studies.

Patients were randomized following admission to hospital with an exacerbation of COPD with mild to moderate respiratory acidosis (pH 7.25–7.35) and respiratory rate greater than 23 breaths/min to receive non-invasive positive pressure ventilation with standard therapy or standard therapy without non-invasive positive pressure ventilation. This was conducted within the hospital ward setting and not in either a high-dependency unit or an ICU. The non-invasive positive pressure ventilation used had an initial inspiratory pressure of 10 cmH$_2$O increasing to 20 cmH$_2$O and expiratory pressure of 5 cmH$_2$O, with a target duration of 24 h on the first day, 16 h on the second day, 8 h on the third day and then discontinuation. Oxygen was supplemented to maintain the patients' SaO$_2$ at 85–90%.

An economic analysis (incremental cost-effectiveness analysis) compared the costs of treatment with and without non-invasive positive pressure ventilation and the primary end-point was the hospital mortality rate.

There were 236 patients randomized. The non-invasive positive pressure ventilation group required less intubation (15% and SD = 7) compared with the group without non-invasive positive pressure ventilation (27% and SD = 8) (P <0.02). There was 10% (SD = 5.5) mortality in the non-invasive positive pressure ventilation arm and 20% (SD = 7.3) mortality in the control arm (P <0.05), but the length of hospital stay was similar at 10 days (P-value not significant).

The non-invasive positive pressure ventilation group had an overall reduction of costs of £49 362 ($78 741 or 73 109 Euros) predominantly through less use of ICUs. The incremental cost-effectiveness ratio was –£645 per death avoided (95% CI = –£2310 to £386). The authors estimated that a typical UK hospital serving 250 000 providing a non-invasive positive pressure ventilation service (estimated treating 56 patients per year with non-invasive positive pressure ventilation) avoids six deaths and three to nine admissions to an ICU per year, with an associated cost reduction of £12 351–53 078 per year.

In summary, non-invasive positive pressure ventilation given on the wards for exacerbations of COPD with respiratory acidosis (pH 7.25–7.35) reduced the need for intubation by 44% and halved the hospital mortality rate. Non-invasive positive pressure ventilation as predicted is cost-effective and the main cost saving is less use of intensive care facilities.

Randomized controlled trial of home-based care of patients with chronic obstructive pulmonary disease

Hermiz O, Comino E, Marks G, Daffurn K, Wilson S, Harris M. *BMJ* 2002; **325**(7370): 938

BACKGROUND. This randomized, controlled trial was set out to evaluate whether limited community-based care following hospital admission with exacerbations of COPD reduced subsequent admission to hospital.

INTERPRETATION. The brief intervention after acute care improved patients' knowledge of COPD, but failed to prevent subsequent presentation and readmission to hospital.

Comment

This study addressed the important problem of patients frequently being readmitted to hospital following an admission with an exacerbation of COPD (in 1996–1997 84% patients presenting to hospital were admitted and 34% re-presented within a 12-month period in this Australian study). The aim of the study was to evaluate the impact of limited home visiting by a community nurse on patients recently discharged from hospital with an exacerbation of COPD. The belief was that such an approach would improve patients' knowledge about the disease, improve their quality of life and reduce re-presentation to hospital.

Patients following admission to hospital with an exacerbation of COPD were randomized into an intervention arm versus usual care. The intervention arm involved a home visit by a community nurse within 1 week of hospital discharge. There was both verbal and written education on the disease. Advice was given about smoking cessation, management of activities of daily living and energy conservation, exercise, understanding and use of drugs, health maintenance and early recognition of signs that require medical intervention. In addition, if the nurses identified problems they referred patients to other services such as home care and their general practitioner (GP) was informed. There was a second home visit 1 month later and the nurses reviewed their progress and need for follow-up. Usual care comprised discharge to GP care with or without specialist follow-up, but there was no routine nurse follow-up. There was a baseline assessment and 3-month follow-up in both groups.

The main end-points studied were the frequency of re-presentation to hospital, changes in disease-specific health status (St George's Respiratory Questionnaire), knowledge and frequency of the use of GP, and nurse visits by 3 months post-intervention.

There were complete data on 67 patients in the intervention arm and 80 in the non-intervention arm. The mean age was 67 years in both arms of the study and 45% in the intervention arm and 39% in the control arm required the assistance of others to care for them. There was no assessment of lung function including FEV_1, but the assumption is that these patients had advanced COPD. The baseline of the two arms of the study was not significantly different.

In the intervention arm at 3 months the patients knew more about their disease, the role of vaccination and factors that prevented the condition worsening. Despite this only 54% knew the name of their disease in the intervention arm compared with 33% in the control arm ($P = 0.04$). In addition, 85% in the intervention arm knew when to seek help compared with 69% in the control arm ($P = 0.07$).

There was no significant difference in the number of visits to a GP in both arms of the study (90% visited their GP in the intervention arm with a mean number of 6.06 visits and 94% in the control arm visited their GP with a mean number of 5.54 visits).

There was no significant difference in the percentage that smoked or received vaccination (in the intervention arm 22% still smoked and only 72% received influenza vaccination compared with 33% that still smoked and 75% who received influenza vaccination in the control arm). There was no significant difference in health status or hospitalization at 3 months between the groups (24% hospitalized in the intervention arm and 18% in the control arm).

In summary, this study with nurse intervention following hospital admission improved patients' knowledge but had no impact on subsequent hospital admission at 3 months and had no impact on overall health status. It is likely that, to achieve efficacy, this nursing intervention should be supplemented with other services such as pulmonary rehabilitation, dietetics and occupational therapy, which may subsequently have a greater impact. In addition, interventions earlier in the disease may have greater impact.

Home hospitalization of exacerbated chronic obstructive pulmonary disease patients

Hernandez C, Casas A, Escarrabill J, *et al.*; CHRONIC Project. *Eur Respir J* 2003; **21**(1): 58–67

BACKGROUND. In order to facilitate early hospital discharge, programmes for facilitating hospital at home using respiratory specialist nurses have been developed. Studies to date have revealed that hospital at home in selected COPD patients is safe and cost-effective. The aim of this study was to assess whether home hospitalization would reduce emergency room relapses, improve health-related quality of life and improve patient self-management.

INTERPRETATION. The comprehensive home care intervention in selected COPD exacerbations appeared to be cost-effective and achieved better outcomes (at 8 weeks) at lower costs than conventional care. The better outcomes included lower rates of short-term relapses requiring emergency room admissions, improvement in health-related quality of life, a higher degree of patient satisfaction and an important positive impact on knowledge of the disease and patient self-management.

Comment

Due to the increasing shortage of medical beds newer methods have been devised for treating patients at home. This randomized, controlled trial evaluated the efficacy of home hospitalization compared with conventional care.

A total of 222 COPD patients were randomized to home care or conventional care. Patients were excluded if they had chest radiograph changes, acute confusion, an impaired level of consciousness, arterial pH <7.35, admission from a nursing home, the presence of neoplasia, poor social conditions, significant medical co-morbidities, illiteracy, no telephone at home or were not living in the healthcare area.

During home hospitalization a specialist nurse delivered integrated care with an 8-week follow-up period. An immediate or early discharge from hospital was encouraged. Such patients had tailored therapy and nursing support following discharge over an 8-week period (maximum of five home visits or telephone calls, which were unlimited). The first home visit was planned within 24 h of discharge. The nurses gave advice on medication, dietary advice and upper and lower limb skeletal muscle exercises. In the control arm there was no specialist nurse support either in hospital or in the community.

The main end-points in the study were emergency room relapses, heath-related quality of life (St George's Respiratory Questionnaire) and patient self-management.

A total of 222 COPD patients were randomized to home care (121 patients with mean $\pm$ SD = age 71 $\pm$ 10 years and mean FEV_1 at 8 weeks' follow-up 43% predicted) and conventional care (101 patients with mean age 70 $\pm$ 9 years and mean FEV_1 at 8 weeks' follow-up 41% predicted).

Sixty-eight per cent of patients in the home hospitalization group were discharged within 24 h compared with 38.6% ($P < 0.001$) in the control group. There was a mean number of home visits of 1.66 $\pm$ 1.03 over the 8-week period in the home hospitalization group and the mean number of telephone calls was 2.33 $\pm$ 2.05.

Home hospitalization over the 8-week period led to reduced emergency room visits (0.13 $\pm$ 0.43) compared with those in the conventional arm (0.31 $\pm$ 0.62) ($P = 0.01$) and improved health-related quality of life (St George's Respiratory Questionnaire) (−6.9 versus −2.4) (a four-point reduction is a clinically significant improvement) ($P = 0.05$).

At 8 weeks a greater percentage had a better knowledge of the disease (58 versus 27%) ($P < 0.01$), better compliance on inhalation technique (81 versus 48%) ($P < 0.001$) and rehabilitation at home (51 versus 21%) ($P < 0.01$).

The costs with home hospitalization were 62% of the costs of conventional care (1255 Euros in the home hospitalization group versus 2033 Euros in the control group) ($P = 0.003$) essentially due to fewer days of in-patient hospitalization (mean $\pm$ SD = 1.7 $\pm$ 2.3 days) compared with those with conventional care (4.2 $\pm$ 4.1 days) ($P < 0.001$).

However, at 8 weeks there was no significant difference in mortality (4.1% in the home hospitalization group and 6.9% in the control group) and there was no significant difference in the percentage of in-patient hospital admissions (20% in the home hospitalization group and 27.7% in the control group).

In summary, the comprehensive home care intervention in selected COPD exacerbations appeared to be cost-effective and achieved better outcomes (at 8 weeks) at lower costs than conventional care. The better outcomes included lower rates of short-term relapses requiring emergency room admissions, improvement in health-related quality of life, a higher degree of patient satisfaction and an important positive impact on knowledge of the disease and on patient self-management. However, this home-based support is only applicable for COPD exacerbations that can be safely treated at home after careful clinical assessment. In addition, respiratory nurse specialists with medical back-up, close liaison with community physicians/GPs and extra equipment, for example nebulizers, for treating patients at home needs to be in place and there is a need for good social support at home.

References

1. Global Initiative for Chronic Obstructive Lung Disease. *Global Strategy for the Diagnosis, Management and Prevention of Chronic Obstructive Pulmonary Disease.* National Heart, Lung and Blood Institute (NHLBI)/World Health Organisation workshop report. Bethesda, NHLBI, April 2001; update of management sections, available on-line at www.goldcopd.com, accessed 1 July 2003.

2. Niewoehner DE, Erbland ML, Deupree RH, Collins D, Gross NJ, Light RW, Anderson P, Morgan NA, for the Department of Veterans Affairs Cooperative Study Group. Effect of systemic glucocorticoids on exacerbations of COPD. *N Engl J Med* 1999; **340**: 1941–7.

3. Davies L, Angus RM, Calverley PM. Oral corticosteroids admitted to hospital with exacerbations of COPD: a prospective randomised controlled trial. *Lancet* 1999; **354**: 456–60.

Overall conclusion

The 25 papers selected for this section have made important contributions to the management of patients with COPD. Chapter 5 on pharmacological treatments for stable COPD has six key papers. Inhaled corticosteroids did not attenuate the decline in FEV_1, but attenuated the decline in health status and reduced the number of exacerbations in patients with an FEV_1 <50% predicted. Withdrawal of inhaled corticosteroids led to a more rapid onset and higher recurrence rate of exacerbations and a significant deterioration in aspects of health-related quality of life over a 6-month period. If long-term treatment is advocated the benefits should outweigh the side effects. The GOLD guidelines currently recommend long-term treatment with inhaled corticosteroids for patients with COPD with an FEV_1 <50% predicted with frequent exacerbations.

There were two 1-year studies that compared combination therapy (a long-acting β_2 agonist combined with an inhaled corticosteroid) with monotherapy with the two agents and placebo in patients with moderate and severe COPD. Combination therapy led to improved symptoms, improved FEV_1, reduced exacerbation frequency and a trend for improvement in health status compared with placebo. In addition, combination therapy improved the symptoms of breathlessness and FEV_1 compared with monotherapy (long-acting β_2 agonist or inhaled corticosteroid).

The next study compared 6 months' treatment with the long-acting anticholinergic tiotropium with the long-acting β_2 agonist salmeterol and placebo in patients with moderate and severe COPD. Compared with placebo, tiotropium led to improved symptoms, improved FEV_1, reduced exacerbations and improved health-related quality of life. Further studies are needed in order to determine whether there would be added efficacy with combination treatments with long-acting β_2 agonists and inhaled corticosteroids.

The final paper in Chapter 5 assessed the anti-inflammatory response with the phosphodiesterase inhibitor cilomilast. This agent is a potential alternative anti-inflammatory to inhaled corticosteroids, but large, multicentred studies are needed in order to assess its clinical efficacy and how it compares with inhaled corticosteroids.

Chapter 6 was on oxygen therapy. The first paper confirmed that oxygen supplementation before or after submaximal exercise derived no physiological or symptomatic benefit in patients with severe COPD with oxygen desaturation on exercise. The next paper confirmed that combination treatment with medroxyprogesterone acetate and acetazolamide could effectively improve minute ventilation and improve daytime blood gases and nocturnal oxygenation. Long-term studies are needed to assess its tolerability and whether these agents can delay the need for long-term oxygen therapy and improve outcomes. The final paper in Chapter 6 was a 3-month study that confirmed that pulsed nitric oxide along with long-term oxygen therapy was safe and improved pulmonary haemodynamics. Long-term studies are needed.

Chapter 7 was on pulmonary rehabilitation and four papers were included. Pulmonary rehabilitation can improve exercise capacity and breathlessness and lower extremity training was an important component. The benefits of rehabilitation tend to wane over a period of 1–2 years and there is therefore a need for further research on how to maintain the benefits with rehabilitation. The next paper evaluated the efficacy of a limited 1-year maintenance rehabilitation programme following 2 months' formal pulmonary rehabilitation. There were modest benefits only with maintenance of exercise tolerance during the 1-year limited programme and the benefits waned when rehabilitation stopped. Further work is needed in order to establish how best to maintain the benefits long term with rehabilitation. The next paper found that proportional assisted ventilation over a 6-week period was useful in patients with severe COPD and allowed greater training intensities and maximum exercise capacity. Larger studies are needed to establish its role. The final paper demonstrated that carbohydrate supplementation when universally prescribed did not enhance the rehabilitation of patients with COPD, although in subgroup analysis patients that had a normal body mass index benefited from carbohydrate supplementation. Larger studies are needed to establish the benefits of rehabilitation with nutritional support.

Chapter 8 included papers on lung volume reduction surgery and transplantation. These papers on lung volume reduction surgery have helped guide the clinician as to whom should be considered for lung volume reduction surgery. Prior to consideration for lung volume reduction surgery patients should have optimization of their medical therapy, be non-smoking and have undergone pulmonary rehabilitation. Lung volume reduction surgery is not without risk and there has been an increased mortality particularly in patients with an FEV$_1$ ≤20% predicted and either homogeneous emphysema on computed tomography scanning or a carbon monoxide gas transfer ≤20% predicted and in patients with diffuse emphysema or emphysema predominantly in the lower lobes with an exercise capacity >25 W for women and >40 W for men.

The patients thought to benefit most are patients with heterogeneous predominant upper lobe emphysema, patients with an FEV$_1$ 21–45% predicted, evidence of hyperinflated lung fields with an elevated total lung capacity ≥100% predicted and residual volume ≥150% predicted in patients without respiratory failure. These selected patients can have long-term functional improvements in exercise tolerance, have improved health-related quality of life and less mortality. Along with the potential benefits with surgery, patients should be aware of the potential morbidity and mortality from lung volume reduction surgery (5–7% 90-day mortality). Finally, lung volume reduction surgery is costly, at least over a 3-year period. However, the procedure may be cost-effective if the benefits with lung volume reduction surgery can be maintained over a longer time such as 5–10 years, but this requires long-term prospective follow-up.

Lung transplantation can improve both functional capacity and health-related quality of life although its impact on survival is less clear. In view of this, patients have to be selected very carefully. Patients should have severe irreversible airflow obstruction with preference given to patients that have respiratory failure that requires long-term oxygen therapy as such patients have the poorest prognosis. Currently the age limits for single lung transplantation are <65 years and <60 years for bilateral lung transplantation.

Lung transplantation, although it can significantly improve exercise capacity and improve quality of life, is associated with significant morbidity and mortality. The morbidity associated with transplantation relates to lifelong immunosuppression, invasive investigations and the treatment of complications such as infection and lung rejection. There is an initial high mortality in the first 30 days (between 5 and 15%) and by 5 years it is around 40–50%. Therefore, patients that are selected should have advanced COPD with an expected poor prognosis with life expectancy <2 years. There continues to be a drive to improve both morbidity and mortality with lung transplantation, which will be helped by newer and more effective immunosuppressive agents and the prompt treatment of both infection and rejection. In light of the lack of donor organs, there has been increased interest in single lung transplantation. The study reviewed, however, revealed that bilateral lung transplantation had a superior 5-year survival compared with single lung transplants without any increase in hospital stay, ICU stay or mechanical ventilation. Bilateral lung transplantation would seem the preferred option but the lack of donor organs is likely to hinder this.

Chapter 9 is on exacerbations of COPD and explores the use of methylxanthines, systemic corticosteroids and non-invasive positive pressure ventilation and explores the treatment of COPD at home. There is currently no evidence base for the use of methylxanthines for exacerbations of COPD, but there were a small number of studies with few patients. Further studies are needed to assess their role in severe exacerbations.

Oral corticosteroids were found to be beneficial for community exacerbations in patients with severe COPD in improving breathlessness and FEV_1 and reducing relapse rates. This study would support the GOLD guidelines recommendation that patients managed as outpatients should be treated with a 10-day course of oral corticosteroids in patients with COPD with a baseline FEV_1 <50% predicted. The next study was a systematic review of systemic corticosteroids in exacerbations of COPD and confirmed that systemic steroids improved lung function quicker and were associated with a shorter length of hospital stay and had reduced relapse rates in patients with severe COPD that required hospital admission. This study would support the GOLD guidelines recommendation that patients managed as inpatients should be treated with a 10–14-day course of oral corticosteroids.

Non-invasive positive pressure ventilation confers advantages in patients with severe exacerbations of COPD that have respiratory failure with acidosis pH <7.35, with reduced intubation rates, length of hospital stay and mortality rates and is cost-effective. The GOLD recommendations for non-invasive positive pressure ventilation include an exacerbation of COPD with respiratory failure (pH <7.35 and $PaCO_2$ >6 kPa or >45 mmHg) and a respiratory rate >25 breaths/min.

The penultimate paper in Chapter 9 explored the benefits of community nurse follow-up following an exacerbation of COPD requiring hospital admission. This improved the patient's knowledge of COPD, but had no impact on subsequent hospital admission or overall health status at 3 months. The final study investigated treating COPD exacerbations at home with a hospital-supported discharge. The hospital-supported discharge led to improved outcomes at 8 weeks and at lower costs than conventional care. The better outcomes included lower rates of short-term relapses requiring emergency room admissions, improvement in health-related quality of life, a higher degree of patient satisfaction and an important positive impact on knowledge of the disease and on patient self-management. However, this home-based support is only applicable for COPD exacerbations that can be safely treated at home after careful clinical assessment. In addition, respiratory nurse specialists with medical back-up, close liaison with community physicians/GPs and extra equipment, for example nebulizers, for treating patients at home need to be in place and there is a need for good social support at home.

Part III

Pulmonary fibrosis

Pulmonary fibrosis

J SIMPSON

Introduction

Two general developments in the last few decades have had an enormous impact on the understanding of diffuse parenchymal lung diseases (DPLDs) (formerly referred to as interstitial lung diseases or ILDs). The first concerned the application of high-resolution computed tomography (HRCT) and other new imaging techniques to the study of DPLD, allowing significant conclusions to be drawn about the underlying disease processes and their prognoses [1]. The second and more recent major development concerned the histological reclassification of the idiopathic interstitial pneumonias (IIPs) in 1998 [2,3]. The importance of the reclassification lies in the recognition that a heterogeneous group of DPLDs could be carefully grouped as conditions with relatively distinct clinical characteristics, prognoses and responses to treatment. This is particularly relevant to idiopathic pulmonary fibrosis (IPF), which has a particularly poor prognosis (median survival typically being around 3 years) [4]. The majority of this section focuses on the renewed interest in IPF, which should in general be considered a progressive disease with no effective treatment at the present time other than successful lung transplantation. However, this section was written at a time of anticipation among physicians who manage IPF, as the results of a large, multicentre, randomized, controlled trial of interferon-γ_{1b} (IFN-γ_{1b}) for IPF were due to be published in January 2004. The considerable interest stems from a previous, small report describing an effect of IFN-γ_{1b} in IPF [5]. Preliminary reports from the multicentre trial have been discussed at international meetings, but in the absence of a full publication at the time of writing this will not be discussed further. Instead the reader is advised to watch out for the full publication.

For the reasons described above, recent years have seen renewed interest in the DPLDs and this is reflected in the publication of many important papers adding to the understanding of these interesting conditions. Unfortunately, one of the by-products of the reclassification of the IIPs has been a confusing and often seemingly impenetrable terminology, which seems to be laid down faster than collagen itself. This language labyrinth unfortunately justifies a brief section on its own. If you are familiar with the reclassification I strongly suggest you skip the following few paragraphs: however, if you are not, get a strong cup of coffee and come back in a minute.

Figure III.1 outlines the modern classification of DPLD. Please note that, when considering the second line of Fig. III.1, this section will deal with examples from the first box (drug-induced DPLD, e.g. amiodarone lung and DPLD associated with connective tissue disease, e.g. rheumatoid lung) and the third box (e.g. sarcoidosis and hypersensitivity pneumonitis). However, the greatest emphasis will be on the IIPs, the group of diseases reclassified histologically in 1998. It is in some ways frustrating that the term IIP was coined and it should be noted that there is no clear evidence to support an infective aetiology for these conditions: the term pneumonia is being used in its strictest pathological sense rather than in the common use of the term implying infection. Of the IIPs IPF is the commonest and responsible for the highest mortality and morbidity.

A brief outline of the IIPs to be covered will be provided below, with particular emphasis on IPF and the importance of the pathological term usual interstitial pneumonia (UIP), followed by a short list of synonyms.

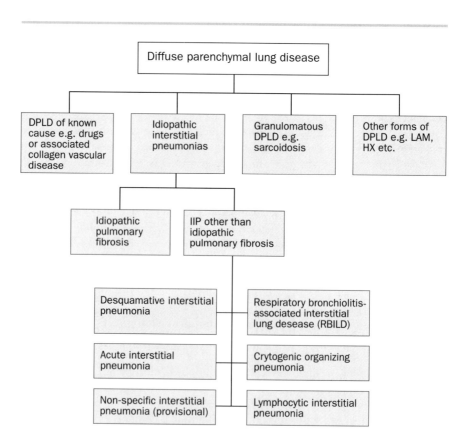

Fig. III.1 Modern classification of diffuse parenchymal lung diseases, with particular emphasis on the idiopathic interstitial pneumonias. LAM, lymphangioleiomyomatosis; HX, histiocytosis X. Source: Adapted from [3].

1. IIPs: these are ILDs for which no cause can be identified (i.e. drugs, connective tissue diseases and relevant environmental or occupational exposures must be rigorously excluded in order to diagnose an IIP) that can be classified according to clinical and histological appearances.

2. IPF (which was previously called cryptogenic fibrosing alveolitis or CFA in the UK): this is the archetypal IIP. Recent diagnostic criteria for IPF have been published in a joint statement from the American Thoracic Society and European Respiratory Society |4| and these are referred to at intervals in the section. IPF is generally a disease of the elderly, occurring more commonly in men and with an appalling prognosis (median survival typically being 3 years). IPF is invariably associated with a histological pattern called UIP. This is a common source of confusion and it is important to be aware that (i) while all cases of IPF have UIP on lung biopsy, UIP need not equal IPF because UIP may be associated with asbestosis, connective tissue diseases such as rheumatoid disease, etc. Thus only *idiopathic* UIP is diagnostic of IPF, emphasizing the initial requirement for constructive dialogue between clinician and pathologist. (ii) the important converse of this is that the only IIP to have the histological features of UIP is IPF and (iii) UIP is one of only two histological patterns among the IIPs which does not give its name to the associated clinical diagnosis (the other exception concerns the rare condition acute interstitial pneumonia). That is, an IIP with histology showing UIP gives a clinical diagnosis of IPF, an IIP with histology showing non-specific interstitial pneumonia 'NSIP' gives a clinical diagnosis of idiopathic NSIP, an IIP with histology showing desquamative interstitial pneumonia 'DIP' gives a clinical diagnosis of idiopathic DIP, etc. A further point to make about IPF is that, prior to reclassification, the term IPF (or CFA) usually, with the benefit of hindsight, contained the other IIPs shown in Fig. III.1. Therefore, if one reads a pre-1998 paper on 'IPF' the first question must be 'is this really IPF or are there other IIPs (which have a better outlook than true IPF) in this cohort?'

3. NSIP: NSIP is a histological pattern and is sometimes divided into cellular and fibrotic NSIP. It should be noted that the histological appearances of NSIP can be found in a variety of conditions including connective tissue diseases. However, when we talk about NSIP in this section it should be assumed that we are referring to idiopathic NSIP (which is an IIP, as shown in Fig. III.1) unless it is specifically stated that the NSIP is associated with a connective tissue disease. Clinically, idiopathic NSIP may mimic IPF, but it is important to discriminate between the two because NSIP in general has a much better prognosis (this is particularly true of cellular NSIP).

4. DIP: DIP is a distinctive histological pattern and gives its name to the clinical diagnosis of idiopathic DIP. This IIP has a particularly good prognosis and response to treatment.

5. Hierarchy of histological patterns in IIP: it is increasingly recognized that more than one histological IIP may be present in the lung at any time |6|. It is generally

accepted that any evidence of UIP overrides any other pathology noted. For example, if a patient with no evidence of connective tissue disease, relevant environmental exposure or relevant drugs goes to lung biopsy and two simultaneous biopsies are taken, one showing NSIP and the other UIP, then UIP is the definitive pathological diagnosis as the subsequent course of the disease is much more likely to follow that of IPF.

Synonyms

Here the preferred terms are given first: DPLD/ILD, IPF/CFA and hypersensitivity pneumonitis/extrinsic allergic alveolitis.

Overview of the section

The aim of this section is to highlight recent papers relating to a variety of DPLDs. The main problems in this field traditionally relate to establishing diagnosis, difficulties in predicting prognosis and the absence of effective treatments (particularly for IPF). Therefore, an attempt has been made to concentrate on these aspects. The section includes papers relating to sarcoidosis and hypersensitivity pneumonitis, but the main emphasis is on the IIPs and particularly IPF given the proliferation of interest in this inexorable, progressive condition for which no ideal treatment exists. This section is therefore divided into three chapters covering the genetics of fibrotic lung disease, the IIPs with particular emphasis on IPF and miscellaneous DPLDs.

It is worth noting that many fewer randomized, controlled trials will be found in this section than in others. Because of the reclassification of the IIPs on histopathological grounds, the recent landmark studies of IPF have by necessity been retrospective analyses of databases assembled prospectively in the last 20 years (i.e. authors have gone back and picked out all lung biopsies reclassified as IPF or NSIP and then looked at the available clinical data accumulated for those patients). Only original articles have been selected for this section, but the reader should be aware that several excellent overviews of DPLDs have been published recently [3,4,7].

How to take key messages from this section

The section is written so that the key messages can be extracted by reading only the Background and Interpretation sections. The Comment section for each paper is designed for the reader who would like more detailed information without necessarily going to the original paper. The Comment sections therefore generally start with an outline of the methods used followed by a more detailed description of the results and then an attempt to outline the strengths and potential limitations of each study before ending with a short conclusion. It should be noted that the papers in this section were specifically chosen because of their significant contribution to the field and the discussion of methodological limitations is simply designed to provide a feel for how broadly the results can be generalized to other clinical settings.

References

1. Ellis SM, Hansell DM. Idiopathic interstitial pneumonias: imaging–pathology correlation. *Eur Radiol* 2002; **12**: 610–26.

2. Katzenstein ALA, Myers JL. Idiopathic pulmonary fibrosis. Clinical relevance of pathologic classification. *Am J Respir Crit Care Med* 1998; **157**: 1301–15.

3. American Thoracic Society and European Respiratory Society. American Thoracic Society/European Respiratory Society international multidisciplinary consensus classification of the idiopathic interstitial pneumonias. *Am J Respir Crit Care Med* 2002; **165**: 277–304.

4. American Thoracic Society. Idiopathic pulmonary fibrosis: diagnosis and treatment. International Consensus Statement. *Am J Respir Crit Care Med* 2000; **161**: 646–64.

5. Ziesche R, Hofbauer W, Wittmann K, Petkov V, Block LH. A preliminary study of long-term treatment with interferon gamma-1b and low-dose prednisolone in patients with idiopathic pulmonary fibrosis. *N Engl J Med* 1999; **341**: 1264–9.

6. Flaherty KR, Travis WD, Colby TV, Toews GB, Kazerooni EA, Gross BH, Jain A, Strawderman III RL, Flint A, Lynch III JP, Martinez FJ. Histopathologic variability in usual and nonspecific interstitial pneumonias. *Am J Respir Crit Care Med* 2001; **164**: 1722–7.

7. American Thoracic Society. Statement on sarcoidosis. *Am J Respir Crit Care Med* 1999; **160**: 736–55.

10

Genetics of fibrotic lung disease

Introduction

It is widely accepted that most diffuse parenchymal lung diseases (DPLDs) of unknown aetiology are the product of exposure to (unidentified) environmental influences in a genetically susceptible host. This has led to the search for polymorphisms in genes encoding proteins of critical importance to inflammation and fibrogenesis, particularly in conditions such as sarcoidosis and idiopathic pulmonary fibrosis (IPF). This is a developing field that is limited in part by the fact that DPLDs are relatively rare and by the difficulties in dissecting out 'clean' and distinctive disease phenotypes in conditions such as IPF (which can behave quite differently in individual patients with regard to survival, high-resolution computed tomography [HRCT] appearances, etc., thereby suggesting the existence of distinct clinical phenotypes requiring better definition). This chapter begins with an extremely elegant dissection of a genetic polymorphism in Löfgren's syndrome, which is related to sarcoidosis |**1**|. The beauty of this paper lies in the extremely well-defined phenotype studied. Attention then turns to some of the polymorphisms showing promise in attempts to dissect out the pathogenesis of IPF.

C-C chemokine receptor 2 and sarcoidosis. Association with Löfgren's syndrome
Spagnolo P, Renzoni EA, Wells AU, *et al. Am J Respir Crit Care Med* 2003; **168**: 1162–6

BACKGROUND. The mechanisms regulating the pathogenesis of sarcoidosis remain unclear. Associations with human leukocyte antigen (HLA) haplotypes argue for a genetic predisposition. It seems logical that the genetic component may result in aberrant immune responses to one or more (as yet unidentified) environmental antigens. For this reason much interest has focused on genes regulating the function of monocytes and T lymphocytes. One such gene encodes C-C chemokine receptor 2 (*CCR2*), which plays a key role in the recruitment of monocytes, dendritic cells and memory T cells. This study aimed to determine whether polymorphisms in the *CCR2* gene were associated with sarcoidosis.

INTERPRETATION. Five single nucleotide polymorphisms (SNPs) in the *CCR2* gene were significantly associated with Löfgren's syndrome (the constellation of fever, bihilar lymphadenopathy, erythema nodosum and polyarthralgia) in a Dutch Caucasian population. Furthermore, a single haplotype containing four of these SNPs was identified, the frequency of which was significantly and independently associated with Löfgren's syndrome, but not with other forms of sarcoidosis. The approach taken in this study has far-reaching implications for the understanding of Löfgren's syndrome and for unravelling mechanisms of pathogenesis in other inflammatory disorders.

Comment

The population studied comprised 137 unrelated white Dutch patients with sarcoidosis, with 167 controls being drawn from donors attending the Dutch Blood Transfusion Service. The patients were subdivided into 47 patients with Löfgren's syndrome and 90 patients with histologically proven sarcoidosis. The study made use of the recent identification of eight discrete SNPs in the *CCR2* gene. Using sequence-specific primers to perform polymerase chain reactions (PCR) they were able to detect whether polymorphisms were present at each of the eight relevant alleles. Five polymorphisms in the *CCR2* gene were found with significantly higher frequency in Löfgren's syndrome than in the controls or in the 90 patients with forms of sarcoidosis other than Löfgren's syndrome. Furthermore, the eight polymorphisms in the *CCR2* gene gave rise to nine identifiable haplotypes and, interestingly, four of the allelic polymorphisms associated with Löfgren's syndrome were unique to one specific haplotype. Not surprisingly, this haplotype was strongly associated with Löfgren's syndrome, but not with other forms of sarcoidosis (Table 10.1). When assessing Table 10.1, note that haplotype 1 is the 'native' haplotype, while haplotype 2 contains the four polymorphisms, which are identified at positions −6572 (which is in the promoter region of the gene), 3000 (in exon 2), 3547 (3′ untranslated region) and 4385 (3′ untranslated region). The HLA haplotype DRB1*0301–DQB1*0201 was also associated with Löfgren's syndrome, but when this haplotype was corrected for, carriage of CCR2 haplotype 2 retained a significant association with Löfgren's syndrome. The presence of both haplotypes (CCR2 haplotype 2 and the DRB1*0301–DQB1*0201 haplotype) was found in 82% of patients with Löfgren's syndrome, but only 36% of controls and 25% of patients with sarcoidosis other than Löfgren's syndrome.

   This is an extremely elegant study providing new insights into Löfgren's syndrome, but also demonstrating beautifully the potential of hypothesis-driven identification of genetic polymorphisms in inflammatory disease. It should be noted that five out of the 47 patients with Löfgren's syndrome had neither CCR2 haplotype 2 nor the DRB1*0301–DQB1*0201 haplotyope, but at a recent international conference the authors suggested they have data implicating a third haplotype in Löfgren's syndrome, which, in combination with the other two, can account for 100% of cases of the disease. This would be an incredible landmark, allowing the authors to hone in on the mechanisms driving the pathogenesis of Löfgren's syndrome. The publication of these data is awaited with enormous interest.

   The authors pointed out that none of the polymorphisms on CCR2 haplotype 2 can be directly implicated, either alone or in combination, in the pathogenesis of

Table 10.1 C-C chemokine receptor 2 haplotype carriage frequencies in Löfgren's syndrome, non-Löfgren sarcoidosis, and control subjects

Haplotype	SNPs' position								Löfgren (n = 47)	Non-Löfgren sarcoidosis (n = 90)	Control subjects (n = 167)
	-6928	-6752	190	3000	3547	3610	3671	4385			
1	G	G	G	G	C	G	C	A	27 (57%)	62 (69%)	122 (73%)
2	G	A	G	A	T	A	C	T	35 (74%)*†	34 (38%)	63 (38%)
3	G	G	G	G	C	G	G	A	12 (26%)	18 (20%)	42 (25%)
4	T	G	G	G	C	A	C	A	3 (6%)	10 (11%)	17 (10%)
5	G	G	A	G	C	G	C	A	4 (9%)	9 (10%)	15 (9%)
6	T	G	G	G	C	G	C	A	2 (4%)	6 (7%)	7 (4%)
7	G	G	A	G	C	A	C	A	3 (6%)	2 (2%)	5 (3%)
8	G	G	G	G	C	G	G	A	1 (2%)	3 (3%)	5 (3%)
9	T	G	G	G	C	G	G	A	0	3 (3%)	3 (2%)

Numbers represent haplotype carriage frequencies with percentages in parentheses. SNPs, single nucleotide polymorphisms.
* P <0.0001 Löfgren vs. non-Löfgren sarcoidosis, polytomous logistic regression; † P <0.0001 Löfgren vs. control subjects, polytomous logistic regression.
Source: Spagnolo et al. (2003).

Löfgren's syndrome at the present time. They may be no more than markers for unidentified polymorphisms in the *CCR2* gene or for polymorphisms on adjacent genes through linkage disequilibrium. Nevertheless, the obvious starting point in investigating the mechanism is to assess the effect of these polymorphisms on the function of the CCR2 molecule. The temptation is to postulate that aberrant CCR2 production results in inappropriate recruitment of monocytes in response to specific infection, which in turn leads to inappropriate clearance of infection and inappropriate interaction with host immune cells. It should be noted that no functional data are presented in the study being discussed.

A considerable strength of the study is that Löfgren's syndrome has a distinctive and well-defined phenotype. It is less easy to define other distinct phenotypes across the spectrum of sarcoidosis. The inference from this is that the 'sarcoidosis other than Löfgren's syndrome' group contains genetically and phenotypically distinct subgroups that cannot be teased out at present. It is a pity that this group was not broken down further in any way in this study, for example to separate out those with exclusively pulmonary sarcoidosis from those with extrapulmonary manifestations. However, the study was probably too small to make these further distinctions. It will also be very interesting to determine whether these genetic associations are conserved in non-Caucasian patients with Löfgren's syndrome, why some patients carrying these polymorphisms do not go on to develop clinical Löfgren's syndrome and whether there are differences among patients whose Löfgren's syndrome persists and those in whom there is spontaneous remission.

In summary, this was an immensely important study paving the way for a full dissection of the pathogenesis of Löfgren's syndrome. The challenge ahead is to pick out distinctive phenotypes in more severe sarcoidosis and identify candidate disease-associated genes in which to screen for polymorphisms.

Transforming growth factor-β_1 gene polymorphisms are associated with disease progression in idiopathic pulmonary fibrosis

Xaubet A, Marin-Arguedas A, Lario S *et al. Am J Respir Crit Care Med* 2003; **168**: 431–5

BACKGROUND. Transforming growth factor-β_1 (*TGF-β_1*) has a variety of pro-fibrotic properties, is found in high concentrations in the lungs of patients with IPF and can induce profound fibrosis in the lungs of experimental animals |2,3|. For these reasons the *TGF-β_1* gene is a logical candidate in which to explore the frequency and effects of genetic polymorphisms in patients with IPF. This study therefore aimed to determine the frequency of two known *TGF-β_1* gene polymorphisms among patients with IPF and the influence of these on disease progression.

INTERPRETATION. An SNP in exon 1 of the *TGF-β_1* gene was associated with a decline in the alveolar–arterial oxygen tension difference ($P(A–a)O_2$) in IPF. This observation needs to be confirmed in larger series.

Comment

This study used standard techniques (PCR and analysis of restriction fragment length polymorphisms) to identify polymorphisms at two distinct loci in exon 1 of the $TGF\text{-}\beta_1$ gene. In the first, a T $\rightarrow$ C substitution at position 869 resulted in a leucine to proline change in codon 10, while in the second a G $\rightarrow$ C substitution at position 915 resulted in an arginine to proline change in codon 25. The allelic frequencies were determined in 128 unrelated patients with IPF and in 140 unrelated controls (73 cadaveric renal allograft donors and 67 'healthy subjects'). The diagnosis of IPF was established in keeping with American Thoracic Society and European Respiratory Society criteria, being confirmed by lung biopsy in 60 out of 128 patients (no HRCT data were provided). The patients had a baseline forced vital capacity (FVC) of 69% predicted and diffusing capacity for carbon monoxide ($D_{L_{CO}}$) of 56% predicted. Pulmonary function tests and $P(A\text{--}a)O_2$ were followed serially in 110 patients (but not in surviving controls) over a mean of 30 months.

No differences in genotypic or allelic frequencies were noted for the G $\rightarrow$ C substitution at position 915 when comparing patients and controls. Similarly, in the patient group the substitution did not predict for any change in disease progression. However, the T $\rightarrow$ C substitution at position 869 proved more interesting. Once again the genotypic and allelic frequencies were similar in the patients and controls (allelic frequencies showed codon 10 to contain leucine in 58% of the controls and 59% of the patients, with proline in 42% of the controls and 41% of the patients). However, among the patients with IPF the presence of proline at codon 10 was associated with a significant deterioration in $P(A\text{--}a)O_2$ (Table 10.2).

This is a fascinating result, providing tantalizing evidence that genetic predictors of disease progression can be defined and reinforcing the central position for TGF-β_1 in the pathogenesis of IPF. It adds TGF-β_1 to a list of important genes with polymorphisms associated with IPF [4,5], combinations of which have been associated with disease progression [6]. However, a number of cautions are required in interpreting

Table 10.2 Changes in pulmonary function tests between carriers and non-carriers of Pro allele in codon 10 during follow-up study

	Pro⁺	Pro⁻	P-value
Patients with IPF, n	70	40	
FVC, %	−0.60 ± 1.36*	−0.11 ± 1.43	0.053
$D_{L_{CO}}$, %	−1.05 ± 2.49*	−0.76 ± 1.37	n.s.
$P(A\text{--}a)O_2$ mmHg	0.42 ± 0.68†	−0.17 ± 0.81	0.002

FVC, forced vital capacity; $D_{L_{CO}}$, diffusion capacity of the lung for carbon monoxide; n.s., not significant.
* Values are expressed as the percentage of change in absolute values with respect to initial assessment divided by the follow-up in months.
† Values are expressed as the difference in pressure (mmHg) at the initial assessment and the end of the follow-up, divided by the follow-up in months.
Source: Xaubet et al. (2003)

the data, principal among which are two themes central to most studies of this type. These relate to the small size of the study and to the difficulties in ascertaining distinct phenotypes within IPF, given that this disease is characterized histologically and at HRCT by temporal and spatial heterogeneity and that the clinical course may vary considerably from one patient to another. Given these considerations it would have been useful to know the diagnostic criteria for the 68 patients without lung biopsies. The issue of phenotypic heterogeneity in IPF poses a significant problem to future studies of this kind. As an aside, it is interesting that 2003 also saw the publication of a paper demonstrating that a polymorphism in the promoter region of the plasminogen activator inhibitor type-1 gene was associated with well-characterized non-specific interstitial pneumonia but not IPF [7].

Another issue of importance in the study by Xaubet et al. relates to the age of the controls. The authors concluded that the polymorphism at position 869 was not associated with the risk of development of IPF because the allelic frequencies were similar in the patients and controls, but it should be noted that the average age of the controls was around 34 years and clearly some 34 year olds could still go on to develop IPF. It is also plausible that smoking may interact with the TGF-β_1 polymorphism to influence disease progression, but no smoking data were provided. Finally, the intriguing results from this study infer that the polymorphism at position 869 results in a functional change in the TGF-β_1 molecule. One of the challenges ahead would appear to be the isolation of the mutant TGF-β_1 molecule and subsequent analysis of its pro-fibrotic effects. In the meantime it would be useful to know the distribution and concentration of TGF-β_1 in the lungs of patients with the mutant allele who have IPF, but no data on this subject have yet been provided. These are awaited with interest.

Overall, the conclusion must be that this study suggests a fascinating potential for genetic variants of TGF-β_1 to influence disease progression in IPF. However, this must be confirmed in larger studies in which the phenotypic characteristics of patients must be rigorously defined and which have the power to investigate the suspected critical interplay between multiple candidate genes in the pathogenesis of IPF.

References

1. American Thoracic Society. Statement on sarcoidosis. *Am J Respir Crit Care Med* 1999; **160**: 736–55.
2. Khalil N, Parekh TV, O'Connor R, Antman N, Kepron W, Yehaulaeshet T, Xu YD, Gold LI. Regulation of the effects of TGF-beta 1 by activation of latent TGF-beta 1 and differential expression of TGF-beta receptors (T beta R-I and T beta R-II) in idiopathic pulmonary fibrosis. *Thorax* 2001; **56**: 907–15.

3. Sime PJ, Xing Z, Graham FL, Csaky KG, Gauldie J. Adenovector-mediated gene transfer of active transforming growth factor-beta 1 induces prolonged severe fibrosis in rat lung. *J Clin Invest* 1997; **100**: 768–77.

4. Whyte M, Hubbard R, Meliconi R, Whidborne M, Eaton V, Bingle C, Timms J, Duff G, Facchini A, Pacilli A, Fabbri M, Hall I, Britton J, Johnston I, Di Giovine F. Increased risk of fibrosing alveolitis associated with interleukin-1 receptor antagonist and tumor necrosis factor-α gene polymorphisms. *Am J Respir Crit Care Med* 2000; **162**: 755–8.

5. Zorzetto M, Ferrarotti I, Trisolini R, Agli LL, Scabini R, Novo M, De Silvestri A, Patelli M, Martinetti M, Cuccia MC, Poletti V, Pozzi E, Luisetti M. Complement receptor 1 gene polymorphisms are associated with idiopathic pulmonary fibrosis. *Am J Respir Crit Care Med* 2003; **168**: 330–4.

6. Pantelidis P, Fanning GC, Wells AU, Wellsh KI, Du Bois RM. Analysis of tumor necrosis factor-α, lymphotoxin-α, tumor necrosis factor receptor II, and interleukin-6 polymorphisms in patients with idiopathic pulmonary fibrosis. *Am J Respir Crit Care Med* 2001; **163**: 1432–6.

7. Kim KK, Flaherty KR, Long Q, Hattori N, Sisson TH, Colby TV, Travis WD, Martinez FJ, Murray S, Simon RH. A plasminogen activator inhibitor-1 polymorphism and idiopathic interstitial pneumonia. *Mol Med* 2003; **9**: 52–6.

11

Idiopathic interstitial pneumonias with particular emphasis on idiopathic pulmonary fibrosis

Introduction

The reclassification of the idiopathic interstitial pneumonias (IIPs) was discussed in the Introduction to this section. This chapter begins by discussing two papers providing significant advances in the understanding of the pathology of IIPs. Attention will then turn to the very important question of whether accurate, non-invasive predictors of poor prognosis can be identified for the IIPs. The importance of this rests with the fact that no good treatment exists for IPF and accurate prognostic indicators would allow us, where appropriate, to refer for early lung transplantation or for good palliative care. Equally, we may be able to avoid unnecessary administration of potentially toxic treatments in patients with a good prognosis. Furthermore, we would considerably advance further research into the condition by identifying groups of patients with defined prognoses. A variety of potential prognostic indicators for IPF have been studied recently including physiological indices derived from pulmonary function tests, exercise testing, bronchoalveolar lavage and high-resolution computed tomography (HRCT) and these are considered in turn.

Thereafter the emphasis turns to papers providing information on the survival of patients with IPF admitted to an intensive care unit (ICU) and then proceeds to consideration of small studies of antifibrotic treatments in advanced IPF.

Usual interstitial pneumonia; histologic study of biopsy and explant specimens

Katzenstein ALA, Zisman DA, Litzky LA, Nguyen BT, Kotloff RM. *Am J Surg Pathol* 2002; **26**: 1567–77

BACKGROUND. Pathological examination of an adequate biopsy specimen remains the final arbiter for diagnosis in IIP. This view stems from the fact that careful pathological classification stratifies patients with IIP into distinct diagnostic categories with characteristic prognoses and response to treatment |1|. Despite this biopsies cannot be expected to provide definitive answers in all cases. This partly reflects a lack of understanding of the pathological natural history of IPF and other IIPs. In particular, it is rare to have the opportunity for examining two temporally distinct pathological specimens from the same patient during life. This study, from one of the leading authorities on the pathology of IIPs, took advantage of the availability of sequential lung biopsy and explant specimens from patients with interstitial lung disease (ILD). The aim was to refine the diagnostic criteria for usual interstitial pneumonia (UIP) and, in view of the increasing recognition that features of more than one IIP can co-exist at any given time |2|, to determine the extent to which a diagnosis of UIP is potentially confounded by additional pathological features.

INTERPRETATION. In 20 cases where explants confirmed the presence of UIP only 50% of corresponding earlier lung biopsies unequivocally diagnosed UIP, with a further 25% showing 'difficult' UIP and 25% not consistent with UIP. Interestingly most biopsies and explants diagnostic for UIP also contained areas consistent with non-specific interstitial pneumonia (NSIP) and desquamative interstitial pneumonia (DIP). In such cases it is known that UIP determines prognosis |2|. The concern arising from this study is that random sampling error led to diagnostically (and prognostically) important areas of UIP being missed in 25% of biopsies, with simultaneous pathology making diagnosis difficult in another 25%. The authors emphasize that the single most useful diagnostic pathological feature of UIP was a patchwork appearance on low-power light microscopy characterized by abrupt change between adjacent areas of normal lung and honeycombing or other pathological features of UIP.

Comment

This study compared initial lung biopsy samples with the matching lung specimen removed at the time of lung transplantation in 21 patients with a mean age of 58 years (median time between biopsy and transplant 26 months). Four patients had a history of possibly relevant occupational exposure, one had scleroderma and one had polymyositis. Two chest physicians gave an opinion as to the likely clinical diagnosis (HRCT was available for 20 patients). The explant specimen was reviewed initially without knowledge of the biopsy specimen and the explant diagnosis was taken to be definitive in all cases. Both specimens were studied specifically for features of UIP (e.g. honeycombing and the characteristic patchwork appearance of alternating normality and abnormality), NSIP and DIP. In eleven cases biopsies had been taken from more than one lobe: in these cases each specimen was examined. In all cases, any evidence of UIP established this as the diagnosis, irrespective of the presence or extent of simultaneous NSIP or DIP.

For the 21 explants, the diagnosis was UIP in 20 and NSIP in one (the patient with scleroderma). The presence of honeycombing or NSIP-like features were graded 1–3 corresponding to less than 10%, 10–50% or more than 50% of the specimen, respectively, while DIP-like features, if present, were classified as focal or prominent. The main findings are shown in Table 11.1 and a few key points should be noted. First, only 50% of explant-proven UIP was easily diagnosed as UIP at biopsy. Secondly, for

Table 11.1 Pathologic findings in biopsy and explant specimens

Case no.	Biopsy				Explant			
	Patchwork pattern	HCC	NSIP-like areas	DIP-like RXn	HCC	NSIP-like areas	DIP-like RXN	Dx
Group I. Biopsy diagnosis: straightforward UIP								
2	+	2+	1+	No	3+	1+	Focal	UIP
3	+	2+	1+	No	2+	1+	Focal	UIP
4	+	2+	2+	Focal	3+	1+	Focal	UIP
5	+	1+	2+	Prom.	3+	2+	Focal	UIP
8	+	2+	1+	Focal	3+	2+	No	UIP
9	+	1+	1+	Prom.	3+	1+	Prom.	UIP
15	+	1+	0	Focal	3+	2+	Focal	UIP
18	+	2+	1+	Focal	3+	2+	Prom.	UIP
20	+	2+	1+	Focal	3+	3+	Prom.	UIP
21	+	1+	0	Focal	2+	2+	Prom.	UIP
Group II. Biopsy diagnosis: difficult UIP								
10	+ (superimposed DAD)	2+	0	0	3+	2+	Prom.	UIP
12	+	0	3+	Prom.	2+	0	Focal	UIP
16	+ (superimposed BOOP)	2+	1+	Prom.	3+	2+	Focal	UIP
17	+	1+	2+	Prom.	3+	0	Focal	UIP
19	+	3+ (95%)	1+	Prom.	2+	2+	Prom.	UIP
Group III. Biopsy diagnosis: NSIP								
11	0	1+	3+	Prom.	3+ (Atypical)	2+	Prom.	NSIP
Group IV. Non-diagnostic biopsies								
1	0 (interstitial fibrosis)	1+ (+ scarring)	2+	Prom.	2+	1+	Focal	UIP
13	0 (interstitial fibrosis)	1+ (+ scarring)	2+	Prom.	3+	2+	Focal	UIP
6	0 (inadequate, apical scar)	0	0	0	1+	2+	Focal	UIP
7	0 (honeycomb change only)	3+ (100%)	0	0	3+ (80%)	0	Focal	UIP
14	0 (normal lung)	0	0	0	3+	0	Focal	UIP

The extent of honeycomb change and NSIP-like areas was graded from 1+ to 3+ (<10%, 10–50% and >50%, respectively), whereas DIP-like reaction were graded as focal or prominent (prom.). HCC, honeycomb change; NSIP, nonspecific interstitial pneumonia; DIP, desquamative interstitial pneumonia; Rxn, reaction; Dx, diagnosis; UIP, usual interstitial pneumonia; DAD diffuse alveolar damage; BOOP, bronchiolitis obliterans-organizing pneumonia.
Source: Katzenstein et al. (2002).

the 20 cases of proven UIP, the clinical diagnosis was of possible or definite IPF in 18. Thirdly, NSIP- and DIP-like areas were extremely common in cases of UIP, occasionally representing more than 50% of the sampled area. Fourthly, in retrospect, biopsies accurately diagnosed UIP in all cases where a patchwork pattern was identified at low-power light microscopy. All five biopsies in the series that failed to detect UIP were characterized by the absence of this pattern and in each case there was circumstantial evidence to suggest that the surgeon may have taken a suboptimal piece of lung for diagnostic purposes. Fifthly, in addition to the patchwork pattern already described, UIP was attended by honeycombing and fibroblastic foci (FF) in all explants and the co-existence of these features makes the diagnosis straightforward. However, it is extremely interesting that the one case of NSIP in this study also had scanty evidence of FF and honeycombing.

Given the importance of lung biopsy in patients for whom a confident clinical diagnosis of IPF cannot be made, this study is extremely significant. It clearly reinforces the message that UIP is characterized by spatial and temporal heterogeneity (i.e. different stages of the disease are represented simultaneously and adjacently in tissue specimens), but emphasizes that the histological interfaces between these stages are characteristically abrupt. It also documents the common simultaneous presence of UIP, NSIP and DIP. This has a number of important implications if UIP is not to be missed. The first is that surgeons must take decent sized biopsies, if possible from more than one lobe, avoiding areas that look macroscopically normal or terminally scarred. The second is that pathologists should make a comprehensive search for UIP before making a diagnosis of NSIP/DIP, particularly if the clinical features make IPF more likely. Finally, the data give us valuable insights into the natural history of UIP. The inevitable question is whether NSIP precedes UIP. The authors considered this unlikely given that NSIP is a characteristically uniform process (i.e. it seems unlikely that a homogeneous histological pattern should change to the characteristically heterogeneous pattern of UIP) and that NSIP was not diagnosed on any of the biopsies from patients shown to have UIP at explant.

Relatively few technical issues need to be addressed in interpreting the study. However, it should be noted that these patients were relatively young and that we have no information on the treatment they received for their disease or of drugs that might have induced ILD. Secondly, it is not clear whether the biopsies were initially examined blind to the result of the corresponding explant. Finally, we are not told the size of the biopsies taken by the surgeons nor whether the inadequate lung biopsies (cases 1, 6, 7, 13 and 14 in Table 11.1) were targeted using HRCT-derived information. However, these considerations are relatively minor and this study should be seen as an important addition to the understanding of the pathology and natural history of IPF.

Fibroblastic foci in usual interstitial pneumonia. Idiopathic versus collagen vascular disease

Flaherty KR, Colby TV, Travis WD, *et al. Am J Respir Crit Care Med* 2003;
167: 1410–15

BACKGROUND. The histological entity of FF has generated a huge amount of interest in recent years. FF are aggregates of spindle-shaped fibroblasts set in a loose stroma often beneath hyperplastic alveolar lining cells |1|. They are a characteristic feature of UIP where they are associated with active fibrosis and high numbers of FF have been associated with a poor prognosis |3|. Less is known about the importance of FF in collagen vascular disease (CVD)-associated ILD. There is some controversy as to whether CVD-associated ILD has a prognosis similar to IIPs, but the overall prognosis appears better in CVD-associated ILD. However, NSIP seems to be more commonly represented in CVD-associated ILD than among IIPs |4| and this may explain the more favourable prognosis in CVD-associated ILD. A different and important question is whether idiopathic UIP has the same prognosis as CVD-associated UIP. The hypothesis of this study was that patients with CVD-associated UIP would indeed have a better prognosis and that the survival difference would correlate with the prevalence of FF.

INTERPRETATION. Patients with biopsy-proven CVD-associated UIP had significantly improved survival as compared with idiopathic UIP (i.e. IPF), although it should be noted that the group of patients with CVD was very small and heterogeneous with respect to primary diagnosis. FF were identified with significantly increased frequency in idiopathic UIP and constituted the single best discriminator between biopsies from patients with CVD-associated UIP and idiopathic UIP. This observation requires to be confirmed in prospective studies but hints at different determinants of pathogenesis and disease progression in CVD lung disease and IPF even when matched for the presence of UIP. This has clear implications for our future understanding of the natural history of ILD.

Comment

These data come from one of the groups with the most experience of IIP worldwide. As in other papers described later in this chapter, the authors made use of an established US database of IPF compiled between 1989 and 2000. Unfortunately it is much less clear how the small number of patients with CVD came to lung biopsy, what proportion of those who did had UIP (as opposed, for example, to NSIP) or indeed the criteria on which their primary rheumatological diagnosis was made. Two expert pulmonary pathologists graded the tissue for each biopsy available on the basis of the number of FF identified, scoring these using a system whereby 0 = absent, 1 = mild, 2 = moderate and 3 = marked. The level of (independent) agreement between the pathologists was very high. All patients had an HRCT that was independently reviewed and scored for the presence of fibrosis and alveolitis by expert radiologists. The patients also had detailed lung function tests.

The authors described 99 patients with idiopathic UIP and nine with CVD-associated UIP, for whom the primary diagnoses were rheumatoid arthritis ($n = 4$), polymyositis ($n = 2$), systemic sclerosis ($n = 1$), systemic lupus erythematosus ($n = 1$) and mixed connective tissue disease ($n = 1$). In general the two groups had similar baseline characteristics (including equivalent degrees of fibrosis on HRCT), but patients with CVD-associated UIP were significantly younger, with a shorter duration of symptoms at the time of biopsy and higher on a percentage as predicted total lung capacity (as well as trends to better preservation of diffusing capacity for carbon monoxide [D_{Lco}] and forced vital capacity [FVC]). Survival was significantly better among patients with CVD-associated UIP (Fig. 11.1). Interestingly, the FF score was significantly higher among patients with idiopathic UIP and, in univariate logistic regression analysis for the prediction of idiopathic UIP over CVD-associated UIP, the FF score was identified as the most discriminatory parameter. The authors also constructed univariate Cox proportional hazard models for identifying predictors of survival. In this setting the FF score was a predictor of survival only when all patients were considered together, but not when idiopathic UIP was considered alone.

This study benefited from the well-established IPF database used and from the enormous expertise of the authors in diffuse parenchymal lung disease. However, potential limitations of the study can be identified and may influence its interpretation. In particular it is impossible to say whether the patients with CVD-associated UIP were representative of the population from which they were drawn. One of several hints that they may not be is that there were more males than females, which

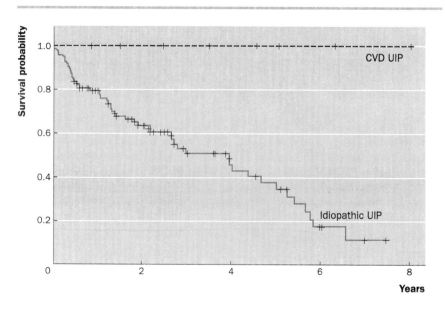

Fig. 11.1 Kaplan–Meier survival curves in patients with CVD UIP and idiopathic UIP (log-rank test, $P = 0.005$). Source: Flaherty et al. (2003).

would be unexpected for such a cohort (curiously there were more females in the UIP group, which is against the trend in the published literature). Furthermore, it seems highly likely that rheumatoid arthritis-associated UIP behaves differently from systemic sclerosis-associated UIP and systemic lupus erythematosus-associated UIP, etc. Thus, the small numbers in the CVD-associated UIP group generally, and in the subgroups specifically, hinder interpretation of the findings. In addition, it seems likely that the patients with CVD may have received disease-modifying drugs, which may in turn have influenced their lung pathology, yet this is not discussed. The other potential area of concern relates to the FF score. It is impossible to say whether the most appropriate and representative areas of lung were biopsied in CVD: although the HRCT fibrosis and alveolitis scores were similar in the two groups, an HRCT diagnosis of NSIP was more likely in the CVD group. This could imply that there was relatively less basilar disease in the CVD group: we are not told this, nor are we told where the (single) lung biopsies were generally taken from in the CVD group. It is not clear whether there is regional variation in the distribution of FF in CVD-associated UIP, but if there is then sampling error in such a small number of patients may have profoundly influenced the results.

These considerations (particularly the size and heterogeneity of the CVD group) make the data harder to interpret. However, it seems reasonable to conclude that the study adds some weight to the contention that idiopathic UIP has a different natural history from CVD-associated UIP (similar findings have been described for systemic sclerosis-associated UIP |4|). Whether FF have a specific influence on this difference remains unclear and, as the authors pointed out, this requires prospective analysis. The implication is that, despite similar histological pulmonary diagnoses and overall levels of fibrosis (as judged by HRCT), specific factors drive patients into respiratory failure and death in idiopathic UIP (or protect the lung from progressive disease in CVD-associated UIP). Identification of these factors would suggest important novel therapeutic options for IPF.

Idiopathic pulmonary fibrosis. A composite physiologic index derived from disease extent observed by computed tomography

Wells AU, Desai SR, Rubens MB, *et al. Am J Respir Crit Care Med* 2003;
167: 962–9

B A C K G R O U N D. In the study of IPF it would be extremely helpful to have a simple, objective, non-invasive tool for predicting the extent and severity of the disease as well as outcome. Lung function analysis may help in this regard, but is partly limited by the fact that co-existent emphysema elevates lung volumes and further reduces transfer factor independently of IPF. With this in mind, the authors devised a composite physiologic index (CPI) for IPF calculated from the relative weighting of lung function tests independently related to the extent of ILD in a large consecutive cohort of patients with HRCT evidence of IPF (36% of whom had emphysema).

INTERPRETATION. The CPI states that

the extent of disease on HRCT = 91 – (0.65 × % predicted $D_{L_{co}}$) – (0.53 × % predicted FVC) + (0.34 × % predicted FEV_1 [forced expiratory volume in 1 s]).

When compared with individual lung function variables the CPI was more strongly associated with disease severity and more predictive of prognosis. The CPI is a most welcome tool because it corrects for the confounding effects of emphysema in patients with IPF and it describes the severity of lung disease using simple, objective, non-invasive parameters.

Comment

The authors studied 212 consecutive patients with a clinical diagnosis of IPF (the criteria were dependent on HRCT scanning, but not histological confirmation). The average age was 62 years and 76 patients (36%) had co-existent HRCT evidence of emphysema. Patients with connective tissue diseases or relevant environmental exposures were excluded. HRCT scans were scored for the extent of ILD using a validated system operated by two leading authorities in the radiological assessment of IPF. The same radiologists assessed the extent of emphysema on the scans using standard criteria. The pulmonary function tests used in the analysis were derived within 1 month of the initial diagnostic HRCT.

The authors used split-sample testing for deriving their model, i.e. two groups of 106 were formed, each of which was matched for the extent of IPF (approximately 55% lung involvement in each group) and the extent of emphysema (approximately 10% lung involvement in each group). In the first group stepwise regression was used to derive the relative contribution of individual lung function parameters to the extent of IPF on HRCT. In this model the $D_{L_{co}}$, FVC and FEV_1 were independently related to the extent of fibrosis, with a regression coefficient of –0.65 for $D_{L_{co}}$, of –0.53 for FVC and of 0.34 for FEV_1, leading to the calculated CPI as described above. The second group was then used to compare the correlation between disease extent and a variety of parameters including the CPI and individual lung function tests. Finally, both groups were combined when testing the prognostic value of the CPI, individual lung function tests and the extent of disease in relation to mortality.

The CPI correlated more strongly with HRCI-extent of IPF ($r^2 = 0.51$) than any of the individual lung function tests analysed (the next best [negative] correlation was with $D_{L_{co}}$) ($r^2 = 0.37$). In view of the fact that the study patients were not required to have a lung biopsy (hence introducing the theoretical possibility of confounding by other IIPs and particularly NSIP) the authors also examined the correlation between CPI (or individual lung function parameters) and disease extent on HRCT in subgroups comprising 32 separate patients with biopsy-proven UIP, 118 patients with 'typical' HRCT appearances for IPF and 62 patients fulfilling all ATS/ERS criteria for IPF (i.e. either histological diagnosis or bronchoalveolar lavage to exclude alternative diagnoses). The results (Table 11.2) demonstrate that the CPI remained the index most closely correlated with disease extent.

Turning to survival data, the study group had a median survival of 22 months, in

Table 11.2 Univariate correlations between physiologic indices, including the composite physiologic index, and the extent of idiopathic pulmonary fibrosis on computed tomography in patients meeting histologic criteria for a diagnosis of usual interstitial pneumonia, ATS/ERS computed tomography criteria for a diagnosis of idiopathic pulmonary fibrosis and ATS/ERS diagnostic criteria for a diagnosis of idiopathic pulmonary fibrosis

	Diagnosis of UIP at biopsy ($n = 32$)	Confident CT diagnosis of IPF ($n = 118$)	ATS/ERS diagnosis of IPF ($n = 62$)
CPI, r^2, P-value	0.61, 0.0005	0.47, <0.0005	0.39, <0.0005
D_{LCO}, r^2, P-value	0.51, <0.0005	0.31, <0.0005	0.20, <0.0005
K_{CO}, r^2, P-value	0.08, n.s.	0.03, n.s.	0.00, n.s.
FEV_1, r^2, P-value	0.27, 0.002	0.09, <0.001	0.15, 0.001
FVC, r^2, P-value	0.47, <0.0005	0.30, <0.0005	0.34, <0.0005
TLC, r^2, P-value	0.36, <0.0005	0.31, <0.0005	0.24, <0.0005
VA, r^2, P-value	0.41, <0.0005	0.28, <0.0005	0.29 <0.0005
RV, r^2, P-value	0.03, n.s.	0.16 <0.0005	0.04, 0.02
P_{O_2}, r^2, P-value	0.14, 0.05	0.17 <0.0005	0.09, 0.02
A-ag, r^2, P-value	0.14, 0.05	0.10 <0.001	0.07, 0.04

ATS/ERS, American Thoracic Society and the European Respiratory Society; A-ag, alveolar-arterial oxygen gradient; CPI, composite physiologic index; D_{LCO}, diffusing capacity for carbon monoxide; RV, residual volume; TLC, total lung capacity; UIP, usual interstitial pneumonia; VA, alveolar volume; Kcos carbon monoxide transfer coefficient; P_{O_2},.partial pressure of oxygen.
Source: Wells *et al.* (2003).

keeping with published series describing mortality in IPF. Using univariate analysis it was shown that the CPI was the most powerful prognostic determinant (followed by disease extent on HRCT and $D_{L_{co}}$). In addition, prognosis among the patients with biopsy-proven UIP was analysed using proportional hazards models and the CPI was again the most predictive parameter. Interestingly, on this occasion FVC but not $D_{L_{co}}$ was a strong prognostic determinant (this is worth noting when considering the papers that follow on from this one).

On the basis of these findings, the CPI would appear to have great potential as a non-invasive severity index in IPF. The fact that the population of patients with IPF on which the CPI is based contained a representative proportion of emphysema is of great importance. It should be noted that, strictly speaking, the model corrects for the confounding effects of emphysema and not chronic bronchitis and one might argue that the latter common disease may also introduce an obstructive element to lung function testing which may skew spirometry in smokers with IPF. However, the major confounding effect from smoking-related chronic obstructive pulmonary disease is undoubtedly more likely to come from emphysema in view of the potential confounding effects on spirometry, lung volumes and transfer factor and, in any event, correction for chronic bronchitis would probably introduce additional complexity to the score. Instead, the principal methodological question is whether the population was entirely composed of genuine IPF. The authors presented several strands of evidence to suggest that any confounding effect of NSIP or similar conditions is likely to have been small. This seems a valid conclusion and it seems likely that the significant majority of the patients had genuine IPF. Finally, it should be noted that the CPI is not the only available score for assessing disease severity in IPF |5| and further comparisons between such scores are required. However, the simplicity of the CPI as well as its strength in describing disease severity and predicting mortality make it an extremely welcome tool for the study of IPF.

Changes in clinical and physiologic variables predict survival in idiopathic pulmonary fibrosis
Collard HR, King Jr TE, Bartelson BB, Vourlekis JS, Schwarz MI, Brown KK. *Am J Respir Crit Care Med* 2003; **168**: 538–42

Prognostic implications of physiologic and radiographic changes in idiopathic interstitial pneumonia
Flaherty KR, Mumford JA, Murray S, *et al. Am J Respir Crit Care Med* 2003; **168**: 543–8

Fibrotic idiopathic interstitial pneumonia. The prognostic value of longitudinal functional trends
Latsi PI, Du Bois RM, Nicholson AG, *et al. Am J Respir Crit Care Med* 2003; **168**: 531–7

BACKGROUND. As previously discussed simple and reliable prognostic indices in IIP would be extremely welcome so as to provide doctors with information for identifying patients who should be referred for early transplantation and for aiding future research efforts into characterizing distinct phenotypes within IIPs in the hope that new therapies can be developed. The prognostic utility of lung function tests in IIP has been debated for some time. The three papers listed alphabetically above appeared together in the *American Journal of Respiratory and Critical Care Medicine* and all addressed the question of whether serial changes in pulmonary function tests predict outcome in IIP. The first paper dealt with IPF exclusively, while the other two incorporated patients with NSIP.

INTERPRETATION. While the patient characteristics and methodologies differed somewhat in these studies, the emerging picture is that serial measurements of lung function can predict survival in IPF. The strongest predictor appears to be the change in FVC over 6 months, although other variables were predictive of outcome in individual studies.

Comment

These studies come from three of the most important groups contributing to the understanding of the IIPs in recent years. The studies were designed along similar general principles in that each centre holds a database of patients with clinical and lung biopsy evidence of IIP. From these Collard *et al.* drew cases of UIP, Flaherty *et al.* extracted UIP and NSIP and Latsi *et al.* selected UIP and fibrotic NSIP. The patients in the databases were generally collected over periods of 10–20 years up to the end of the last decade. Each group had collected pulmonary function data from their patients. One of the aims in each study was to identify predictors of survival.

The patient groups were broadly similar, particularly in the studies by Collard *et al.* and Flaherty *et al.*, in whom patients with UIP ($n = 81$ and $n = 80$, respectively) had a mean age of around 61 years, an FVC of 67% predicted and $D_{L_{co}}$ of approximately 51% predicted. The median survival times were 4.3 years (Collard *et al.*) and 5.8 years (Flaherty *et al.*). The British patients with IPF ($n = 61$) differed a little in being younger (mean age 55 years), with a lower $D_{L_{co}}$ (47% predicted) and a median survival time of 2.8 years. It therefore appears that the British study contained patients with more aggressive disease. It may be relevant in this regard that the proportion of males with IPF was 85% in the latter study, but 50% (Flaherty *et al.*) and 63% (Collard *et al.*) in the American studies. In each study almost all patients had received treatment for their IIP.

Collard *et al.* and Latsi *et al.* both found a number of baseline physiological variables to be predictive of survival in IPF, with the percentage predicted FVC and percentage predicted $D_{L_{co}}$ being found to have prognostic significance in either study. With regard to serial changes in pulmonary function tests at 6 months Collard *et al.* found a variety of pulmonary function tests to predict survival, with equal predictive value for change in the percentage predicted FVC (hazards ratio [HR] = 0.934) and change in the percentage predicted $D_{L_{co}}$ (HR = 0.935). On the other hand Latsi *et al.* found that change in the percentage predicted FVC and change in the percentage predicted $D_{L_{co}}$ were predictive of survival, but when all pulmonary function tests were entered into a proportional hazards model $D_{L_{co}}$ was the only remaining lung function variable to have independent prognostic determination. In contrast Flaherty *et al.* found a decrease in FVC of greater than 10% to be the only pulmonary function variable with prognostic determination. The FVC data from Collard *et al.* are shown in Fig. 11.2.

The situation after 12 months was less consistent, possibly reflecting loss of patients to follow-up over this period. Generally, Collard *et al.* continued to observe a prognostic value for changes in a variety of physiological parameters and Latsi *et al.* found that the serial changes in lung function were stronger predictors of mortality than they had been at 6 months (particularly $D_{L_{co}}$), while Flaherty *et al.* found that changes in lung function over 12 months added no prognostic information to their models.

It is worth briefly assessing additional data from the British study in relation to $D_{L_{co}}$. The study found that a $D_{L_{co}}$ of below 35% predicted at presentation selected out subgroups of patients with UIP and fibrotic NSIP who had poor prognoses.

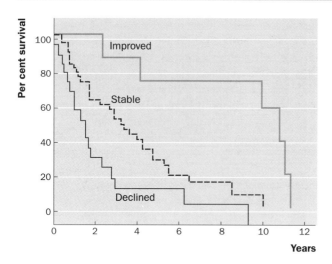

Fig. 11.2 Kaplan–Meier survival estimates for change in FVC % predicted. Six-month change in FVC % predicted. Improved indicates an increase in percent predicted FVC of 10 or greater (*n* = 9). Stable indicates that the change in percentage predicted FVC was less than 10 (*n* = 50), and decline indicates a decrease in percentage predicted FVC of 10 or greater (*n* = 22). Source: Collard *et al.* (2003).

Stratification in the change of $D_{L_{co}}$ (fall of 15% from baseline over 1 year or not) also allowed the identification of a small subgroup of patients with fibrotic NSIP and a larger subgroup of patients with UIP who had similar and particularly poor prognoses (Fig. 11.3). These data are important in defining a subgroup of patients with NSIP with a particularly poor prognosis. It is worth recalling that virtually all patients in these studies were treated and so the inference is that this subset of NSIP is refractory to therapy. The authors therefore emphasized that NSIP is likely to comprise a mixture of heterogeneous phenotypes that require to be dissected out. These specific data also suggest that the change in $D_{L_{co}}$ may be a useful predictor of mortality in appropriate sets of patients.

It is hard to make definitive statements based on these three papers. The emerging trend appears to be that serial lung function can predict mortality in IPF (and probably NSIP), but that further study is required in order to understand this in more detail. In the meantime, the change in FVC over 6 months appears to be the most useful tool available (not least because FVC is such an easy and reproducible measurement to make in practice), but the change in $D_{L_{co}}$ also seems to have great promise and may help identify subsets of patients with fibrotic NSIP who have a poor prognosis. Although the details have not been covered here, it is worth noting that, under specific circumstances, changes in lung function equalled or outperformed histological diagnosis as a predictor of mortality in one of these studies.

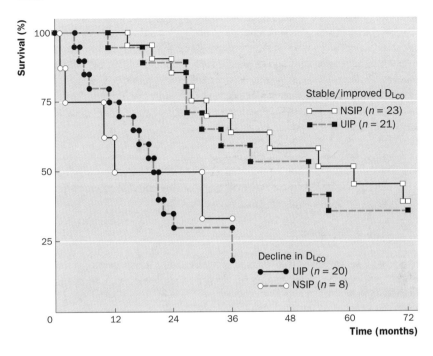

Fig. 11.3 Survival in 72 patients remaining under follow-up at 12 months in relationship to the serial 12-month changes in total gas transfer. Mortality was substantially higher in those with a significant (more than 15%) deterioration in gas transfer ($P < 0.0005$) but did not differ between UIP and NSIP, after D_{LCO} trends had been taken into account. Source: Latsi *et al.* (2003).

Studies like these have greatly improved the understanding of IIPs in recent years. They have the enormous strength of robust diagnosis confirmed by biopsy and the close collaboration of recognized authorities on clinical, radiological and patho-logical manifestations of IIP. However, they have some inevitable limitations, partly because they are necessarily retrospective and partly because of inevitable selection bias. The specialist centres from which the studies derive are likely to attract younger patients. In addition, we cannot assume that all patients with IIP in each catchment area were referred (it is conceivable that the sickest patients may have been treated locally in a palliative setting and this would potentially bias outcome data). In addition, the studies necessarily only included patients with a tissue diagnosis, there-by excluding patients who were considered too frail for surgery or to have significant co-morbidities leading to relative contraindication to a general anaesthetic (these arguments may have particularly applied to the two studies enrolling patients in the early 1980s). Furthermore, in the British study some patients with NSIP did not have more than one biopsy at the time of operation and this leaves the possibility that undetected UIP may have been present elsewhere in the lung, thereby influencing prognosis |2|. In addition, in relatively small studies of survival such as these, a handful of deaths unrelated to IIP could significantly influence the results and information for excluding this possibility is only provided in the paper by Collard *et al.*

However, these limitations do not detract from the important message emerging from these papers, which is that serial lung function (and particularly the change in FVC over 6 months) appears to have an important place in the non-invasive prognostic evaluation of patients with IIP.

Prognostic value of desaturation during a 6-minute walk test in idiopathic pulmonary fibrosis

Lama VN, Flaherty KR, Toews GB, *et al. Am J Respir Crit Care Med* 2003; **168**: 1084–90

B A C K G R O U N D . As described in relation to previous papers in this section a simple and accurate clinical predictor of outcome in IIP would be extremely useful. As oxygen desaturation on exercise is a common accompaniment of IIP, this study aimed to assess the prognostic information provided by a 6-minute walk test in patients with biopsy-proven IPF and NSIP.

I N T E R P R E T A T I O N . Exercise-associated oxygen desaturation to below 88% is common in both IPF and NSIP. The 4-year survival for both diseases was significantly lower among patients with evidence of desaturation on a 6-minute walk test. Furthermore, desaturation remained a significant predictor of survival even after adjustment for the demographic, physiological and histological factors associated with mortality. It therefore appears that the 6-minute walk test has a useful role to play in predicting outcomes in IPF and NSIP.

Comment

This study drew on the comprehensive ILD database compiled by the University of Michigan. In essence the database contains detailed demographic, physiological, radiological and (crucially) lung biopsy data, allowing analysis of outcomes in relation to clinical variables from the database.

In this particular study oxygen desaturation during a standard 6-minute walk test was defined as an oxygen saturation of arterial blood (SaO_2) of 88% or less on exercise. Patients with an SaO_2 of less than 88% at rest were excluded from the study and those who desaturated below 87% during the 6-minute walk test had the test repeated using supplemental oxygen. During a study period of 6 years from January 1996 123 patients with IPF or idiopathic NSIP had a 6-minute walk test, with 18 excluded from analysis because their resting SaO_2 was less than 88%. This left 83 patients with IPF and 22 patients with NSIP.

Desaturation on a 6-minute walk test was identified in 53% of patients with IPF and 36% of patients with NSIP. Among patients with IPF the baseline $D_{L_{co}}$ and resting SaO_2 were predictors of desaturation after adjustment for a variety of demo-graphic, physiological and HRCT indices. Importantly, desaturation was associated with a poorer prognosis in both groups of patients (Fig. 11.4). For IPF the 4-year survival among patients who desaturated on exercise was 35% and the authors made the pertinent point that, in the USA, this is lower than the expected 4-year survival after lung transplantation (approximately 45%). In contrast, the 4-year survival was almost 70% among those with IPF who did not desaturate on exercise in this study. When the authors performed Cox regression analysis they found that desaturation on a 6-minute walk test was a predictor of mortality after adjusting for age, sex, smoking, $D_{L_{CO}}$, FVC, resting SaO_2, histology and CT fibrosis score (hazards ratio ~4.5, i.e. predictive of a greater than fourfold risk of mortality). This analysis persisted when IPF was studied alone and when the definition of desaturation was changed to a fall in SaO_2 of at least 4% relative to the baseline (used by many labora-tories as the accepted definition of desaturation on exercise).

The importance of these data lies in the fact that desaturation strongly predicts mortality even after correction for important confounding variables and the fact that the 6-minute walk test is simple, non-invasive and inexpensive. The size of the study and the robust histological diagnoses are also considerable strengths. The data are broadly consistent with other exercise data in IIP, including recent papers showing that exercise-induced hypoxaemia detected on formal cardiopulmonary exercise testing is a predictor of mortality in IPF |6|. One potentially important practical point

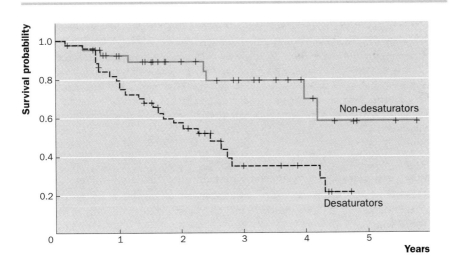

Fig. 11.4 Kaplan–Meier survival curve for patients with UIP grouped by desaturation (oxygen saturation of 88% or less) on a 6-minute walk test ($P = 0.0018$).
Source: Lama *et al.* (2003).

to arise, as described above, is that patients who desaturated on a 6-minute walk test had a prognosis likely to be improved by lung transplant and this should prompt us to consider early referral of such patients to lung transplant facilities.

The potential limitations of this kind of study include selection bias introduced by limiting the study to those patients who had a lung biopsy and by the fact that centres of excellence are likely to receive a skewed population of patients with IPF. As discussed previously, such limitations are inevitable in studies like this, which are specifically dependent upon patients with histological diagnoses (and which have made enormous contributions to the understanding of IIP). In addition, when studying mortality in small groups of patients (particularly those with NSIP), the cause of death should perhaps be taken into account, as it would only take a few deaths unrelated to IIP (e.g. in road traffic accidents) to influence the results significantly. One specific question relating to this study is whether the 6-minute walk test is reproducible in the same patient on consecutive days? However, these minor limitations should not detract from the undoubted importance of these results.

In summary, the 6-minute walk test would appear to be a safe, simple, inexpensive and ultimately very useful addition to our attempts at predicting outcome in IIP.

BAL findings in idiopathic nonspecific interstitial pneumonia and usual interstitial pneumonia
Veeraraghavan S, Latsi PI, Wells AU, *et al. Eur Respir J* 2003; **22**: 239–44

BACKGROUND. As described previously, it remains desirable to identify simple and safe clinical investigations that discriminate between distinct IIPs and can accurately predict prognosis. An inflammatory pattern to bronchoalveolar lavage (BAL) fluid has been described in UIP and in NSIP. Because the inflammatory component of each condition is quite distinct histologically and because they have different prognoses, it is important to establish whether BAL can distinguish each disease and independently predict outcome. This study set out to address these issues, specifically comparing BAL from patients with UIP and patients with fibrotic NSIP who had similar clinical presentations.

INTERPRETATION. The total and differential cell counts in BAL fluid were remarkably similar when comparing UIP and fibrotic NSIP. No prognostic determinants could be identified in BAL fluid.

Comment

This study retrospectively analysed BAL fluid retrieved from patients who went on to have a lung biopsy in keeping with UIP or fibrotic NSIP and who had clinical features including bilateral crackles, restrictive spirometric defect or reduced $D_{L_{CO}}$, a chest X-ray compatible with IPF and no evidence for connective tissue disease or environmental/occupational exposures associated with ILD. The patients studied seem to be derived from the same cohort described by Latsi *et al.* (p. 180). Expert pathologists

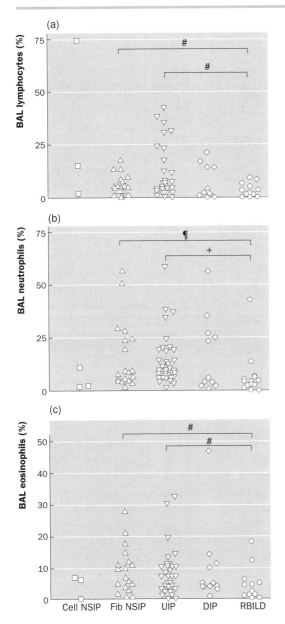

Fig. 11.5 Histograms showing a comparison of BAL (a) lymphocyte, (b) neutrophil and (c) eosinophil percentages between idiopathic cellular NSIP (Cell NSIP), fibrotic NSIP (Fib NSIP), usual interstitial pneumonia (UIP), desquamative interstitial pneumonia (DIP) and respiratory bronchiolitis-associated interstitial lung disease (RBILD). #P = 0.01; ¶P = 0.01; +P = 0.0002 according to Mann-Whitney tests. Source: Veeraraghavan *et al.* (2003).

reviewed biopsy samples and selected out those with UIP and NSIP. In total 74 patients with biopsy-proven evidence for idiopathic UIP or NSIP had BAL fluid retrieved, but 17 were excluded on the grounds that the bronchoscopy was 4 months removed from the time of lung biopsy and a further three were excluded because they had cellular NSIP. Thus, the study group comprised idiopathic UIP ($n = 35$) and fibrotic NSIP ($n = 19$). BAL fluid data were reviewed particularly with regard to the total cell count and differential cell count, both estimated using standard techniques. Survival data and lung function data were collected from the authors' established database.

At the time BAL was performed the two groups of patients were remarkably similar with regard to their mean age (approximately 55 years in each group), mean FVC (approximately 77% predicted in each group), mean $D_{L_{co}}$ (approximately 47% predicted in each group) and the proportion of patients receiving prednisolone with or without an immunosuppressant (approximately 20% in each group). The absolute cell count was similar in each group (202 000/ml for fibrotic NSIP and 240 000/ml for UIP). The differential cell count was also remarkably similar when comparing the two groups, as shown in Fig. 11.5, which incorporates comparative data from patients with DIP, respiratory bronchiolitis-associated ILD and cellular NSIP. Patients were followed up for a median of 3.4 years and, although the mortality associated with UIP was significantly higher (83% as compared with 58% for fibrotic NSIP), no component of BAL fluid was predictive of mortality. Similarly, the BAL findings were not predictive of subsequent changes in lung function.

The authors pointed out that the diagnosis of NSIP appears to encompass a spectrum of patients with variable prognosis. The undoubted strength of this study lies in the fact that both groups of patients were well defined in terms of histology and clinical presentation. Indeed, this appears to be the most comprehensive analysis of BAL findings in a well-defined subset of patients with NSIP to date. It is extremely useful to know that BAL performed at the time of diagnosis can neither distinguish IPF from fibrotic NSIP (presenting like IPF) nor provide prognostic information.

A few methodological limitations potentially exist, most of which have been discussed in relation to the previous four papers discussed. It should be stressed that the authors went to some length to demonstrate that sampling error at biopsy was unlikely. With specific regard to the BAL procedure it is not clear whether BAL fluid retrieval was equally good in both conditions, whether the same lobes were lavaged in each group or whether there was intra- and/or inter-observer variability in the total and differential cell counts. However, it seems unlikely that these considerations would have radically altered the results of the study.

In summary, BAL appears to have nothing to offer either diagnostically or prognostically in distinguishing UIP from fibrotic NSIP presenting in a similar way. This is another useful observation in the search for practical, simple and safe markers of disease in IIP.

Radiological versus histological diagnosis in UIP and NSIP: survival implications

Flaherty KR, Thwaite EL, Kazerooni EA, *et al. Thorax* 2003; **58**: 143–8

BACKGROUND. One of the most important clinical decisions in IIP is whether a lung biopsy is likely to yield prognostic information. In particular, can HRCT provide information that would give adequate prognostic data without recourse to lung biopsy? This study aimed to address the latter question, whilst also determining the accuracy of HRCT in making a diagnosis of NSIP.

INTERPRETATION. In the appropriate clinical setting an HRCT satisfying specific radiological criteria for idiopathic UIP (which must include honeycombing) has 100% specificity and therefore a lung biopsy is not required under these circumstances. In contrast, an HRCT diagnosis of NSIP is associated with a histological diagnosis of UIP in over 50% of cases. Importantly, it seems that a confident HRCT diagnosis of UIP identifies a group with a particularly poor prognosis, whereas patients who have an HRCT consistent with IIP but without 'classical' features of UIP may have quite disparate prognoses defined only by histological information. This suggests that, in the absence of classical UIP on HRCT, a lung biopsy is warranted.

Comment

This study retrospectively assessed data from patients with biopsy-proven UIP or NSIP in the period 1989–2000 who had also had an HRCT scan around the time of biopsy. The pathological diagnosis of NSIP or UIP conformed to pre-defined criteria. In most cases (79%) biopsies were taken from more than one lobe and the presence of UIP in any of the sampled areas confirmed this as the histological diagnosis: this is relevant in that it minimizes the chances of UIP being underestimated in the sample. Importantly, recognized experts made pathological and radiological diagnoses and in particular an HRCT diagnosis was reached using a rigorous process requiring expert consensus. An HRCT diagnosis of UIP required the presence of honeycombing as an absolute criterion.

Ninety-six patients were studied (73 with UIP and 23 with NSIP, of whom 20 had the 'fibrotic' form of NSIP). All patients received some form of therapy at some stage of their disease. Interestingly, only 27 (37%) of the 73 patients with histological UIP were independently considered to have an HRCT diagnosis of definite or probable UIP (Table 11.3). Conversely, all patients with a confident HRCT diagnosis of UIP had histological confirmation (Table 11.3). The authors followed the survival time in all patients and those with UIP on HRCT had a particularly low median survival of 2.1 years. The remaining 69 patients (i.e. those with an HRCT diagnosis of NSIP or appearances which did not allow a clear diagnosis of NSIP or UIP [called 'indeterminate' in Table 11.3]) were subdivided on the grounds of histology. Those with a histological diagnosis of NSIP had a median survival time greater than 9 years

Table 11.3 HRCT consensus diagnosis segregated by final histological diagnosis

Consensus HRCT diagnosis	Histological diagnosis		
	UIP	NSIP	Total
Definite UIP	16	0	16
Probable UIP	11	0	11
Indeterminate	20	5	25
Probable NSIP	17	8	25
Definite NSIP	9	10	19
Total	73	23	96

Source: Flaherty et al. (2003).

(two out of 23 died), while those with a histological diagnosis of UIP ($n = 46$) had a median survival time of 5.8 years.

The emerging picture is that HRCT appears to define two groups of patients with histological UIP each having a very different prognosis (i.e. those with and those without classical HRCT features). Patients in the more favourable prognosis group (i.e. those without honeycombing on HRCT) were more likely to be female, non-smokers and to have had their symptoms for a shorter period. There was also a trend for these patients to be younger with a better-preserved $D_{L_{co}}$. The intriguing question is whether these patients may be more responsive to specific treatments than those with 'burnt out' honeycombing disease.

These data are very robust, yet a few issues may potentially have influenced the results. First, it is not explicitly stated that the cases studied were consecutive. This may not have been the case as a separate paper from the same group, also discussed in this chapter, recruited 99 patients with UIP over the same time period. Second, it appears that the expert radiologists were asked to review HRCTs in which the only available diagnoses were NSIP or UIP: it is hard to extrapolate this situation to 'real life' where many radiologists will not be authorities on ILD and where scans do not come ready packaged with a diagnosis of IIP.

However, the considerations above are relatively minor and this study should be considered as having important pragmatic implications for patients with IIP. In particular, the data strongly suggest that patients with clinical and definitive HRCT evidence of idiopathic UIP do not require lung biopsy and have a particularly poor prognosis. In contrast, patients with an HRCT that is not 'classical' for idiopathic UIP are less homogeneous in diagnostic and prognostic terms and a biopsy would seem to be indicated in this group. The challenge ahead is to determine whether the surprisingly high proportion of patients with histological UIP but without classical HRCT features may be amenable to more effective treatment.

Outcome of patients with idiopathic pulmonary fibrosis admitted to the intensive care unit

Saydain G, Islam A, Afessa B, Ryu J, Scott JP, Peters SG. *Am J Respir Crit Care Med* 2002; **166**: 839–42

BACKGROUND. The significant morbidity and short median survival associated with IPF inevitably mean that a high proportion of patients with limited pulmonary reserve will at some stage present to hospital services in acute-on-chronic respiratory failure. Because IPF is a disease of the elderly it is not uncommonly found in patients with co-morbidities and therefore some patients will have acute non-respiratory presentations. Despite this, very little evidence exists in relation to the outcome of patients with IPF who present acutely to the ICU and this subject was therefore the focus of this retrospective study.

INTERPRETATION. The in-hospital mortality of patients with IPF admitted acutely to an ICU was 60%, as compared with a predicted rate of 26%. Data on mortality were available for 95% of patients in the study and among these 97% died either in hospital or within a few months (median 2 months) of discharge. Respiratory failure was by far the commonest reason for an acute ICU admission and amongst this subgroup progression of IPF appeared to be the commonest cause. The almost universally appalling prognosis described calls into question the indications for ICU admission in this group of patients at the present time.

Comment

This retrospective study collected data on all patients with IPF known to have been admitted to a single US centre's ICU over a period of 67 months between 1995 and 2000. IPF had been established by lung biopsy or (retrospectively) by the ATS/ERS non-biopsy criteria in all patients, all of whom were said to have had compatible lung function tests and HRCT scans. Patients with evidence of CVD, drug toxicity or relevant environmental/occupational exposure were excluded from the analysis as were patients admitted to the ICU simply for electrocardiogram monitoring or for observation after a non-thoracic operation. As such the final cohort of patients analysed appeared to have 'pure' IPF. A variety of clinical parameters were derived from hospital databases, including acute physiology and chronic health evaluation (APACHE) III scores and related predictions of mortality.

There were 38 patients in the cohort for analysis. The median duration of illness from the time of diagnosis was 2 years (but it should be noted that the range went up to 12 years). Interestingly, prior to admission the only immunosuppressive treatments for IPF among these patients were corticosteroids ($n = 20$) and colchicine ($n = 11$, eight of whom were also receiving corticosteroids), with 15 patients on no immunosuppression. Most patients ($n = 24$) had received domiciliary oxygen. Respiratory failure was the reason for ICU admission given for 32 patients (remaining diagnoses were hypotension, gastrointestinal haemorrhage and acute abdomen;

$n = 2$ in each case). No cause was found in 15 of the 32 patients with respiratory failure and these were therefore considered to have progression of IPF. In addition ten were considered to have pneumonia, but this diagnosis was most often made on clinical grounds without recourse to alveolar sampling. A further two patients had pulmonary embolism, two had congestive cardiac failure and two had pneumothorax. The final patient developed respiratory failure after mitral valve surgery. Nineteen patients received mechanical ventilation and 15 asked not to be resuscitated.

Twenty-three patients died in hospital (61%) as compared with a predicted in-hospital mortality of 26%. Another 12 patients died at a median of 2 months from discharge. No follow-up mortality data were available for two of the remaining three patients and the final patient (the patient who had mitral valve surgery) survived for at least 16 months after discharge. Interestingly, septic shock or severe sepsis was only described in two of the 37 patients for whom specific data were available. Five patients (13%) were considered to have developed nosocomial pneumonia in the ICU. No clear predictors of mortality could be detected in this small study.

The strength of this study lies in its being one of the first of its kind and in the confident diagnosis of IPF in most/all patients. The authors made a frank appraisal of the shortcomings of the study, principal among which were its retrospective nature and small sample size. It is also quite likely that the diagnosis of pneumonia in this study was inaccurate in a few cases. Furthermore, it is possible that the severity of illness may have been skewed towards more severe disease, given that the hospital was a regional referral centre. One question not addressed by the paper was whether the in-hospital mortality showed any sign of improvement over the 5 years of the study, i.e. is there anything to suggest that improvements in ICU care give us any optimism for the future in this group of patients? It is also worth noting that we are not specifically told the mortality in the authors' ICU for respiratory failure in patients without IPF over the corresponding period. Finally, in interpreting these data, it must be kept in mind that this US ICU almost certainly admitted a high proportion of patients who, at least in the UK, would have been admitted to a medical high dependency unit for non-invasive ventilation and monitoring. For the British reader this may make the mortality figures still more depressing.

Despite its retrospective nature and size this paper is extremely valuable in providing us with the best evidence yet on which to base our decisions on how/where to manage acutely ill patients with IPF. As the authors pointed out, these data allow us to discuss prognosis with such patients and their relatives based on at least some evidence and it would presently seem appropriate if a proportion of such patients were to opt for palliative management. In the group of patients who choose to be managed aggressively it is essential that relatively large prospective studies are planned in the hope of identifying ways to improve the awful prognosis described in this useful study.

Interferon gamma-1b therapy for advanced idiopathic pulmonary fibrosis

Kalra S, Utz JP, Ryu JH. *Mayo Clin Proc* 2003; **78**: 1082–7

BACKGROUND. As described in the Introduction to this section, the report of clinical benefit with interferon-γ_{1b} (IFN-γ_{1b}) in IPF |7| provoked not only huge interest but a large, multicentre, randomized, placebo-controlled trial, the results of which are, at the time of writing, expected to be published in January 2004 and are awaited with great interest. The study described here emerged from the fact that a proportion of patients will continue to present with IPF more advanced than that addressed in the multicentre trial. The authors pointed out that further information on the effects of IFN-γ_{1b} in patients with relatively advanced IPF is required. Therefore they carried out a retrospective analysis of patients who had specifically opted out of or been excluded from the multicentre trial of IFN-γ_{1b} in IPF.

INTERPRETATION. This study provides no evidence to support the use of IFN-γ_{1b} in the treatment of patients with relatively advanced IPF, although interpretation must be tempered by the fact that this was a retrospective study and had no control arm.

Comment

This study recruited 21 patients, all satisfying the ATS/ERS criteria for IPF, over a period of 27 months from the start of 2000. The patients had either been ineligible or had not given informed consent for a placebo-controlled trial of IFN-γ_{1b} in IPF. Eleven patients had UIP on lung biospsy, nine had features of IPF on HRCT including honeycombing and one had HRCT appearances of IPF without evidence for honeycombing. All patients were prescribed 200 µg of IFN-γ_{1b} given subcutaneously three times a week. Their pulmonary function tests, symptoms and survival were monitored.

The patients had a mean age of 68 years and the median time from diagnosis to starting IFN-γ_{1b} was 1 year. Four patients received low-dose prednisone during the study. Lung function data were incomplete for the group as a whole, but the mean vital capacity was 55% predicted ($n = 20$), mean $D_{L_{co}}$ was 40% predicted ($n = 16$), mean partial pressure of oxygen in arterial blood (PaO_2) breathing room air was 59 mmHg in nine patients tested and mean SaO_2 86% on air in an additional nine patients. Patients took IFN-γ_{1b} for a mean of 8 months, although 33% stopped treatment because of lack of benefit. Adverse effects included minor flu-like symptoms in four patients, but did not require discontinuation of treatment. Only one patient reported an improvement in symptoms, this patient being the only one for whom there appeared to be an improvement in lung function parameters.

Eleven patients in the group died during the study. Those who died tended to be older and to have more severe disease at baseline as compared with survivors, but the differences did not reach statistical significance. A Kaplan–Meier survival curve was constructed for the group (Fig. 11.6). For several reasons it is hard to generalize these

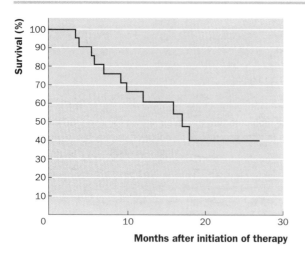

Months after initiation of therapy

Fig. 11.6 Kaplan–Meier survival curve for 21 patients who received IFN-γ_{1b} therapy. Source: Kalra *et al.* (2003).

survival data (for example, this is a very selective group of patients with relatively severe disease, there is no control group and cause of death is not described). Nevertheless, bearing in mind that the median time from diagnosis to treatment with IFN-γ_{1b} was 1 year and that the median survival time in IPF is traditionally reported at approximately 3 years, intuitively it seems unlikely that IFN-γ_{1b} conferred survival advantage in this group. It is tempting to speculate that, in keeping with limited experiences with pirfenidone (see the following study by Nagai *et al.*), advanced IPF may be particularly refractory even to antifibrotic agents, while earlier disease may be more amenable to a slowing of the pathological process. It is also interesting that a recent case series from France described four fatal cases of acute respiratory failure during treatment with IFN-γ_{1b} and prednisolone [8]. At least two of these patients had biopsy-proven IPF, and the acute deterioration was associated with histological diffuse alveolar damage.

The obvious limitations of the study by Kalra *et al.* relate to its retrospective nature, the lack of complete data for parameters such as lung function tests, the small sample size and the lack of a control group. It is a pity that no survival data were provided for comparable patients from the same single tertiary referral centre who were not treated with IFN-γ_{1b}, even allowing for the problems inherent in using historical controls. However, the data are useful. They provide no evidence to support the current use of IFN-γ_{1b} in relatively advanced IPF at the present time.

Open-label compassionate use one year-treatment with pirfenidone to patients with chronic pulmonary fibrosis

Nagai S, Hamada K, Shigematsu M, Taniyama M, Yamauchi S, Izumi T.
Intern Med 2002; **41**: 1118–23

BACKGROUND. The development and evaluation of antifibrotic drugs for IPF is urgently required. Pirfenidone is a pyridone molecule that has been shown to have antifibrotic effects on human lung fibroblasts *in vitro* and to reduce collagen deposition in animal models of bleomycin-induced pulmonary fibrosis. A previous observational, open-label trial of pirfenidone for compassionate use in IPF appeared to stabilize the disease and had an acceptable safety profile |9|. This study by Nagai *et al.* set out to evaluate the efficacy and safety of pirfenidone in patients who, as a group, had evidence for a decline in their lung function and PaO_2.

INTERPRETATION. Pirfenidone was associated with a clear trend towards the stabilization of PaO_2 and radiographic score ($P = 0.05$ in each case) in patients who completed 1 year of treatment. Although these results are encouraging and broadly support previous observations, the open-label nature of this study and the small number of patients enrolled prevent any definitive conclusions from being drawn other than that the results of prospective, randomized, controlled trials of pirfenidone should be awaited with great interest.

Comment

This study enrolled 13 patients for compassionate, open-label administration of pirfenidone. Of these, three patients died with cardiac failure consequent upon progressive pulmonary hypertension within 3 months of starting pirfenidone and were excluded from analysis. Among the remaining ten patients, eight had IPF (seven biopsy proven and one with supportive HRCT, including honeycombing) and two had pulmonary fibrosis associated with systemic sclerosis (one had UIP on lung biopsy and the other had a supportive HRCT, including honeycombing). All patients were male and their mean age was 61 years, mean vital capacity was 55% predicted, mean DL_{co} was 33% predicted and mean PaO_2 measured whilst using supplemental oxygen by nasal cannulae at 1 l/min was 62 mmHg. One patient had aspergilloma at the time of entry despite active infection constituting an exclusion criterion. All ten patients were receiving domiciliary oxygen and five were given simultaneous prednisolone with or without immunosuppressive treatment. The loading dose of pirfenidone was 400 mg, followed by 20 mg/kg/day for 3 days, 30 mg/kg/day for 4 days and then 40 mg/kg/day (in divided doses) for 1 year. The authors gathered data on a chest X-ray score, pulmonary function tests and PaO_2 from 1 year before the start of the trial, then at baseline and at the end of 1 year's treatment. They calculated the rate of change for each variable in the year prior to pirfenidone and compared this to the rate of change in the year during which pirfenidone was given.

No changes in the rate of decline of the patients' lung function parameters were noted. However, the rate of decline in the chest X-ray score appeared to improve ($P = 0.05$). Similarly the patients' resting PaO_2 (with supplemental oxygen by nasal cannulae at 1 l/min) appeared to stabilize on pirfenidone, having deteriorated in all patients in the previous year (Fig. 11.7) ($P = 0.05$). It is almost impossible to work out the patient outcomes after pirfenidone was discontinued, but it would appear that at least six died within a further 2 years. With regard to safety, four patients were diagnosed with pneumonia during pirfenidone treatment but all responded to antibiotics. Five patients developed anorexia early in the course of treatment, three patients developed photosensitivity (but successfully restarted pirfenidone after approximately 1 month) and two patients described malaise/somnolence. However, none of the patients discontinued pirfenidone permanently because of adverse effects.

Significant caution should be exercised in interpreting these data because this was not a randomized, controlled trial and because the numbers enrolled were so small. The apparent arrest in the progression of hypoxaemia and X-ray change seems impressive in the face of an inexorably progressive disease. However, it must be remembered that three patients were not available for analysis because they died early in the course of pirfenidone treatment. We received no data on the course of the PaO_2 or chest X-ray change in these three patients, but it seems certain that these deteriorated. In addition, the authors did not state whether the five patients receiving prednisolone with or without azathioprine had been taking this treatment before the

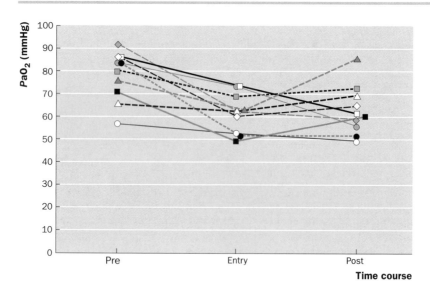

Fig. 11.7 Serial changes in PaO_2 (mmHg) during the study period. The abscissa expresses the time of arterial blood sampling and the ordinate expresses PaO_2 (mmHg) at rest under supplemented oxygen (1.0 l/min via nasal cannula). Source: Nagai (2002).

trial. If this were not the case, these treatments may have influenced the observed results. It is also frustrating that the reader is not told the time from diagnosis to entry in the trial, such that there is no way of knowing whether these patients had unusually progressive disease relative to historical controls. Finally, while the data in this study at least superficially echo the reduced rate of progression of disease noted by Raghu *et al.* |9| in IPF and a trial studying patients with lung fibrosis associated with Hermansky–Pudlak syndrome |**10**|, there is a suggestion that pirfenidone may be most effective if given early in the course of the disease and this may have further prevented the emergence of striking effects in a very small trial such as the one described here.

For all these reasons it is difficult to know how to judge these data. The clear rise in PaO_2 observed in at least two patients (one of whom had systemic sclerosis) is very much against the natural history of pulmonary fibrosis and could potentially be attributable to pirfenidone. Certainly there are biologically plausible reasons to suggest that an effect of pirfenidone would halt the progression of radiographic change and hypoxaemia. It seems reasonable to conclude that the data are interesting enough to justify prospective, randomized, controlled trials of pirfenidone in IPF. Indeed, these are in progress and their final results are awaited with great interest.

References

1. Katzenstein ALA, Myers JL. Idiopathic pulmonary fibrosis. Clinical relevance of pathologic classification. *Am J Respir Crit Care Med* 1998; **157**: 1301–15.

2. Flaherty KR, Travis WD, Colby TV, Toews GB, Kazerooni EA, Gross BH, Jain A, Strawderman III RL, Flint A, Lynch III JP, Martinez FJ. Histopathologic variability in usual and nonspecific interstitial pneumonias. *Am J Respir Crit Care Med* 2001; **164**: 1722–7.

3. King Jr TE, Schwarz MI, Brown K, Tooze JA, Colby TV, Waldron Jr JA, Flint A, Thurlbeck W, Cherniack RM. Idiopathic pulmonary fibrosis. Relationship between histopathologic features and mortality. *Am J Respir Crit Care Med* 2001; **164**: 1025–32.

4. Bouros D, Wells AU, Nicholson AG, Colby TV, Polychronopoulos V, Pantelidis P, Haslam PL, Vassilakis DA, Black CM, Du Bois RM. Histopathologic subsets of fibrosing alveolitis in patients with systemic sclerosis and their relationship to outcome. *Am J Respir Crit Care Med* 2002; **165**: 1581–6.

5. King Jr TE, Tooze JA, Schwarz MI, Brown KR, Cherniack RM. Predicting survival in idiopathic pulmonary fibrosis: scoring system and survival model. *Am J Respir Crit Care Med* 2001; **167**: 1171–81.

6. Miki K, Maekura R, Hiraga T, Okuda Y, Okamoto T, Hirotani A, Ogura T. Impairments and prognostic factors for survival in patients with idiopathic pulmonary fibrosis. *Respir Med* 2003; **97**: 482–90.

7. Ziesche R, Hofbauer W, Wittmann K, Petkov V, Block LH. A preliminary study of long-term treatment with interferon gamma-1b and low-dose prednisolone in patients with idiopathic pulmonary fibrosis. *N Engl J Med* 1999; **341**: 1264–9.

8. Honoré I, Nunes H, Groussard O, Kambouchner M, Chambellan A, Aubier M, Valeyre D, Crestani B. Acute respiratory failure after interferon-γ therapy of end-stage pulmonary fibrosis. *Am J Respir Crit Care Med* 2003; **167**: 953–7.

9. Raghu G, Johnson WC, Lockhart D, Mageto Y. Treatment of idiopathic pulmonary fibrosis with a new antifibrotic agent, pirfenidone; results of a prospective, open-label phase II study. *Am J Respir Crit Care Med* 1999; **159**: 1061–9.

10. Gahl WA, Brantly M, Troendle J, Avila NA, Padua A, Montalvo C, Cardona H, Calis KA, Gochuico B. Effect of pirfenidone on the pulmonary fibrosis of Hermansky–Pudlak syndrome. *Mol Genet Metab* 2002; **76**: 234–42.

12

Miscellaneous diffuse parenchymal lung diseases

Introduction

This chapter will begin by highlighting the difficulties in the diagnosis of sarcoidosis and proceed to an extremely useful guide to the clinical diagnosis of hypersensitivity pneumonitis.

The diagnostic pathway to sarcoidosis
Judson MA, Thompson BW, Rabin DL, *et al.* for the ACCESS Research Group. *Chest* 2003; **123**: 406–12

BACKGROUND. The early detection of sarcoidosis would seem to be a laudible medical aim, so that patients can be monitored for complications and/or deterioration and appropriate treatment instituted as necessary. Because sarcoidosis is a multisystem disorder, it may present in a variety of ways. Thus, sarcoidosis may present to a variety of different specialists and often forms part of a broad differential diagnosis. The potential for diagnostic delay is therefore considerable. This retrospective study aimed to determine the time from presentation to diagnosis in patients with biopsy-proven sarcoidosis and to characterize the factors associated with delays.

INTERPRETATION. Delays in the diagnosis of sarcoidosis are common, taking more than 6 months from the first contact with a physician in almost one- quarter of cases. Respiratory symptoms predict for a greater time to diagnosis and this may reflect delays in performing chest X-rays and/or reluctance to consider sarcoidosis in patients with obstructive spirometry. Physicians need to keep an open mind regarding the possibility of sarcoidosis, particularly in the differential diagnosis of unexplained breathlessness or in respiratory illness that behaves in an atypical way.

Comment

This study was embedded within ACCESS (A Case Control Etiology of Sarcoidosis Study). ACCESS has systematically examined various aspects of sarcoidosis in American patients, adding considerably to understanding of the disease and other publications from the study are very much recommended. A significant strength of

ACCESS is that patients require biopsy evidence of non-caseating granulomatous disease. Biopsies are specifically examined in order to exclude other causes of granulomas (particularly those related to dusts and infections) and diagnostic rigour is therefore built in. In this particular investigation the authors asked patients to identify the time of onset of their symptoms, the time they first saw a doctor (this included primary care and secondary care doctors) and the number of visits leading to a diagnosis of sarcoidosis. They collected a spectrum of demographic and clinical variables contained within the ACCESS database and determined the influence of these on the time to diagnosis.

This investigation enrolled 189 patients. Approximately half of the patients were under 40 years of age, 57% were female and 32% were black. Pulmonary symptoms were present in 52% of all patients (it should be noted that some patients were asymptomatic, with sarcoidosis suggested incidentally on a routine chest X-ray). The diagnosis was made within one visit to a doctor in 15% of cases, with 55% diagnosed within three visits, but 15% of patients remained undiagnosed after six visits. Put another way, 45 and 76% of patients had a diagnosis within 3 months or 6 months of seeing a doctor, respectively, yet the diagnosis took over 1 year in 11% of patients and over 2 years in 8%.

Respiratory symptoms predicted for a greater delay in diagnosis and skin symptoms for a shorter time to diagnosis (Table 12.1), possibly reflecting strong diagnostic 'clues' provided by erythema nodosum and lupus pernio. Interestingly, systemic symptoms, gender, race, income and the type of doctor first seen did not appear to influence the time to diagnosis. Turning specifically to respiratory considerations, a diagnosis taking more than 6 months was associated with a lower forced expiratory volume in 1 s (FEV_1) and with a significantly higher Scadding score on chest X-ray (a Scadding score of 0 = normal, 1 = bihilar lymphadenopathy, 2 = bihilar lymphadenopathy plus pulmonary infiltrates, 3 = pulmonary infiltrates without bihilar lymphadenopathy and 4 = established fibrosis). The inference would appear to be that sarcoidosis is less commonly considered in the presence of an obstructive picture on spirometry and that the reduced diagnostic specificity associated with increasing chest X-ray abnormality leads to sarcoidosis being missed initially.

Table 12.1 Factors affecting the time between first physician visit and diagnosis*

Factors	≤6 mo	>6 mo	P-value†
With pulmonary symptoms	64 (68.8)	29 (31.2)	0.02
Without pulmonary symptoms	72 (83.7)	14 (16.2)	
With skin symptoms	21 (95.5)	1 (4.5)	0.02
Without skin symptoms	115 (73.2)	42 (26.8)	

* Data are presented as No. (%).
† χ^2 test (P <0.05 considered significant).
Source: Judson et al. (2003).

How broadly these data can be generalized is open to debate. The first question is whether the sample was representative of sarcoidosis in the USA? While the sex ratio seemed representative, the authors pointed out that white patients were over-represented and that the group as a whole was wealthy (indeed the power of the study to pick up the influence of poverty on health access seems limited). The second question is how/whether the data can be generalized to countries outside the USA? This is a more difficult question, but given the relative wealth of American healthcare it seems plausible that delays will be still longer in most countries, except those in which sarcoidosis is particularly prevalent. A further difficult question is how many patient–doctor contacts are acceptable in the lead up to a diagnosis of sarcoidosis? This clearly depends on the nature of presentation. Assuming that many patients with breathlessness had stage I or II sarcoidosis, then one might expect that an early chest X-ray in the diagnostic process would have considerably increased diagnostic certainty. The inference may be that delay to a chest X-ray in young patients who had fairly persistent dyspnoea may have played a part in explaining these data. Unfortunately this cannot be tested, as the time to first chest X-ray was not included in the study. On the other hand for the (relatively rare) patient with stage III sarcoidosis, it is easy to imagine how a patient might have two to three visits in primary care before coming to a specialist with a wide differential diagnosis leading to investigations including a transbronchial biopsy, followed by a wait for the results to return, then a discussion of the final diagnosis. In other words a predictable diagnostic pathway could easily take half a dozen visits for stage III sarcoidosis.

A couple of methodological points should also be considered. The study relied on patients' memories for the onset of symptoms, number of visits, timing of diagnosis and type of doctor seen. Patient memory is notoriously inaccurate for this sort of analysis and it is not clear from the paper whether some of this information (number of visits and the time from first visit to diagnosis) was verified from case records. Intuitively it seems likely that most patients would overestimate these variables, which would have implications for the study findings. On the other hand we must bear in mind that this was not a screening study and therefore many more patients from the same catchment areas with persistently undiagnosed sarcoidosis may have been excluded from the study.

Overall, the messages from this study are that all doctors must remain aware of sarcoidosis and that in patients with respiratory symptoms sarcoidosis should be retained in the differential diagnosis when there is evidence of obstructive spirometry. Finally, a lower threshold for a chest X-ray in patients with unexplained breathlessness would have reduced the delay in diagnosis of sarcoidosis in this study.

Clinical diagnosis of hypersensitivity pneumonitis

Lacasse Y, Selman M, Costabel U, *et al.* for the Hypersensitivity Pneumonitis Study Group. *Am J Respir Crit Care Med* 2003; **168**: 952–98

BACKGROUND. The diagnosis of hypersensitivity pneumonitis (which is synonymous with extrinsic allergic alveolitis) remains difficult, partly because the associated symptoms and signs are so non-specific. For these reasons biopsy specimens are often used for improving diagnostic confidence. An accurate clinical prediction rule for hypersensitivity pneumonitis would be of enormous benefit in defining the probability of hypersensitivity pneumonitis. In an important group of patients such a rule might provide sufficient diagnostic confidence to obviate the need for biopsy. This study therefore aimed to develop such a rule for the diagnosis of active hypersensitivity pneumonitis.

INTERPRETATION. The presence or absence of six clinical or laboratory variables appears to allow accurate prediction of the probability of hypersensitivity pneumonitis (Table 12.2). The relevant variables are exposure to a known offending antigen, recurrent episodes of symptoms, symptoms present 4–8 h after exposure, weight loss, crackles on auscultation and precipitating antibodies to the offending antigen. In many cases this rule should allow clinicians to make or exclude the diagnosis of hypersensitivity pneumonitis with less requirement for histology, while in other cases the rule may help identify patients in whom further investigation is warranted.

Comment

This study was performed by many of the foremost world authorities on hypersensitivity pneumonitis. Consecutive adult patients for whom hypersensitivity pneumonitis was in the differential diagnosis were prospectively enrolled in seven centres from seven countries in three continents. The investigators derived information from a history and examination for all patients and requested a battery of investigations including serum precipitating antibodies, high-resolution computed tomography (HRCT) and bronchoalveolar lavage (BAL) with differential cell count.

One considerable difficulty for the study was the absence of an accepted 'gold standard' for the diagnosis of hypersensitivity pneumonitis. The study criteria therefore stipulated that BAL lymphocytosis and HRCT evidence of bilateral ground glass change or poorly defined centrilobular opacities were essential if the diagnosis of hypersensitivity pneumonitis was to be accepted without further investigation. If after HRCT, BAL and further investigation the investigators still felt there was insufficient diagnostic information a lung biopsy was performed. An adjudication panel (comprising four clinicians, one radiologist and one pathologist) reviewed the material on which the investigators had made the final diagnosis for every patient in the study. In the event of disagreement between the host centre and the adjudication panel, an independent radiologist and an independent pathologist provided

Table 12.2 Percentage probability of having hypersensitivity pneumonitis

Exposure to a known offending antigen	Recurrent episodes of symptoms	Symptoms 4–8 h after exposure	Weight loss	Crackles + Serum precipitins +	Crackles + Serum precipitins −	Crackles − Serum precipitins +	Crackles − Serum precipitins −
+	+	+	+	98	92	93	72
+	+	+	−	97	85	87	56
+	+	−	+	90	62	66	27
+	+	−	−	81	45	49	15
+	−	+	+	95	78	81	44
+	−	+	−	90	64	68	28
+	−	−	+	73	33	37	10
+	−	−	−	57	20	22	5
−	+	+	+	62	23	26	6
−	+	+	−	45	13	15	3
−	+	−	+	18	4	5	1
−	+	−	−	10	2	2	0
−	−	+	+	33	8	10	2
−	−	+	−	20	4	5	1
−	−	−	+	6	1	1	0
−	−	−	−	3	1	1	0

All the predictors are dichotomous variables: '−' indicates absent; '+' indicates present.
Source: Lacasse *et al.* (2003).

arbitration. This process resulted in two groups of patients, those with and those without hypersensitivity pneumonitis. The clinical characteristics of the groups were compared and those showing a statistically significant difference were entered into a stepwise logistic regression model for identifying predictors of hypersensitivity pneumonitis, from which the clinical prediction rule was derived. The authors then validated the rule prospectively using a separate cohort of patients satisfying the same entry criteria (i.e. a presentation for which hypersensitivity pneumonitis was in the differential diagnosis).

Over a 3-year period 728 patients were enrolled in the study, 67 of whom were excluded on the grounds of incomplete data. Fifty-five per cent of the remaining 661 patients were female. The first 400 patients were involved in generation of the clinical rule and the remaining 261 in its validation. In total 199 patients were considered to have hypersensitivity pneumonitis. By far the commonest hypersensitivity pneumonitis was pigeon breeder's/bird fancier's disease ($n = 132$). The commonest diagnoses in the 'non-hypersensitivity pneumonitis' group were idiopathic interstitial pneumonia (IIP) ($n = 226$) and sarcoidosis ($n = 52$). In total 18 clinical and laboratory variables were statistically different when comparing patients with or without hypersensitivity pneumonitis, but the stepwise logistic regression model yielded only six significant predictors of hypersensitivity pneumonitis. These parameters made up the clinical prediction rule as illustrated in Table 12.2. A receiver operating characteristics (ROC) curve was constructed and the area under the curve was 0.93. Importantly, in the validation study the area under the ROC curve was 0.90, suggesting useful clinical reproducibility and applicability. When viewing Table 12.2 it should be noted that calculation of the probability of hypersensitivity pneumonitis requires only knowledge of whether each variable is present or absent. It should also be noted that the area under the ROC curve was very similar across all seven centres in the study suggesting the rule can be widely applied.

This comprehensive study represents a significant advance for the diagnosis of hypersensitivity pneumonitis. A considerable strength of the study was the cohort of patients from which hypersensitivity pneumonitis was derived (i.e. from all-comers in whom hypersensitivity pneumonitis was considered in the differential diagnosis, which is exactly the population in which we would wish to use such a rule). The study also went to considerable lengths to ensure as robust a diagnosis as possible for a condition with no diagnostic 'gold standard'. It systematically evaluated the most predictive of a wide range of clinical and laboratory characteristics from a large cohort of patients. The clinical prediction rule relies on simple clinical variables and the clinician need only decide whether they are present or absent. Importantly, the rule has been prospectively validated and seems equivalent across diverse geographical and cultural settings. Therefore, the rule seems applicable to widespread clinical practice.

Whether some cases of atypical hypersensitivity pneumonitis could have been missed in the study obviously remains unknown. In addition, ideally it would have been useful to know more about the defining diagnostic criteria for some of the more difficult cases. For example, it appears that 98 patients with BAL lymphocytosis and compatible HRCT changes were deemed not to have hypersensitivity pneumonitis, yet a maximum of 87 out of the 98 patients appear to have had further investigation such as biopsy. It is therefore unclear why at least twelve of these patients were considered not to have hypersensitivity pneumonitis. Similarly 35 patients were diagnosed with hypersensitivity pneumonitis in the absence of BAL lymphoctosis or compatible HRCT or both, yet only 18 of these appear to have had further investigation in arriving at a diagnosis of hypersensitivity pneumonitis. The independent adjudication system built into the trial makes it likely that these cases did have robust evidence for hypersensitivity pneumonitis, but this evidence is not available to the reader.

However, overall this study should be viewed as an extremely valuable tool in the diagnosis of hypersensitivity pneumonitis. The authors suggested that, in the absence of additional, unexpected clinical findings, a probability of over 90% (or under 10%) should allow the diagnosis to be clinically confirmed (or refuted) without recourse to invasive investigations. An intermediate probability might be best used to help guide us towards the level of investigation we would consider necessary to confirm (or refute) the diagnosis of hypersensitivity pneumonitis.

Overall conclusion

This section has tried to give a flavour of key advances in pulmonary fibrosis made in 2003 and late 2002. Certainly we are considerably further forward in the identification of genes that may be implicated in Löfgren's disease and idiopathic pulmonary fibrosis (IPF). In addition, major advances have been made in dissecting out the features predicting survival in the IIPs and these will help greatly in the clinic in designing important research protocols and in identifying phenotypic subgroups of patients within the blanket diagnoses of IPF or idiopathic non-specific interstitial pneumonia.

Gradually, we are also receiving more information about the terminal stages of IPF, allowing us to make informed decisions about issues such as intensive care unit referral and when to involve palliative care networks.

We have also learned a little more about the potential roles for antifibrotic drugs in IPF. The eagerly anticipated results from the multicentre trial of interferon-γ_{1b} are due for publication in January 2004, just ahead of the time of writing, but already further trials of this drug are planned and the hunt for new antifibrotic treatments will inevitably go on. Indeed, a number of other trials of therapy for IPF are due to report soon and will yield fascinating information.

Finally, a huge number of unanswered questions remain in other diffuse paren-chymal lung diseases (DPLDs) such as pulmonary sarcoidosis and hypersensitivity pneumonitis. The last year has provided us with an extremely useful clinical rule for the diagnosis of hypersensitivity pneumonitis and highlighted difficulties in the diagnosis of sarcoidosis.

In summary, the DPLDs continue to pose significant clinical challenges, but con-certed and organized research efforts are making gradual progress towards better understanding of the pathogenesis and development of new management strategies.

Part IV

Tuberculosis

Tuberculosis

A HILL

Introduction

Tuberculosis (TB) remains a global problem, with the World Health Organization estimating that one-third of the world's population is latently infected with *Mycobacterium tuberculosis* and that TB accounts for approximately 2 million deaths throughout the world annually.

Effective regimens are available in drug-sensitive TB and, if there is compliance with treatment, there should be high cure rates. However, the emergence of multidrug-resistant TB – that is, resistance to at least rifampicin and isoniazid – is an international problem. The approximate prevalence rates for new cases of TB are approximately 1%, but are higher for patients with prior treatment for TB at approximately 9% [1]. In certain regions, for example in Iran, rates over 50% have been reported. Overall the prognosis for multidrug-resistant TB is variable, but successful outcomes can be achieved in approximately 75% if patients are human immunodeficiency virus negative and if patients can be treated with three (preferably five) susceptible drugs, from *in vitro* drug testing, for at least 18 months after conversion to a negative sputum culture [2]. Treatment regimens can be complex and are often associated with a significant side-effect profile. It is recommended that patients should ideally be treated with a directly observed therapy regimen in centres with experience in the management of multidrug-resistant TB.

In order to reduce the burden of TB there has been a focus on treating active TB, rigorous contact tracing and treating latent TB infection and bacilli Calmette–Guérin vaccination in some countries.

Fifteen key papers of clinical relevance were selected from 1 October 2002 to 31 October 2003. The articles have an initial Background section, which is the scientific rationale for the study. An Interpretation section then follows, which is the main message from the paper. There is then a final Comment section. This final Comment section gives a more in-depth account of the paper and, in each paper, the scientific rationale is discussed, there is a summary of the study design/methodology, a summary of the main results and a final conclusion with comments on how this research may impact on clinical practice.

The articles selected have been split into five chapters dealing with the treatment of latent TB, the side effects of first-line anti-TB drugs, investigations for TB, advances in the management of mycobacterial disease and a final chapter on pleural TB.

References

1. World Health Organization/International Union Against Tuberculosis and Lung Disease Working Group on Anti-tuberculosis Drug Resistance Surveillance. Espinal MA, Laszlo A, Simonsen L, Boulahbal F, Kim SJ, Reniero A, Hoffner S, Rieder HL, Binkin N, Dye C, Williams R, Raviglione MC. Global trends in resistance to anti-tuberculosis drugs. *N Engl J Med* 2001; **344**(17): 1294–303.

2. Tahaoglu K, Torun T, Sevim T, Atac G, Kir A, Karasulu L, Ozmen I, Kapakli N. The treatment of multi-drug resistant tuberculosis in Turkey. *N Engl J Med* 2001; **345**(3): 170–4.

13

Treatment of latent tuberculosis

Introduction

Latent tuberculosis (TB) infection is defined as evidence of *Mycobacterium tuberculosis* infection (patients with a strongly positive tuberculin skin test) without evidence of active TB. The identification and treatment of latent infection is central to TB elimination because the development of active TB in these persons can effectively be prevented with treatment, thereby stopping further spread of the disease. Latent *M. tuberculosis* infection is predominantly identified through TB contact tracing, although it can be detected by other routes, for example immigrant screening, pre-employment screening or as part of a bacille Calmette–Guérin vaccination programme. In order to reduce the probability of developing active TB a variety of regimens are recommended internationally for treating latent *M. tuberculosis* infection. Some of the available regimens include 6–9 months' isoniazid therapy, 4 months' rifampicin therapy, 3 months' combination of rifampicin and isoniazid therapy and 2 months' combination therapy with rifampicin and pyrazinamide |**1,2**|. Three papers evaluating the use of isoniazid and rifampicin and pyrazinamide regimens for the treatment of latent TB were selected.

Use of isoniazid for latent tuberculosis infection in a public health clinic

LoBue PA, Moser KS. *Am J Respir Crit Care Med* 2003; **168**(4): 443–7

BACKGROUND. Six to nine months' isoniazid monotherapy has been widely used for the treatment of latent TB. The aim of this study was to determine the adverse effects and treatment completion rates associated with the use of isoniazid at a county TB clinic from 1999 to 2002.

INTERPRETATION. Six months' isoniazid monotherapy for latent TB was safe (0.3% hepatotoxicity), although its effectiveness was limited by suboptimal completion rates (64%).

Comment

Isoniazid has been the most frequently used drug for latent TB. There is concern about the potential hepatotoxicity with isoniazid and the long duration of treatment (≥6 months), which has hindered treatment completion rates.

The authors extracted information from their latent TB treatment database in order to determine the adverse effects and treatment completion rates associated with the use of isoniazid at a county TB clinic.

Hepatotoxicity in this study was defined as liver transaminases more than three times normal in the presence of symptoms compatible with liver injury or more than five times normal in the absence of symptoms.

Outcomes were available for 3788 patients started on isoniazid between 1999 and 2002, all of whom were <49 years old. Overall, 1.3% were human immunodeficiency virus positive (only 4% screened), 0.4% admitted drinking alcohol to excess, 0.2% reported using intravenous drugs, 1.2% were homeless and 2% reported having been in a correctional facility.

This was not a randomized, placebo-controlled trial and so some of the adverse effects may be overestimated. Eighteen per cent experienced one or more adverse effects. The adverse effects reported were 0.3% with hepatotoxicity, 3.4% with rash, 3.1% with itching without rash, 3.5% with nausea and vomiting without hepatotoxicity, 4.6% with abdominal pain without hepatotoxicity, 9% with headache, 4.7% with paraesthesia and 0.4% with dizziness. No hospitalizations or deaths occurred in patients experiencing an adverse effect. Multivariate analysis revealed that female sex, increasing age, homelessness and having spent time in a correctional facility were associated with adverse effects.

Sixty-four per cent completed at least 6 months of isoniazid. Lower completion rates were associated with being homeless, using excess alcohol and having experienced an adverse effect.

In summary, this large study confirmed that isoniazid is a safe therapy for latent TB, but its effectiveness is limited by modest completion rates. The next two studies evaluated the efficacy of the shorter 2-month rifampicin and pyrazinamide regimen, with increased completion rates being expected with the shorter regimen.

Safety of 2 months of rifampin and pyrazinamide for treatment of latent tuberculosis

Stout JE, Engemann JJ, Cheng AC, Fortenberry ER, Hamilton CD. *Am J Respir Crit Care Med* 2003; **167**(6): 824–7

BACKGROUND. Shorter regimens for the treatment of latent TB are being encouraged in order to improve compliance and completion rates. This study assessed the safety of 2 months' combination therapy with rifampicin and pyrazinamide for the treatment of latent TB.

INTERPRETATION. This observational study revealed that approximately 5% of patients treated with the 2-month rifampicin and pyrazinamide regimen developed hepatotoxicity. From the previous study hepatotoxicity occurred in <1% with 6 months' isoniazid therapy. The completion rates were suboptimal even with the 2-month regimen with rifampicin and pyrazinamide (approximately 68%). The rifampicin and pyrazinamide regimen for latent TB infection may be useful for high-risk, traditionally non-adherent patient groups, patients that have not tolerated isoniazid and patients that have been in contact with a known case of isoniazid-resistant TB. If this regimen is used it is advised that there is careful monitoring for toxicity during treatment.

Comment

Shorter regimens for the treatment of latent TB infection are being promoted in order to simplify regimens and ultimately improve compliance and completion rates. In addition, rifampicin and pyrazinamide combination therapy is an alternative regimen in patients that have not tolerated isoniazid or patients that have been in contact with a patient with known isoniazid-resistant TB. Safety is an imperative and this study assessed the safety of 2 months' combination therapy with rifampicin and pyrazinamide for the treatment of latent TB.

Patients with latent TB infection were recruited. Latent TB infection was defined as a positive Mantoux skin test in the absence of active TB by clinical and radiological evaluation. The patients selected had no prior treatment for latent or active TB. The patients were treated with 60 days of daily rifampicin (10 mg/kg with a maximum daily dose of 600 mg) plus pyrazinamide (20 mg/kg with a maximum daily dose of 2000 mg) or 16 doses of twice weekly rifampicin (10 mg/kg with a maximum dose of 600 mg) plus pyrazinamide (50 mg/kg with a maximum dose of 4000 mg). The main outcomes were treatment completion rates and the side effects with rifampicin and pyrazinamide.

Confirmed hepatitis due to the anti-TB drugs was defined as elevation of one or both of the transaminases aspartate animotransferase and alanine animotransferase to greater than five times the upper limit of normal with one or more accompanying clinical symptoms (nausea, vomiting, abdominal pain or jaundice) and if the transaminases returned to baseline after cessation of rifampicin and pyrazinamide. Asymptomatic transaminase elevation to more than ten times the upper limit of normal, which rose with therapy and resolved after rifampicin and pyrazinamide discontinuation, was also classified as confirmed hepatitis. Suspected hepatitis was defined as two or more symptoms or signs of hepatitis in the absence of laboratory testing.

There were 114 patients treated for latent TB infection with rifampicin and pyrazinamide for 2 months: 60.5% of these patients were homeless and at least 17% drank alcohol to excess, defined as more than three alcoholic drinks daily and 8% had a history of viral hepatitis or chronic liver disease.

Overall, 67.5% completed a full 2-month course of rifampicin and pyrazinamide. No patients died or were hospitalized due to drug side effects. The most common side effects were gastrointestinal disturbance in 12% and drug rash in 8%. Most patients (80%) that experienced gastrointestinal disturbance or drug rash were able to resume therapy.

Four of the 114 (3.5%) patients developed hepatitis on therapy and another two had symptoms consistent with hepatitis, but did not report for laboratory testing (total confirmed plus suspected hepatitis rate 5.3%) (95% CI = 2.0–11.1%). No patient who developed hepatitis had a history of viral hepatitis or liver disease and none had been previously treated with isoniazid.

In summary, despite the shorter 2-month regimen with rifampicin and pyrazinamide there was only a 67% completion rate. Side effects were common, predominantly gastrointestinal disturbance, drug rash and hepatotoxicity, but there were no hospitalizations or deaths.

Pyrazinamide and rifampin versus isoniazid for the treatment of latent tuberculosis: improved completion rates but more hepatotoxicity

McNeill L, Allen M, Estrada C, Cook P. *Chest* 2003; **123**(1): 102–6

BACKGROUND. The aim of this study was to evaluate the completion rates and incidence of hepatotoxicity of the shorter regimen of rifampicin and pyrazinamide for latent TB infection as compared with isoniazid therapy.

INTERPRETATION. This study revealed that the risk of hepatitis in patients receiving rifampicin and pyrazinamide for the treatment of latent TB infection is increased threefold as compared to patients receiving isoniazid. When patients were monitored more intensively, severe hepatotoxicity did not develop. However, the completion rates were slightly improved in the shorter 2-month regimen with rifampicin and pyrazinamide (71%) compared with isoniazid (59%), although this just failed to reach conventional statistical difference ($P = 0.07$).

Comment

Shorter regimens for the treatment of latent TB infection are being promoted in order to simplify regimens and ultimately improve compliance and completion rates. It is also an alternative regimen in patients that have not tolerated isoniazid or patients that have been in contact with a patient with known isoniazid-resistant TB. Safety is an imperative and this study assessed the safety of 2 months' combination therapy with rifampicin and pyrazinamide compared with 6 months' isoniazid for the treatment of latent TB infection.

This was a prospective study of 224 patients in a community setting between 1999 and 2001 who were treated with self-administered daily rifampicin and pyrazinamide for 2 months or daily isoniazid for 6 months for latent TB. This was not a randomized, controlled trial. Patients were offered the rifampicin and pyrazinamide 2-month treatment regimen unless there were contraindications (active hepatitis or on medications metabolized through the cytochrome P450 pathway) or if isoniazid was preferred (contact lens users, jail inmates, oral contraceptive users not willing to change or children <14 years).

Patients received daily rifampicin (10 mg/kg/day with a maximum of 600 mg/day) and pyrazinamide (15 mg/kg/day with a maximum of 2 g/day) for 2 months or daily isoniazid at a dose of 300 mg/day and pyridoxine at a dose of 50 mg/day for 6 months.

The main outcome measures were treatment completion and hepatotoxicity (a fourfold increase in alanine transaminase) or severe hepatotoxicity (a 40-fold increase in alanine transaminase).

One hundred and ten patients were treated with rifampicin and pyrazinamide (mean age 38.8 ± 17.4 years) whilst 114 patients received isoniazid (mean age 34.7 ± 17.3 years). Treatment was completed by 71% in the rifampicin and pyrazinamide group and by 59% in the isoniazid group, although this just failed to reach conventional statistical significance ($P = 0.07$).

Hepatotoxicity (alanine transaminase >160 U/l, a greater than fourfold rise) was documented in 13% of patients in the rifampicin and pyrazinamide group and in 4% of patients in the isoniazid group ($P = 0.03$). The onset of hepatotoxicity occurred within the first 4 weeks in 93%. None of the acquired hepatotoxicity required a liver transplant and there were no deaths.

Severe hepatotoxicity (alanine transaminase >1600 U/l, a greater than 40-fold rise) occurred in 5% receiving rifampicin and pyrazinamide prior to instituting intensive monitoring (previously liver function tests monitored at baseline and 1 and 2 months). Once more intensive monitoring of liver enzymes was implemented (baseline and 2, 4 and 8 weeks), severe hepatotoxicity did not occur in any of 67 patients.

In summary, although this was a prospective study it was not a randomized, controlled trial. This study revealed that the risk of hepatitis in patients receiving rifampicin and pyrazinamide for the prevention of latent TB is increased threefold as compared to patients receiving isoniazid. When patients were monitored more intensively, severe hepatotoxicity did not develop. However, the completion rates were better in the shorter 2-month regimen with rifampicin and pyrazinamide compared with isoniazid, although this just failed to reach conventional statistical difference.

Conclusion

Isoniazid monotherapy for 6–9 months has remained the commonest regimen for the treatment of latent TB. There has been increased interest in the shorter 2-month regimen with rifampicin and pyrazinamide. Hepatotoxicity with this regimen is more frequent than with isoniazid monotherapy and, disappointingly, there has been no significant improvement in completion rates. These studies are similar to the study last year by Jasmer *et al.* confirming not only increased hepatotoxicity, but an increased frequency of drug rash with 2 months' combined therapy with rifampicin and pyrazinamide compared with 6 months' isoniazid monotherapy [3]. Again, the completion rates were not significantly different (Table 13.1).

Currently it would seem advisable to reserve this shorter 2-month regimen with rifampicin and pyrazinamide for patients intolerant of isoniazid, patients in contact with a known case of isoniazid resistance or patients where there is concern with

Table 13.1 Outcomes for the two groups: patients taking rifampicin plus pyrazinamide compared with patients taking isoniazid alone

	Rifampicin plus pyrazinamide	Isoniazid alone
Number	307	282
Hepatotoxicity (%)[a]	7.7***	1
Discontinuation because of hepatotoxicity (%)	5.8*	1
Skin rash (%)	6**	2
Completed treatment (%)	61	57

[a]Serum alanine transaminase >250 U/l or more than five times normal.
*P <0.05; **P <0.01; ***P <0.005.

compliance. If the 2-monthly regimen is used it would be recommended for there to be regular monitoring of the liver function tests during treatment.

References

1. American Thoracic Society/Centers for Disease Control and Prevention/Infectious Diseases Society of America. Treatment of tuberculosis. *Am J Respir Crit Care Med* 2003; **167**(4): 603–62.

2. Targeted tuberculin testing and treatment of latent tuberculosis infection. This official statement of the American Thoracic Society (ATS) was adopted by the ATS Board of Directors, July 1999. This is a Joint Statement of the American Thoracic Society and the Centers for Disease Control and Prevention (CDC). This statement was endorsed by the Council of the Infectious Diseases Society of America (IDSA), September 1999, and the sections of this statement. *Am J Respir Crit Care Med* 2000; **161**(4 Pt 2): S221–47.

3. Jasmer RM, Saukkonen JJ, Blumberg HM, Daley CL, Bernardo J, Vittinghoff E, King MD, Kawamura LM, Hopewell PC, Short-course Rifampicin and Pyrazinamide for Tuberculosis Infection (SCRIPT) Study Investigators. Short-course rifampicin and pyrazinamide compared with isoniazid for latent tuberculosis infection: a multi-centre clinical trial. *Ann Intern Med* 2002; **137**(8): 640–7.

14

Side effects of first-line antituberculosis drugs

Introduction

There are two papers in this chapter. The first paper reviews the incidence of major side effects with first-line antituberculosis (anti-TB) drugs (rifampicin, isoniazid, ethambutol and pyrazinamide). The paper following reviews the clinical and genetic risk factors for the development of hepatotoxicity whilst on anti-TB drugs.

Incidence of serious side effects from first-line antituberculosis drugs among patients treated for active tuberculosis

Yee D, Valiquette C, Pelletier M, Parisien I, Rocher I, Menzies D. *Am J Respir Crit Care Med* 2003; **167**(11): 1472–7

BACKGROUND. The aim of this study was to investigate the incidence of major side effects (defined as any adverse reaction that resulted in discontinuation of one or more drugs and/or that directly resulted in hospitalization) from first-line anti-TB drugs among patients treated for TB.

INTERPRETATION. The incidence of pyrazinamide-induced hepatotoxicity and rash during treatment for active TB was substantially higher than with the other first-line anti-TB drugs (isoniazid and rifampicin) and higher than previously recognized.

Comment

Adverse reactions to one of the first-line drugs for TB (rifampicin, isoniazid, ethambutol and pyrazinamide) can have important implications, including morbidity, potential mortality and healthcare costs. The aim of this study was to investigate the incidence of major side effects from first-line anti-TB drugs among patients treated for active TB.

Patients that were treated for active TB in a single centre (Montreal, Canada) between 1990 and 1999 were analysed. A major side effect was defined as any adverse reaction that resulted in discontinuation of one or more drugs and/or that directly resulted in hospitalization.

Drug-induced hepatitis was considered if the transaminases were normal before therapy, increased during therapy and returned to normal after discontinuation of the responsible drug. Hepatitis was defined as liver transaminases greater than three times the upper limit of normal in the presence of symptoms such as anorexia, nausea, vomiting or abdominal pain or transaminases greater than five times the upper limit of normal in the absence of symptoms. A drug was defined as responsible for the side effect if the symptoms and signs resolved after withdrawal with or without recurrence after rechallenge.

Overall 430 patients were treated between 1990 and 1999 and 91% had pulmonary TB. The mean age was 40.3 years, 88% were foreign born (42% in Asia) and 4% had human immunodeficiency virus (HIV), but HIV status was not recorded in 61% of cases.

Eighty-eight per cent had TB fully sensitive to first-line drugs and 2% had multidrug-resistant TB, which is resistance at least to rifampicin and isoniazid. Ninety-five per cent took self-administered therapy.

The overall mortality was 4%, but none of the deaths were attributable to side effects from the anti-TB treatment. Nine per cent had major side effects (46% due to rash or drug fever, 26% due to hepatitis, 24% due to severe gastrointestinal upset, 2% due to visual toxicity and 2% due to arthralgia).

All except one developed a major side effect within the first 60 days of treatment and this was often sooner in females and older patients ($\geq$60 years). Following the development of the major side effect, 43% required hospital admission for a median of 16 days. In addition, 78% that developed a major side effect required more clinic and home visits. The total duration of therapy was 380 $\pm$ 209 days for patients with major side effects compared with 228 $\pm$ 111 days for the remainder (P <0.001).

As the drugs were used for variable time intervals, the side effects were expressed as events per 100 person-months of treatment in order to allow effective comparisons between the first-line drugs. Overall the incidence of side effects was higher with pyrazinamide compared with other first-line drug (incidence = 1.48 and 95% confidence interval [CI] = 1.36–1.6) events per 100 person-months of treatment compared with isoniazid (incidence = 0.49 and 95% CI = 0.42–0.55), rifampicin (incidence = 0.43 and 95% CI = 0.37–0.49) and ethambutol (incidence = 0.07 and 95% CI = 0.04–0.10) events per 100 person-months.

Overall the incidence of hepatitis was higher with pyrazinamide compared with other first-line drug (incidence = 0.52 and 95% CI = 0.45–0.59) events per 100 person-months of treatment compared with isoniazid (incidence = 0.18 and 95% CI = 0.14–0.22), rifampicin and ethambutol zero events per 100 person-months (Fig. 14.1). The patients that developed drug-induced hepatitis all had normal pre-treatment liver function tests and there was no history of alcohol abuse. Ninety-two per cent were symptomatic and all had transaminases greater than five times normal.

Overall the incidence of drug rash was higher with pyrazinamide compared with other first-line drug (incidence = 0.60 and 95% CI = 0.52–0.68) events per 100 person-months of treatment compared with isoniazid (incidence = 0.15 and

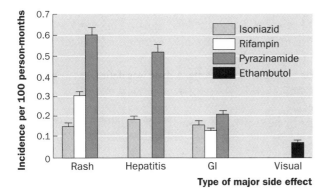

Fig. 14.1 Incidence of serious side-effects by type and drug. GI, gastrointestinal. Source: Yee *et al.* (2003).

95% CI = 0.11–0.18), rifampicin (incidence = 0.30 and 95% CI = 0.25–0.35) and ethambutol zero events per 100 person-months (Fig. 14.1).

The occurrence of any major side effect was associated with female sex (adjusted hazard ratio [HR] = 2.5 and 95% CI = 1.3–4.7), age over 60 years (adjusted HR = 2.9 and 95% CI = 1.3–6.3), being born in Asia (adjusted HR = 2.5 and 95% CI = 1.3–5.0) and HIV-positive status (adjusted HR = 3.8 and 95% CI = 1.05–13.4).

Pyrazinamide-associated adverse events were associated with age over 60 years (adjusted HR = 2.6 and 95% CI = 1.01–6.6) and being born in Asia (adjusted HR = 3.4 and 95% CI = 1.4–8.3), whereas rifampicin-associated adverse events were associated with age over 60 years (adjusted HR = 3.9 and 95% CI = 1.02–14.9) and HIV-positive status (adjusted HR = 8.0 and 95% CI = 1.5–43). Isoniazid-associated adverse events were associated with age 35–39 years versus <35 years (adjusted HR = 3.4 and 95% CI = 1.1–10.3) and drug resistance (adjusted HR = 3.4 and 95% CI = 1.1–10.9).

In summary, there was a 9% occurrence of major side effects in this study of patients treated for TB with first-line drugs. The incidence of major side effects, that is that led to hospitalization or discontinuation of therapy, particularly hepatitis and rash, was highest with pyrazinamide and was associated with female sex, age ≥60 years, being born in Asia and HIV infection. The authors found rechallenging responsible drugs to be unsuccessful, but the data regarding this were not complete and there was insufficient information regarding the rechallenge process, so firm conclusions from this study should not be made regarding rechallenging. The consequences of developing a major side effect led to increased hospitalization, home and clinic visits and prolonged therapy.

Evaluation of clinical and immunogenetic risk factors for the development of hepatotoxicity during antituberculosis treatment

Sharma SK, Balamurugan A, Saha PK, Pandey RM, Mehra NK. *Am J Respir Crit Care Med* 2002; **166**(7): 916–19

BACKGROUND. The aim of this study was to investigate clinical and/or genetic risk factors for the development of hepatotoxicity in 346 North Indian patients with TB undergoing anti-TB treatment.

INTERPRETATION. The risk of hepatotoxicity from first-line anti-TB drugs is influenced by both clinical and genetic factors.

Comment

Hepatotoxicity is a frequent complication in patients being treated for TB, being more frequent in Indian studies at 11.5% (95% CI = 9.5–13.5%) compared with 4.3% (95% CI = 3.4–5.3%) in Western studies [1].

Though several risk factors for the development of hepatotoxicity due to anti-TB drugs have been established (older age, female sex, poor nutritional status, high alcohol state, pre-existing liver disease, chronic viral hepatitis, hypoalbuminaemia and extensive TB), the involvement of genetic factors is not fully established.

The authors studied the major histocompatibility complex (MHC) class II alleles and clinical risk factors for the development of hepatotoxicity in 346 North Indian patients with TB undergoing anti-TB treatment.

The MHC class II alleles and clinical risk factors for the development of hepatotoxicity were studied. The definition of drug-induced hepatotoxicity in this study was the normalization of liver function after withdrawal of the TB treatment and the presence of at least one of the following criteria: a five or greater rise over the upper limit of the normal range in serum aspartate aminotransferase and/or alanine aminotransferase, serum bilirubin >1.5 mg/dl, any rise in aspartate aminotransferase and/or alanine aminotransferase together with anorexia, nausea, vomiting and jaundice and the absence of serologic evidence of infection with hepatitis A, B, C or E.

Overall 346 patients with TB were studied, all of whom had negative serologic tests for hepatitis A, B, C and E and HIV. None had co-morbid illnesses such as gastrointestinal, renal and cardiac disease or liver cirrhosis. All were treated with standard first-line drugs (rifampicin, isoniazid, pyrazinamide and ethambutol).

Fifty-six of these patients developed drug-induced hepatotoxicity. All had negative auto-antibodies (rheumatoid factor, antinuclear antibodies, antineutrophil cytoplasmic antibodies and anti-double-stranded DNA antibodies). The remaining 290 patients did not develop drug-induced hepatotoxicity.

In multivariate logistic regression analysis, older age (odds ratio [OR] = 1.2 and 95% CI = 1.01–1.04), moderately/far advanced disease (OR = 2.0 and 95% CI = 1.0–4.0), serum albumin ≤ 3.5 g/dl (OR $= 2.3$ and 95% CI $= 1.1$–4.8), the absence of HLA-DQA1*0102 (OR $= 4.0$ and 95% CI $= 1.1$–14.3) and the presence of HLA DQB1*0201 (OR $= 1.9$ and 95% CI $= 1.0$–3.9) were independent risk factors for drug-induced hepatotoxicity.

In summary, the results of this study in patients with TB with no significant co-morbidities and no viral hepatitis or HIV suggest that a genetic influence associated with the MHC class II region, in particular the DQ locus, is implicated in the development of drug-induced hepatotoxicity. In addition, clinical factors were important including advancing age, more extensive disease and pre-treatment hypoalbuminaemia. Thus, the risk of hepatotoxicity from anti-TB drugs is influenced by clinical and genetic factors.

Reference

1. Steele MA, Burk RF, Desprez RM. Hepatitis with isoniazid and rifampicin: a metanalysis. *Chest* 1991; **99**: 465–71.

15

Investigations for tuberculosis

Introduction

The standard investigation for pulmonary tuberculosis (TB) is three spontaneous sputum samples for a TB smear and culture. If patients do not produce sputum then samples can be obtained by either inducing sputum with hypertonic saline or by a bronchoalveolar lavage via the bronchoscope. Samples can be smear negative and formal cultures take several weeks. There has been increased interest in adjunctive measurements for aiding the diagnosis of TB. There are two papers in this chapter. The first paper evaluates the use of serum pro-calcitonin in the diagnosis of pulmonary TB. Pro-calcitonin is normally produced in the C cells of the thyroid gland and is the precursor of calcitonin. Normally all pro-calcitonin is cleaved and none is released in the bloodstream and, therefore, pro-calcitonin levels are usually undetectable (<0.1 ng/ml). However, during severe infections the pro-calcitonin level may increase to over 100 ng/ml and is probably produced by extra-thyroid tissues. The first paper selected evaluated whether serum pro-calcitonin is a useful diagnostic tool in the diagnosis of lower respiratory tract infections and TB. The paper that follows evaluated the investigation of choice for patients with suspected pulmonary TB who are either sputum smear negative or do not produce sputum.

Pro-calcitonin as a diagnostic tool in lower respiratory tract infections and tuberculosis

Polzin A, Pletz M, Erbes R, *et al. Eur Respir J* 2003; **21**(6): 939–43

B A C K G R O U N D . Serum pro-calcitonin has been recognized to be a useful marker in severe pneumonia. The aim of this study was to assess the diagnostic significance of serum pro-calcitonin concentrations in lower respiratory tract infections and TB.

I N T E R P R E T A T I O N . Using the current cut-off level of 0.5 ng/ml, serum pro-calcitonin concentration is not a useful parameter for the diagnosis of lower respiratory tract infections (acute exacerbation of chronic bronchitis, community-acquired pneumonia, hospital-acquired pneumonia and TB). Serum pro-calcitonin is not a useful test for the diagnosis of pulmonary TB.

Comment

The diagnostic significance of serum pro-calcitonin concentrations in lower respiratory tract infections and TB is not known, but has been shown to be a useful marker in severe systemic bacterial infections such as sepsis. A prospective analysis was therefore performed in patients with acute exacerbation of chronic bronchitis, community-acquired pneumonia, hospital-acquired pneumonia and TB and their serum pro-calcitonin levels compared with those of patients with non-infectious lung diseases (controls).

This was a prospective study in four patient groups (acute exacerbation of chronic bronchitis, community-acquired pneumonia, hospital-acquired pneumonia and pulmonary TB) and a control group with non-infectious lung disease such as fibrosing alveolitis and sarcoidosis. All patients with TB were smear positive and had infiltration and/or cavitation on a chest radiograph. A blood sample was taken on the first day after the onset of clinical symptoms before treatment was started (pro-calcitonin, C-reactive protein and white cell count).

One hundred and twenty-nine patients were included, 25 with hospital-acquired pneumonia (mean age 63.1 years), 26 with community-acquired pneumonia (mean age 63.1 years), 26 with acute exacerbations of chronic bronchitis (mean age 64.5 years), 27 with pulmonary TB (mean age 45.2 years) and 25 controls (mean age 48.4 years).

The median pro-calcitonin concentrations in the hospital-acquired pneumonia (0.46, 95% CI = 0.27–0.62), community-acquired pneumonia (0.22, 95% CI = 0.13–0.31), acute exacerbation of chronic bronchitis (0.19, 95% CI = 0.13–0.22) and pulmonary TB (0.14, 95% CI = 0.13–0.19) groups and the controls (0.11, 95% CI = 0.09–0.15) were not elevated in relation to the cut-off level of 0.5 ng/ml.

None of the patients with acute exacerbation of chronic bronchitis, pulmonary TB patients or the controls had serum pro-calcitonin concentrations >0.5 ng/ml, while ten of the 25 hospital-acquired pneumonia patients and one of the 26 community-acquired pneumonia patients had serum pro-calcitonin concentrations >0.5 ng/ml. Three groups (hospital-acquired pneumonia, community-acquired pneumonia and acute exacerbation of chronic bronchitis) had higher median pro-calcitonin concentrations, but below the usual cut-off level, compared with the controls (P <0.05), whereas this was not seen for patients with pulmonary TB.

The median C-reactive protein concentrations were higher in three of the groups (hospital-acquired pneumonia, community-acquired pneumonia and pulmonary TB) compared with the controls (P <0.01), whereas this was not seen for patients with acute exacerbation of chronic bronchitis.

The median white cell counts were higher in three of the groups (hospital-acquired pneumonia, community-acquired pneumonia and acute exacerbation of chronic bronchitis) compared with the controls (P <0.01), whereas this was not seen for patients with pulmonary TB.

In summary, relative to the current cut-off level of 0.5 ng/ml, serum pro-calcitonin concentration was not a useful parameter for the diagnosis of lower respiratory tract infections, including pulmonary TB. The authors suggested lowering the cut-off point, but for patients with TB, serum pro-calcitonin was not a useful test and could not differentiate TB from other lower respiratory tract infections. This study highlighted that serum pro-calcitonin was not a useful test for the diagnosis of active TB.

Induced sputum and bronchoscopy in the diagnosis of pulmonary tuberculosis

McWilliams T, Wells AU, Harrison AC, Lindstrom S, Cameron RJ, Foskin E.
Thorax 2002; **57**(12): 1010–14

BACKGROUND. The aim of this study was to compare the efficacy of three induced sputum samples with bronchoscopy for the diagnosis of active pulmonary TB. This comparison was made in patients who produced no sputum or had smear-negative sputum.

INTERPRETATION. Three times-daily induced sputum samples are the recommended next tests in patients being investigated for active TB who produce no sputum or have smear-negative sputum and negate the need for routine bronchoscopy with bronchoalveolar lavage.

Comment

The normal investigation for patients with suspected active pulmonary TB is sending three early morning sputum samples for TB microscopy and culture. Samples can be obtained from patients who do not produce sputum by inducing sputum using hypertonic saline (from 3 to 5%) or bronchoalveolar lavage with bronchoscopy.

There has been increased interest in the use of inducing sputum that is less invasive. This study compared the efficacy of three induced sputum samples with bronchoscopy for the diagnosis of active pulmonary TB in patients who produce no sputum or have smear-negative sputum.

This was a prospective study of patients with possible active pulmonary TB. Patients either produced no sputum or smear-negative sputum. Bronchoscopy was only performed if at least two induced sputum samples were smear negative.

There were 129 patients in this study of median age 38 years. Twenty-seven patients (21%) had smear-negative and TB culture-positive specimens. Thirteen patients were culture positive on induced sputum alone, one patient was culture positive on bronchoscopy alone and 13 were culture positive on both tests.

Induced sputum positivity was more prevalent when chest radiographic appearances showed any features of active TB (20 out of 63 or 32%) than when appearances suggested inactivity (one out of 44 or 2%) (*P* <0.005). Induced sputum was more sensitive than bronchoscopy in diagnosing active TB in this study (*P* <0.005). Six of the 26 patients who were culture positive from the induced sputum samples were positive on one test, seven were positive on two tests and 13 were positive on all three samples.

The induced sputum costs ($370 for three induced sputum samples) were approximately one-third those of bronchoscopy ($1196). There was no account taken for the indirect costs for the three daily induced sputum samples.

In summary, for a patient being investigated for suspected active TB who produces no sputum or has smear-negative sputum the authors suggested that the most effective next strategy is to perform three induced sputum tests over three consecutive days that would avert the routine need for bronchoscopy.

Taking the process a step back, the normal investigation for pulmonary TB is to obtain samples for TB smear and culture. This study did not address whether induced sputum was superior to spontaneous sputum in diagnosing TB. Spontaneous sputum collection is less invasive and the recommended first approach is to send three spontaneous sputum samples for TB smear and culture. In non-sputum producers the next approach is to obtain samples by either induced sputum or bronchoalveolar lavage via the bronchoscope. The authors suggested that, from this study, three induced sputum samples over three consecutive days is the most effective next strategy that would avert the routine need for bronchoscopy. Multiple samples improved the diagnostic yield, with three samples being superior to one or two samples, a similar finding to the results of Al-Zahrani *et al.* |1|. Further studies are needed in order to determine whether there would be similar efficacy with collecting samples over a shorter time period than three consecutive days.

Overall the advantages of induced sputum are that it is a less invasive test and incurs lest cost. However, it requires expertise in the process of inducing sputum with hypertonic saline and appropriate training would be needed. In addition, in view of the high risk of nosocomial TB, induced sputum should be carried out in a negative pressure room and appropriate protective masks should be worn.

Reference

1. Al Zahrani K, Al Jahdali H, Poirier L, Rene P, Menzies D. Yield of smear, culture and amplification tests from repeated sputum induction for the diagnosis of pulmonary TB. *Int J Tuberc Lung Dis* 2001; 5: 855–60.

16

Advances in the management of mycobacterial disease

Introduction

Five papers were selected for this chapter. There has been increased interest in developing simpler regimens in order to improve tuberculosis (TB) completion rates. In view of the long half-life of rifapentine, this has allowed the development of a once-weekly treatment in combination with isoniazid. Unfortunately this regimen had increased failure or relapse rates compared with standard regimens (reviewed last year in *The Year in Respiratory Medicine 2003* [YIRM 2003]) |**1**|. The first paper was a pharmacokinetic study that evaluated the reasons for the reduced efficacy of the once-weekly rifapentine and isoniazid regimen in the continuous phase for pulmonary TB, that is after the first 2 months' initiation phase. The next two papers explored the efficacy of adjunctive treatment with interleukin-2 (IL-2) and arginine in patients with pulmonary TB. The rationale for these adjunctive treatments are discussed in the relevant papers. Traditionally patients with multidrug-resistant TB are treated in hospital using considerable healthcare resources and causing significant social isolation for patients. The next paper explored an alternative management strategy examining the efficacy of outpatient-supervised therapy for multidrug-resistant TB. The final paper examined the 5-year outcome for patients treated for *Mycobacterium malmoense* with rifampicin and ethambutol with or without isoniazid for 2 years. This was an extension of the paper from the Research Committee of the British Thoracic Society (BTS) in 2001 and was reviewed in YIRM 2003 |**2**|.

Low isoniazid concentrations and outcome of tuberculosis treatment with once-weekly isoniazid and rifapentine
Weiner M, Burman W, Vernon A, *et al.*; Tuberculosis Trials Consortium.
Am J Respir Crit Care Med 2003; **167**(10): 1341–7

B A C K G R O U N D . Studies have revealed that the once-weekly combination therapy of rifapentine with isoniazid had higher relapse or failure rates compared with twice-weekly combination therapy with rifampicin and isoniazid in the continuation phase of TB treatment. The aim of this pharmacokinetic study was to evaluate whether insufficient concentrations of rifapentine or isoniazid were responsible for the increased relapse or

failure rates. The authors studied human immunodeficiency virus (HIV) sero-negative patients with either failure (n = 4), relapse (n = 35) or cure (n = 94) who were recruited from a comparative treatment trial |1|.

INTERPRETATION. In the once-weekly regimen with rifapentine and isoniazid, low isoniazid concentrations were associated with failure or relapse whereas there was no association with rifapentine. In order to achieve highly active once-weekly therapy with rifapentine a drug with a consistently greater area under the concentration–time curve than isoniazid may be needed.

Comment

There has been a drive to simplify regimens for the treatment of TB in order to improve compliance and treatment completion rates. However, it is important that these simplified regimens are safe and efficacious.

The long half-life of rifapentine allowed therapy with a once-weekly regimen. The study by the Tuberculosis Trials Consortium |1| revealed that the once-weekly combination therapy of rifapentine with isoniazid had higher relapse or failure rates compared with twice-weekly combination therapy with rifampicin and isoniazid in the continuation phase (that is after the initial 2 months' initiation phase) of TB treatment.

Patients with relapse, failure and cure were selected from this latter study to take part in a pharmacokinetic study evaluating whether low concentrations of rifapentine or isoniazid were responsible for the increased failure or relapse rates.

The authors studied HIV sero-negative patients with either failure (n = 4), relapse (n = 35) or cure (n = 94) from the trial of 1004 patients in HIV sero-negative patients that compared once-weekly rifapentine and isoniazid with a twice-weekly combination of rifampicin and isoniazid in the continuation phase of TB treatment.

Pharmacokinetic studies were carried out in these selected patients (the mean area under the curve concentration during 12 h after dosing was thought to be more important than the peak concentration).

The primary end-point in the study was the area under the curve concentration–time curve for 12 h after the dose of isoniazid, rifampicin and rifapentine.

All the isoniazid pharmacokinetic parameters in the once-weekly rifapentine and isoniazid-treated group (the mean area under the curve concentration during 12 h after dosing, maximal concentration and half-life) were lower among patients with failure or relapse compared with cases that were cured. The median area under the curve concentration for isoniazid was 36 µg/h/ml in failure/relapse versus 56 µg/h/ml in control cases (P = 0.005).

In the twice-weekly rifampicin and isoniazid regimen, the isoniazid area under the curve concentration was not significantly different among patients with failure or relapse compared with cases that were cured. Similarly both the rifampicin and rifapentine area under the curve concentrations were not significantly different among patients with failure or relapse compared with cases that were cured.

In proportional hazard regression analysis after adjustment with known risk factors for failure or relapse, such as a positive sputum culture at 2 months, the isoniazid pharmacokinetic parameters retained their association with failure or relapse, whereas neither rifampicin nor rifapentine was associated with treatment outcome.

Isoniazid acetylator status, as determined by the N-acetyltransferase type 2 geno-type, was associated with the outcome with once-weekly isoniazid and rifapentine. The presence of N-acetyltransferase type 2 genotypes that more rapidly metabolize isoniazid was associated with failure or relapse (P <0.05). This was not seen in the twice-weekly regimen with rifampicin and isoniazid.

In summary, the study supports the suggestion that isoniazid plays a role in the reduced efficacy of the once-weekly rifapentine and isoniazid regime. Therefore, a drug with a consistently greater area under the concentration–time curve than iso-niazid may be needed in order to achieve highly active once-weekly therapy with rifapentine.

Randomized trial of adjunctive interleukin-2 in adults with pulmonary tuberculosis

Johnson JL, Ssekasanvu E, Okwera A, *et al.*; Uganda–Case Western Reserve University Research Collaboration. *Am J Respir Crit Care Med* 2003; **168**(2): 185–91

BACKGROUND. The aim of this study was to assess whether the addition of recombinant human IL-2 to standard TB treatment enhanced the rate of killing of tubercle bacilli in HIV sero-negative adults that had smear-positive, drug-susceptible pulmonary TB.

INTERPRETATION. IL-2 did not enhance bacillary clearance or lead to an improvement in symptoms in HIV sero-negative adults with drug-susceptible pulmonary TB.

Comment

Effective T cell function is central in controlling TB. IL-2 is a cytokine produced by activated T lymphocytes and has a central role in the activation and expansion of T cells. There is frequently deficient IL-2 cell proliferation and decreased IL-2 receptor generation in patients with TB. The hypothesis was that adjunctive treat-ment with IL-2 would enhance the cell-mediated immune response in TB and increase the rate of killing of tubercle bacilli and these effects may be most evident during early treatment, when the bacillary load is high in patients with drug-susceptible TB.

The authors conducted a randomized, controlled trial to evaluate the safety, microbiologic and immunologic effects of IL-2 in HIV sero-negative adults with smear-positive, drug-susceptible pulmonary TB.

Ninety-five HIV sero-negative adults (age 18–50 years) with smear-positive culture-confirmed pulmonary TB were recruited from Uganda. Patients previously treated for TB were excluded and only patients that were fully sensitive to first-line drugs were included in the study. The patients were all treated with 2 months of daily rifampicin, isoniazid, ethambutol and pyrazinamide followed by 4 months' combination therapy with rifampicin and isoniazid. The patients were randomized to receive twice-daily intradermal injections of 225 000 IU recombinant human IL-2 or placebo (5% dextrose) as an adjunct to the above therapy in the first 30 days. The patients were followed up for 1 year after initiation of the TB therapy.

The primary end-points in the study were the proportions of patients with sputum culture conversion (culture positive to negative) after 1 and 2 months of treatment and the safety and tolerability of the recombinant human IL-2.

Forty-eight patients were randomized to receive IL-2 and 47 received placebo. There were no treatment failures or deaths. There was one relapse in each group, which was the same isolate and none had acquired drug resistance.

After 1 month, the proportion of patients for whom sputum culture converted to negative was 17% for the IL-2 group compared with 30% in the control group ($P = 0.14$). After 2 months 77% in the IL-2 group were culture negative compared with 85% of those receiving placebo ($P = 0.29$).

There were no differences in weight gain and no improvement in fever, cough and chest pain between groups.

There was no dose reduction or discontinuation in the group receiving IL-2. Local pain, tenderness on palpation, erythema, ecchymoses and temporary hyperpigmentation at the injection site occurred more frequently ($P < 0.01$) in the patients receiving IL-2.

In summary, immunotherapy with IL-2 was generally safe and well tolerated. However, immunotherapy during the first 30 days of TB treatment did not enhance bacillary clearance or improve the symptoms in HIV sero-negative adults with drug-susceptible pulmonary TB. Further studies are needed in order to assess the role of immunotherapy with IL-2 in HIV-positive patients with pulmonary TB and in patients with multidrug-resistant TB.

Arginine as an adjuvant to chemotherapy improves clinical outcome in active tuberculosis
Schon T, Elias D, Moges F, *et al. Eur Respir J* 2003; **21**(3): 483–8

BACKGROUND. The hypothesis of this study was that patients with active TB would be prone to developing deficiency of the amino acid arginine due to increased catabolism and reduced energy intake and this could limit one of the mycobactericidal pathways, the production of nitric oxide from arginine. The aim of this randomized, controlled study was to study the efficacy of arginine as an adjuvant to standard anti-TB treatment.

INTERPRETATION. Adjuvant treatment with 1 g/day arginine for 4 weeks in HIV-negative patients with active pulmonary TB led to improvements in symptoms and sputum conversion (sputum smear positive to three consecutive negative smears for TB) at 8 weeks. However, this positive effect with arginine was not seen in patients with active pulmonary TB who were HIV positive.

Comment

Nitric oxide is thought to be involved in the host defence against TB. Patients with TB exhibit increased catabolism and reduced energy intake and the hypothesis for this study was that restoring a relative deficiency in the amino acid arginine, the substrate for mycobactericidal nitric oxide production, would improve the clinical outcome of TB by increasing nitric oxide production.

Patients with smear-positive pulmonary TB ($n = 120$) were given arginine or placebo for 4 weeks in addition to conventional anti-TB treatment in a randomized, double-blind study. This was a study carried out in Ethiopia and there were sputum smears using Ziehl Neelson staining, but no TB cultures were carried out.

The anti-TB treatment regimen used was 2 months of rifampicin, isoniazid, pyrazinamide and ethambutol or streptomycin followed by 6 months of isoniazid and ethambutol. In the first 4 weeks of treatment the patients were randomized to receive 1 g/day arginine or placebo. All treatment was supervised.

The primary outcomes in this study were sputum conversion from smear-positive TB to three consecutive negative smears for TB, weight gain and clinical symptoms after week 8.

One hundred and twenty patients with smear-positive pulmonary TB were recruited and there was a high HIV prevalence (52.5%) in this study. Twenty-four received arginine (mean age 28.8 years) and 32 received placebo (mean age 29.9 years) in the HIV-negative group while 33 received arginine (mean age 29.1 years) and 26 received placebo (mean age 30.8 years) in the HIV-positive group.

The group of HIV-negative patients who received supplemental arginine had increased sputum conversion at 8 weeks (100% compared with 84% in the placebo group) ($P < 0.05$) and a reduced prevalence of cough (25% compared with 66% in the placebo group) ($P < 0.05$). There was no significant difference from placebo in weight gain.

The arginine level in the arginine-treated group increased from 100.2 µM at baseline (range 90.5–109.9 µM) to 142.1 µM (range 114.1–170.1 µM) at 2 weeks compared with the placebo group with 105.5 µM (range 93.7–117.3 µM) at baseline and 95.7 µM (range 82.4–108.9 µM) at 2 weeks.

There was no improvement with arginine in the HIV-positive patients. Subgroup analysis demonstrated that the patients most likely to benefit were HIV-negative patients who were depleted in arginine with baseline serum arginine concentrations <103.0 µM.

In summary, in this study arginine was beneficial as an adjuvant treatment in HIV-negative patients with active pulmonary TB, which was most likely mediated by increased production of nitric oxide. This is an interesting finding and supports the suggestion that arginine may be a useful adjunct to conventional anti-TB treatment. It is unlikely that this adjunct to treatment will be used in clinical practice until this small preliminary study is confirmed with larger multicentred studies. It will be important in these studies that formal TB cultures are part of these studies in order to confirm the diagnosis of *Mycobacterium tuberculosis* with certainty.

Community-based therapy for multidrug-resistant tuberculosis in Lima, Peru

Mitnick C, Bayona J, Palacios E, *et al. N Engl J Med* 2003; **348**(2): 119–28

BACKGROUND. Treatment for multidrug-resistant TB is normally recommended in centres with experience in multidrug-resistant TB, often requiring prolonged treatment in hospital. The aim of this study was to evaluate community-based therapy for multidrug-resistant TB in a poor section of Lima, Peru.

INTERPRETATION. Community-based, outpatient treatment of multidrug-resistant TB can yield high cure rates in patients who tolerate treatment with five drugs that patients were susceptible to from *in vitro* drug susceptibility tests for at least 18 months.

Comment

Traditionally patients with multidrug-resistant TB should ideally be treated in centres with experience of multidrug-resistant TB. Patients usually have supervised treatment in hospital for many months, usually until the patients are deemed non-infectious, that is when their TB cultures have converted to negative. The aim of this study was to assess the efficacy of community-based, outpatient treatment.

The authors described 75 patients who received ambulatory treatment with individualized regimens for chronic multidrug-resistant TB. A retrospective review of their charts was carried out (August 1996 to February 1999) and predictors of poor outcomes were identified.

The patients received supervised therapy on an outpatient basis. They were treated with at least five drugs that patients were susceptible to from *in vitro* drug susceptibility tests for at least 18 months. A parenteral agent was administered for at least 6 months after culture conversion, that is a change from TB culture positive to culture negative. Treatment was terminated after twelve or more consecutive negative cultures.

Probable cure was defined as at least 12 months of consecutive negative cultures during therapy. Treatment failure was defined as the presence of a positive culture after 6 months of treatment. Withdrawal of therapy was defined by ≥ 1 month of missed therapy in the first year or ≥ 2 months of missed therapy in the second year. Relapse was defined as two or more positive cultures after completion of treatment among patients whose treatment outcome was probable cure.

Seventy-five patients with multidrug-resistant pulmonary TB with a median age of 26.8 years were treated. The infecting strains of *M. tuberculosis* were resistant to a median of six drugs. Only one out of 65 patients tested was HIV positive. Eighty-six per cent had a low body mass index (BMI) (<20 kg/m^2 in men and <18.5 kg/m^2 in females), 37% had a low haematocrit and 23% had a history of homelessness, imprisonment, other institutionalization or addiction to drugs or alcohol. The patients were treated with a median of six drugs for a median of 23 months.

Eighty-eight per cent managed to take therapy for ≥4 months. The other 12% died within the first 4 months (three with massive haemoptysis, five with respiratory failure and one of unknown cause). Overall 83% of the 66 patients who completed ≥4 months of therapy were probably cured at the completion of treatment. Eight per cent withdrew from therapy and 8% died while receiving therapy (two with respiratory failure, one with multi-organ failure and two of unknown cause). There was only one treatment failure. The patients were followed for a median of 40 months after therapy and there was only one relapse or reinfection with multidrug-resistant TB, which was 23 weeks after completion.

In univariate analysis a low haematocrit (hazard ratio [HR] = 5.17 and 95% confidence interval [CI] = 2.03–13.17) (P <0.001) and low BMI (HR = 5.13 and 95% CI = 1.68–15.69) (P = 0.004) were associated with a poor outcome during therapy and follow-up. In a multiple Cox proportional hazards regression model, the predictors of the time to treatment failure or death were a low haematocrit (HR = 4.09 and 95% CI = 1.35–12.36) and possibly a low BMI (HR = 3.23 and 95% CI = 0.90–11.53) (P = 0.07).

In summary, community-based, outpatient treatment of multidrug-resistant TB can yield high cure rates if patients are able to tolerate the cocktail of drugs usually for at least 18 months. This was a very effective programme for treating multidrug-resistant TB out in the community and all therapy was directly supervised. Patients will clearly prefer this outpatient regimen and it will have significant cost benefits compared with inpatient treatment. However, community treatment is only feasible if supervised therapy can be provided at home, there are adequate social circumstances at home, there is effective community back-up and there is no significant concern about the spread of disease in the patient's home environment.

Pulmonary disease caused by *Mycobacterium malmoense* in HIV-negative patients: 5-year follow-up of patients receiving standardized treatment

Research Committee of the British Thoracic Society. *Eur Respir J* 2003; **21**(3): 478–82

BACKGROUND. This prospective study examined the long-term outcome and 5-year follow-up of patients receiving standardized treatment for pulmonary disease caused *by* **M. malmoense** in HIV-negative patients.

INTERPRETATION. Pulmonary disease caused by *M. malmoense* is a serious condition that is associated with high morbidity and mortality. Rifampicin and ethambutol, with or without isoniazid, cured only 42% of patients at 5 years. The results of standard susceptibility tests did not correlate with the bacteriological response of the disease to antimycobacterial therapy. There is a need for more effective regimens that will reduce the mortality and failure of treatment/relapse rates, but, in addition, attention should be directed at improving the management of co-morbid conditions and improving the general health of the patient.

Comment

This randomized, controlled trial |2| confirmed that 2 years of rifampicin and etham-butol proved equivalent to 2 years of rifampicin, ethambutol and isoniazid after 3 years' follow-up after treatment ended for patients with *M. malmoense*.

The patients recruited for this study were ≥16 years old, had two or more positive sputum cultures for *M. malmoense* and had radiological changes compatible with mycobacterial pulmonary disease. All were HIV negative. The patients were random-ized to receive 2 years' daily therapy with 600 mg of rifampicin (450 mg if <50 kg) and 15 mg/kg ethambutol or triple therapy with rifampicin, ethambutol and isoni-azid. After completing treatment the patients were followed for 3 years.

Failure of treatment was defined as remaining culture positive for *M. malmoense* for >21 months. Patients with negative cultures in the last 3 months of treatment and whose sputum remained culture negative in the subsequent 3 years were classed as cured.

In over 5 years a total of 106 patients were recruited to the study. Their mean age was 58 years (range 24–89 years). A total of 58% were male, 55% previously or at the time of the study had other lung diseases (chronic obstructive pulmonary disease, asthma, old, healed TB and bronchiectasis) and 20% had worked in jobs involving dust.

Sputum was positive on direct smear in 58% and cavitation was seen on the chest radiographs of 74%, the majority having cavities of ≥2 cm in diameter. Forty-eight per cent showed bilateral disease and disease was confined to the upper zone(s) in 30%.

As stated in the introduction this randomized, controlled trial showed equiva-lence independent of the treatment regimen. A total of 59% of patients were alive at 5 years, 42% of whom completed treatment and were alive and cured. Thirty-four per cent died, 11% of whom (four out of 36 deaths) died from *M. malmoense*. The causes of death in the other 32 patients were not attributed to *M. malmoense* and they died from a variety of causes (respiratory failure, lung cancer, pneumonia, ischaemic heart disease, cerebrovascular disease, rectal cancer and suicide). Ten per cent failed treatment or relapsed after the end of treatment, but there was no correlation between the failure of treatment/relapse and *in vitro* resistance. The outcome was unknown in 7% (Table 16.1).

Cavitation was still present in 76% of 50 patients radiographed after 5 years, com-pared with 74% of all 106 patients at entry.

In summary, pulmonary disease caused by *M. malmoense* is a serious condition that is associated with high morbidity and mortality. There was equivalence regard-less of whether 2 years' daily combination with rifampicin and ethambutol or rifampicin, ethambutol and isoniazid was used. However, rifampicin and etham-butol, with or without isoniazid, only cured 42% of patients at 5 years. The results of standard susceptibility tests did not correlate with the bacteriological response of the disease to chemotherapy.

There is a need for more effective regimens that will reduce the mortality and failure of treatment/relapse rates, but, in addition, attention should be directed at

Table 16.1 *Mycobacterium malmoense (M. malmoense)* pulmonary disease: results during and after treatment

	R and E	R, E and H	Total
Patients *n*	52	54	106
Outcome unknown	3	4	7 (7)
Alive at 5 yrs	32	21	63 (59)
Deaths			
All causes	17	19	36 (34)
M. malmoense	1	3	4 (4)
Failures of treatment and relapses	6	5*	11* (10)
Completed treatment allocated and alive and cured after 5 yrs	20	24	44 (42)

Data presented as *n* or *n* (%). R, rifampicin; E, ethambutol; H, isoniazid. *One patient died.
Source: The Research Committee of the British Thoracic Society (2003).

improving the management of co-morbid conditions and improving the patients' general health. The results from a randomized, controlled trial conducted by the BTS with rifampicin and ethambutol and the addition of either ciprofloxacin or clarithromycin and/or the addition of *Mycobacterium vaccae* are currently awaited.

References

1. Benator D, Bhattacharya M, Bozeman L, Burman W, Cantazaro A, Chaisson R, Gordin F, Horsburgh CR, Horton J, Khan A, Lahart C, Metchock B, Pachucki C, Stanton L, Vernon A, Villarino ME, Wang YC, Weiner M, Weis S; The Tuberculosis Trials Consortium. Rifapentine and isoniazid once a week versus rifampicin and isoniazid twice a week for treatment of drug-susceptible pulmonary tuberculosis in HIV-negative patients: a randomised clinical trial. *Lancet* 2002; **360**(9332): 528–34.
2. The Research Committee of the British Thoracic Society. First randomised trial of treatments for pulmonary disease caused by *Mycobacterium avium intracellulare, Mycobacterium malmoense,* and *Mycobacterium xenopi* in HIV negative patients: rifampicin, ethambutol and isoniazid versus rifampicin and ethambutol. *Thorax* 2001; **56**(3): 167–72.

17

Pleural tuberculosis

Introduction

Patients with pleural tuberculosis (TB) usually present with a unilateral pleural effusion and there may or may not be associated parenchymal abnormalities. The combination of a pleural aspirate and pleural biopsy gives the highest diagnostic yield for diagnosing pleural TB and allows the exclusion of other pathologies such as cancer.

The pleural aspirate should be sent for measurement of pH, protein and glucose (in tuberculous empyema the pH is <7.2, the protein is >30 g/l and the pleural glucose:blood glucose ratio is <0.5). The pleural fluid should be sent for routine smear and culture in order to exclude a complicated parapneumonic effusion or empyema, for a TB smear and culture and for cytology (a predominant lymphocytosis is seen in a tuberculous pleural effusion). The pleural biopsy should be sent in normal saline for smear and TB culture and in formaldehyde for histological examination (examining for evidence of granulomas with central caseating necrosis with/without the identification of *Mycobacterium tuberculosis*).

Alternative methods have been used for investigating pleural TB and the first paper selected investigated the use of induced sputum in the diagnosis of pleural TB in patients with and without parenchymal abnormalities. Alternatively researchers have investigated whether adenosine deaminase and interferon-γ (IFN-γ) from pleural fluid may be also useful adjuncts to the investigation of pleural TB. However, they are not currently available for routine clinical testing.

The majority of human immunodeficiency virus (HIV)-negative patients with TB pleural effusion have adenosine deaminase concentrations from pleural fluid >47 U/l, due principally to the monocytes producing adenosine deaminase isoenzyme 2. However, increased concentrations of adenosine deaminase have been found in patients with other conditions such as non-tuberculous empyema and rheumatoid arthritis-related pleural effusions. In addition, lower concentrations have been found in patients with acquired immune deficiency syndrome who have TB-related pleural effusions. However, a recent study by Jimenez Castro *et al.* [1] has shown that adenosine deaminase concentrations <40 U/l excluded TB in 99% of patients with lymphocytic pleural effusions. The gold standard remains pleural aspiration and pleural biopsy for microbiological confirmation with sensitivity tests and to exclude other diagnoses. Adenosine deaminase measurement from pleural fluid is not available for routine clinical testing, but may be a useful adjunct to the other pleural fluid and biopsy results. The next paper selected explored the measurement of IFN-γ from pleural fluid and its utility for the diagnosis of pleural TB.

The final paper was a randomized, controlled study that assessed the efficacy of pleural drainage (pigtail drainage) as an adjunct to anti-TB treatment in TB pleural effusion.

Yield of sputum induction in the diagnosis of pleural tuberculosis

Conde MB, Loivos AC, Rezende VM, *et al. Am J Respir Crit Care Med* 2003;
167(5): 723–5

BACKGROUND. The aim of this study was to evaluate the diagnostic yield of acid-fast bacilli smear and culture prospectively for *M. tuberculosis* using sputum induction in the work-up of patients with suspected pleural TB.

INTERPRETATION. The yield of induced sputum cultures is high in patients suspected of having pleural TB, even in those cases with no pulmonary parenchymal abnormalities on a chest radiograph (induced sputum TB culture positive in 55%). Combining the use of pleural fluid, pleural biopsy and induced sputum, the use of induced sputum on its own led to an early diagnosis (smear positive on direct smear) in 2% of cases and a later diagnosis following TB cultures in 15% of cases.

Comment

Investigation of pleural TB is a common clinical problem. A chest radiograph will normally reveal a unilateral pleural effusion that may occur in the presence or absence of pulmonary parenchymal disease.

The pleural fluid associated with TB contains a relatively small number of organisms. The conventional investigations are a pleural aspirate and a blind pleural biopsy. The aim of this study was to assess the value of induced sputum for TB smear and culture in the investigation of pleural TB.

One hundred and thirteen adult patients (age 18 years old and over) who were clinically and radiologically suspected as having pleural TB were studied. None were able to expectorate sputum spontaneously.

All patients studied had a clinical assessment, HIV test, pleural aspirate, pleural biopsy (five samples, two of which were for TB smear and culture and three for histological assessment) and induced sputum using hypertonic saline. The samples were stained with Ziehl Neelsen stain, Grocot's methenamine silver stain and samples were cultured on Lowenstein Jensen and Sabouroud medium. In addition, pleural biopsy samples were stained with haematoxylin and eosin and the rest of the pleural fluid stained with Papanicolaou.

A diagnosis of pleural TB was made on the growth of *M. tuberculosis* on pleural fluid and/or tissue culture, granulomatous inflammation on the pleural biopsy or a presumptive diagnosis after a clinical and radiological improvement following 3 months' anti-TB treatment.

Pleural TB was diagnosed in 84 patients (71 HIV sero-negative). The patients' mean age was 37.2 ± 14.6 years. Ninety-six per cent had pleural effusions less than half a hemithorax. The majority (76%) had no pulmonary parenchymal abnormalities. All pleural fluids were exudative and 84% were lymphocytic effusions (differential counts from pleural fluid analysis revealed >80% lymphocytes).

Histopathologic examination of the pleural biopsy tissue had the highest diagnostic yield (78%). The bacteriologic yield for TB cultures was 62% for the pleural tissue and 52% for induced sputum cultures, but only 12% for pleural fluid cultures (Table 17.1).

On direct smear, the samples were smear positive in 17% for pleural tissue and 12% for induced sputum, but only 2% for pleural fluid (Table 17.1).

Combining the use of pleural fluid, pleural biopsy and induced sputum, the use of induced sputum on its own led to an early diagnosis (smear positive on direct smear) in 2% of cases and a later diagnosis following TB cultures in 15% of cases.

The yield of induced sputum culture for *M. tuberculosis* was 55% (35 out of 64) in patients with a normal radiograph (except for the pleural effusion) and 45% (nine out of 20) in those with evidence of parenchymal disease suggestive of pulmonary TB ($P = 0.6$). There were no serious adverse effects with sputum induction.

In summary, the pleural aspirate and biopsy remain the gold standards for the diagnosis of suspected TB-related pleural effusion. It helps exclude other potential diagnoses such as non-TB parapneumonic effusions or cancer, but also helps to obtain bacterial confirmation of *M. tuberculosis* with sensitivity results.

Table 17.1 Yield of diagnostic methods in 84 cases of tuberculous pleural effusions

Method of diagnosis	Total ($n = 84$)	HIV seronegative ($n = 71$)	HIV seropositive ($n = 13$)	P-value*
Presumptive diagnosis	5 (6)	5 (7)	0	1.0
Pleural biopsy tissue	78 (93)	65 (91)	13 (100)	0.58
Bacteriologic diagnosis	52 (62)	42 (59)	10 (77)	0.36
AFB smear positive	14 (17)	9 (13)	5 (38)	0.06
Culture for *M.tb* positive	52 (62)	42 (59)	10 (77)	0.36
Histologic diagnosis	66 (78)	54 (76)	12 (92)	0.28
Pleural fluid	10 (12)	7 (10)	3 (23)	0.18
AFB smear positive	2 (2)	1 (1)	1 (8)	0.28
Culture for *M.tb* positive	9 (11)	7 (10)	2 (15)	0.62
Sputum induction	44 (52)	34 (48)	10 (77)	0.10
AFB smear positive	10 (12)	7 (10)	3 (23)	0.18
Culture for *M.tb* positive	44 (52)	34 (48)	10 (77)	0.10

AFB, acid fast bacilli; *M.tb*, *Mycobacterium tuberculosis*.
* P-value of the yield of diagnostic methods between HIV-seronegative and HIV-seropositive tuberculous pleural patients.
n, number of cases (%).
Source: Conde *et al.* (2003).

The study reminds us of the low yield from direct smear results from pleural fluid, pleural biopsy or induced sputum, which reflects the low bacterial load in patients with TB pleural effusions. Both histology and TB cultures reveal the greatest diagnostic yield, but the results from TB cultures can take up to 8 weeks. Independent of the presence or absence of pulmonary parenchymal abnormalities, induced sputum can be a useful adjunct to the investigation.

A strategy of sending the combination of spontaneous sputum if present, induced sputum if there is no spontaneous sputum, pleural fluid and pleural biopsies for TB smear, culture and histology should lead to an improved diagnostic yield for the investigation of TB-related pleural effusions.

Interferon gamma levels in pleural fluid for the diagnosis of tuberculosis

Villena V, Lopez-Encuentra A, Pozo F, *et al. Am J Med* 2003; **115**(5): 365–70

BACKGROUND. The aim of this large study (595 cases) was to assess the utility of IFN-γ levels from pleural fluid, including identification of the best cut-off for the diagnosis of tuberculous pleural effusions.

INTERPRETATION. Elevated pleural IFN-γ levels (>3.7 IU/ml) are valuable in diagnosing pleural TB. Patients with pleural effusion due to haematological neoplasms occasionally have levels slightly above the cut-off.

Comment

The diagnosis of TB pleural effusion can be difficult. This study assessed the value of the measurement of IFN-γ from pleural fluid in determining whether it helped in the diagnosis of pleural TB.

The authors prospectively studied 595 patients that had pleural effusions. The diagnosis of pleural TB was based on positive cultures from fluid or tissue, granulomas seen on histology from the pleural biopsy in the absence of other pleural granulomatous diseases, patients with a diagnosis of extra-pleural TB that had responded to anti-TB treatment or patients ≤40 years who responded clinically to anti-TB treatment who had either a positive skin test or ≥95% lymphocytes in their pleural fluid.

There were 595 patients with a median age of 65 years. There were 82 patients with TB pleural effusion and 513 with non-tuberculous pleural effusions (231 had neoplasms, 89 had parapneumonic effusions, 75 had transudates, 68 were miscellaneous and 50 were of unknown aetiology).

IFN-γ levels were measured blindly by radioimmunoassay. A cut-off of 3.7 IU/ml yielded a sensitivity of 0.98 (95% confidence interval [CI] = 0.91–1.00) and a specificity of 0.98 (95% CI = 0.96–0.99). The areas under the receiver operating characteristic curves and the test's sensitivity and specificity were similar among patients of different ages and by the percentage of lymphocytes in the pleural fluid.

The cut-off of 3.7 IU/ml yielded twelve false-positive results (seven with cancer, five of whom had haematological malignancies, three of whom had para-pneumonic effusions and two of whom had transudates with values >3.7 IU) and two false-negative results. There were few patients studied with connective tissue disease, vasculitis or other granulomatous disease apart from TB.

In summary, this study supports the diagnostic use of IFN-γ from pleural fluid for the diagnosis of pleural TB and that a concentration >3.7 IU/ml strongly supports the diagnosis.

If pleural TB is suspected, pleural aspiration and biopsy still remain the first-line tests, not only for confirming the diagnosis and excluding other pathologies that can mimic TB, but also for obtaining bacterial confirmation of *M. tuberculosis* with sensitivity results. However, it is true to say that direct smears are often unhelpful in pleural TB and that normally a more definitive result comes from histology and TB cultures. Both IFN-γ or adenosine deaminase from pleural fluid may be useful adjunct investigations at baseline, which should be additive to the pleural fluid and biopsy results, allowing the clinician to treat with more confidence. At present, however, the measurement of IFN-γ or adenosine deaminase from pleural fluid is not available for routine clinical testing.

Pigtail drainage in the treatment of tuberculous pleural effusions: a randomized study
Lai YF, Chao TY, Wang YH, Lin AS. *Thorax* 2003; **58**(2): 149–51

BACKGROUND. The aim of this randomized, controlled study was to assess the efficacy of pleural drainage (pigtail drainage) as an adjunct to anti-TB treatment in TB pleural effusion.

INTERPRETATION. Compared with anti-TB treatment alone, pleural drainage as an adjunct with anti-TB treatment led to quicker relief of breathlessness, but had no impact on the symptoms (dyspnoea, cough, night sweating, fatigue, appetite, pleurisy and general well-being) plotted on the visual analogue scale (from 1 week to 6 months) or forced vital capacity (FVC) or residual pleural thickening at the end of treatment (6 months).

Comment

The conventional treatment for TB pleural effusions is 6 months' anti-TB treatment (assuming fully sensitive, an initial 2 months' treatment with rifampicin, isoniazid, ethambutol and pyrazinamide followed by 4 months of rifampicin and isoniazid). Residual pleural thickening is a common sequala, approximately 50%, being evident post-treatment. To try and reduce this sequala some advocate the addition of oral corticosteroids, but this approach has little evidence base to back this recommendation. This randomized, controlled study evaluated the efficacy of draining the pleural effusion with a pigtail drain over standard anti-TB treatment.

Sixty-one patients with tuberculous pleurisy were divided into two groups:

30 patients received pigtail drainage combined with anti-TB drug treatment and 31 received only anti-TB drugs.

The end-points in this study were the number of days fever and breathlessness persisted after treatment initiation, the change in the visual analogue score on symptoms (dyspnoea, cough, night sweating, fatigue, appetite, pleurisy and general wellbeing), FVC and assessment of residual pleural thickening at 6 months, the end of treatment.

The median age was 61.5 years (standard deviation [SD] 17.7 years) and 93% had a pleural effusion more than one-third of a hemithorax.

Although the duration of dyspnoea was significantly shortened by the use of pigtail drainage (median 4 days and interquartile range [IQR] 4–5 days versus 8 days and IQR 7–16 days) (P <0.001) in patients treated with anti-TB medication only, there was no effect on the duration of fever (median 0 days and IQR 0–6 days for the pigtail group and median 0 days and IQR 0–5 days for the group treated with anti-TB medication only).

A comparison of the combined mean ($\pm$SD) visual analogue scale scores showed no significant difference between the groups after 1 week of treatment (57.1 $\pm$ 33.2 for pigtail drainage versus 68.5 $\pm$ 44.7 for anti-TB medication only or at any time during the follow-up period). The incidence of residual pleural thickening of more than 10 mm in the group treated with pigtail drainage and anti-TB drugs was 26% compared with 28% in the group receiving drug treatment only. The incidences of residual pleural thickening levels of more than 2 mm in the two groups were 50 and 51%, respectively. No statistical difference between the two groups in terms of FVC was found at 6 months, the end of treatment (median 85.5% and IQR 69–94% of predicted for the pigtail drainage group versus median 88% and IQR 78–96% of predicted for the drug treatment only group).

All patients were cured with 6 months' therapy. There was no morbidity related to pigtail drainage.

In summary, this randomized, controlled trial revealed that anti-TB treatment alone was effective in the treatment of pleural TB. In clinical practice, the pleural effusions normally resorb with anti-TB treatment without the need to insert an intercostal chest drain. However, intercostal chest drains should be used if there is a clinical need to relieve breathlessness.

Reference

1. Jimenez Castro D, Diaz Nuevo G, Perez-Rodriguez E, Light RW. Diagnostic value of adenosine deaminase in nontuberculous lymphocytic pleural effusions. *Eur Respir J* 2003; 21(2): 220–4.

Overall conclusion

The 15 papers selected for this section have been clinically useful in the management of patients with TB. Chapter 13 has three papers on treatment for latent TB. The World Health Organization estimated that one-third of the world is latently infected with *M. tuberculosis* and clinicians regularly treat patients with latent TB in clinical practice. The most widely used treatment has remained 6–9 months' isoniazid therapy. Although this therapy is safe with a small risk of hepatotoxicity, the length of treatment is cumbersome and treatment completion rates are thus suboptimal. In light of this there has been a drive for shorter regimens and there has been much interest in the 2-month regimen with rifampicin and pyrazinamide. Unfortunately the side effects are greater with this shortened regimen, in particular hepatotoxicity and again the completion rates are still suboptimal. If this regimen is used then it would be recommended that there is closer monitoring, in particular liver function test measurements, whilst on therapy. This regimen will likely be favoured by patients due to the shorter course, clinicians are likely to use it if the patient requires supervision of therapy and it will be used in patients who are intolerant of isoniazid or who have been in contact with a known case of isoniazid-resistant TB. There needs to be continuing research into simpler regimens in order to improve treatment completion rates.

Chapter 14 investigated the side effects from the first-line anti-TB drugs, including the risks of hepatotoxicity. The main offender appears to be pyrazinamide and this agent is more likely to cause side effects, in particular drug rash and hepatotoxicity, than rifampicin, isoniazid or ethambutol. Hepatotoxicity caused by the anti-TB drugs is due to both clinical and genetic factors.

Chapter 15 explored the role of serum pro-calcitonin and induced sputum in the diagnosis of pulmonary TB. Although serum pro-calcitonin has been found to have a role in the diagnosis of ventilator-associated pneumonia, its measurement was not useful in cases with TB and did not help differentiate TB from other lower respiratory tract illness. Three spontaneous sputum samples should be sent for TB smear and culture in patients with suspected pulmonary TB. If there is no sputum production, then there is evidence that three, daily, induced sputum samples should be sent for TB smear and culture. This strategy was found to be less invasive, more effective and less costly than bronchoscopy with bronchoalveolar lavage.

Chapter 16 was on advances in the management of mycobacterial disease. There has been a new treatment strategy for patients in the continuation phase of TB treatment, that is after the initial 2 months' initiation phase. The long half-life of rifapentine has allowed a once-weekly regimen with 600 mg of rifapentine and 15 mg/kg (maximum 900 mg) isoniazid. Unfortunately this regimen had higher relapse or failure rates compared with the standard treatment of twice-weekly rifampicin and isoniazid. Pharmacokinetic studies have revealed that the problem relates to inadequate concentrations of isoniazid and other alternative agents may be required if the once-weekly rifapentine regimen is to be successful. The next two papers explored the efficacy of adding interleukin-2 (IL-2) and arginine to standard TB treatment in patients with smear-positive pulmonary TB. IL-2 was not additive to standard treatment and does not have a role in the current management of HIV-negative cases with pulmonary TB. Further studies are needed in HIV-positive cases with pulmonary TB and in cases with multidrug resistant-TB. The preliminary study with arginine replacement suggested that arginine replacement may be beneficial particularly in TB cases that were arginine deficient. This is an interesting small study, but it is not likely to change clinical practice until there are further larger studies. The next paper treated multidrug-resistant TB cases in the community using supervised therapy. In patients that were able to complete treatment there were high cure rates. Currently clinicians managing patients with multidrug-resistant TB in many countries manage these cases as inpatients in hospital until the cases are non-infectious with negative TB cultures. This uses considerable healthcare resources and causes significant social isolation for the patient. This outpatient regime could be modelled in other countries if the community back-up is available for supervised therapy, there is adequate social support and there are adequate home circumstances to limit spread of the disease. The final paper in this chapter was the 5-year outcome of treatment of *Mycobacterium malmoense*. We wait with interest the results of whether there are improved outcomes with treatment with rifampicin and ethambutol and either ciprofloxacin or clarithromycin with or without *Mycobacterium vaccae* from the British Thoracic Society study.

Chapter 17 was on pleural TB. If pleural TB is suspected, pleural aspiration and biopsy still remain the first-line tests, not only for confirming the diagnosis and excluding other pathologies that can mimic TB, but also for obtaining bacterial confirmation of *M. tuberculosis* with sensitivity results.

There is usually a low yield from direct smear results from pleural fluid, pleural biopsy or induced sputum, which reflects the low bacterial load in patients with TB pleural effusions. Both histology and TB cultures reveal the greatest diagnostic yield, but the results from TB cultures can take up to 8 weeks. Independent of the presence or absence of pulmonary parenchymal abnormalities, induced sputum can be a useful adjunct to the investigation. A strategy of sending the combination of spontaneous sputum if present, induced sputum if there is no spontaneous sputum, pleural fluid and pleural biopsies for TB smear, culture and histology should lead to an improved diagnostic yield for the investigation of TB-related pleural effusions.

Both IFN-γ or adenosine deaminase from pleural fluid may be useful adjunct investigations at baseline, which should be additive to the pleural fluid and biopsy results, allowing the clinician to treat with more confidence. At present, however, the measurement of IFN-γ or adenosine deaminase from pleural fluid is not available for routine clinical testing.

Part V

Pneumonia and its causes

Pneumonia and its causes

J SIMPSON

Introduction

Pneumonia is a significant problem throughout the world, particularly at the extremes of life. Over 2 million children under the age of 5 years die with pneumonia every year |**1**|, largely in developing countries. While improvement of this damning statistic is partly dependent on politicians, pharmaceutical companies and healthcare organizers, it is beholden upon the medical profession to improve the prevention, diagnosis and treatment of pneumonia. However, the problems caused by pneumonia are clearly not exclusive to developing countries. 'Pneumonia and influenza' together made up the seventh commonest cause of all deaths in the USA in 1999, becoming still more important among the elderly |**2**|. The attendant health costs are enormous |**3**|.

This depressing outlook is now haunted by the increasing global spread of antibiotic resistance. While this problem is particularly important in the hospital environment, there is no doubt that antibiotic resistance among community-acquired infection is increasing. Indeed, the rates of penicillin resistance among isolates of *Streptococcus pneumoniae*, the principal cause of community-acquired pneumonia, have been described at over 50% in specific locations |**4**|.

The mortality associated with pneumonia and the spread of antibiotic resistance were of course well recognized in late 2002. What the medical community could not anticipate was the emergence of severe acute respiratory syndrome (SARS), a new highly infectious form of pneumonia with a significant associated mortality |**5**|. The rapid identification of the causative agent, which is discussed later in this section (p. 267), should be regarded as a significant scientific breakthrough of 2003. It is interesting to reflect that the study of pneumonia over the last 50 years has been characterized by the emergence of newly identified pathogens from *Mycoplasma pneumoniae*, to the first outbreak of Legionnaire's disease, infections such as *Pneumocystis carinii* pneumonia associated with the human immunodeficiency virus (HIV) epidemic, the emergent antibiotic-resistant nosocomial pneumonias and now SARS. Within this fascinating array of pathogens we must not forget the influenza pandemics that cost millions of lives as a consequence of secondary pneumonia in the last century.

Against this background a huge amount of basic and clinical research is required in order to advance understanding of the biology of pneumonia, with the aim of improving prevention and treatment. It is important to recognize that refinements in vaccines in recent years have generated great promise with regard to the prevention of influenza and streptococcal disease. Further understanding of host–pathogen interactions and of the adaptive immune response is required, but vaccine programmes are particularly attractive options for the future because they can potentially prevent antibiotic-resistant as well as antibiotic-sensitive pneumonia. It should also be emphasized that the last few years have seen a more systematic approach to clinical research into community-acquired pneumonia. As a result of this we can expect further evidence-based guidelines regarding which patients can be safely managed at home and how to stratify management for those patients at risk of death from pneumonia.

This section was written with the above considerations in mind. The aim was to cover a variety of clinical problems across a spectrum of pathogens (bacteria, viruses and fungi) in different age groups (but concentrating mainly on adult pneumonia) and in different settings (nosocomial and community-acquired pneumonia). The emphasis is deliberately on the prevention and treatment of pneumonia. Only original articles have been selected, reporting randomized, controlled trials where possible. However, the reader should be aware that several important consensus statements and comprehensive reviews of pneumonia have been published recently |**6–9**|.

The section is divided into four chapters: Prophylaxis and vaccination against infection, Viral infections and their treatment, Community-acquired pneumonia and Miscellaneous respiratory infections (incorporating nosocomial and aspiration pneumonia).

How to take key messages from this section

The chapters are written so that the key messages can be extracted by reading only the Background and Interpretation sections. The Comment section for each paper is designed for the reader who would like more detailed information without necessarily going to the original paper. The Comment sections therefore generally start with an outline of the methods used, followed by a more detailed description of the results, then an attempt to outline the strengths and potential limitations of each study, ending with a short conclusion. It should be noted that the papers in this section were specifically chosen because of their significant contribution to the field and the discussion of methodological limitations is simply designed to give a feel for how broadly the results can be generalized to other clinical settings.

Similarly, given that infection is such a huge topic, Table V.1 was compiled in the hope that readers who are looking for a specific theme (e.g. the paediatrician, the geriatrician or the virologist) can identify papers of interest without having to trawl through the whole section.

Table V.1 Studies covered in this section

Authors	Page	Study design	Age group	Setting	Disease studied	Organism(s) studied
Mussini et al.	251	Multicentre RCT	Adults	Italy	HIV	P. carinii
Stark et al.	253	Prospective birth cohort study	Infants	USA	Lower respiratory illness	Fungi
Klugman et al.	255	RCT	Infants	South Africa	HIV	S. pneumoniae
Jackson et al.	258	Retrospective cohort study	65 or older	USA	Pneumococcal bacteraemia and pneumonia	S. pneumoniae
Nichol et al.	262	Observational, multiregion	65 or older	USA	Pneumonia, ischaemic heart disease, stroke	Influenza
Kaiser et al.	265	Pooled data from RCTs	Adults	Multinational	Influenza and its complications	Influenza
Kuiken et al.	267	Retrospective cohort study	Adults	Multinational	SARS	SARS-CoV
Ho et al.	269	Retrospective cohort study	Adults	Hong Kong	SARS	SARS-CoV
Schaaf et al. and Gallagher et al.	273	Case–control study	Adults	Germany and Ireland	Sepsis and pneumonia	S. pneumoniae
Rello et al.	276	Retrospective cohort study	Adults	Spain	Severe CAP	Organisms isolated by microbiology
MASCOT investigators	279	Multicentre RCT	Children	Pakistan	Non-severe CAP	No specific organism
Fine et al.	281	RCT	Adults	USA	CAP	No specific organism
Torres et al.	284	RCT	Adults	Multinational	CAP	No specific organism
Root et al.	286	RCT	Adults	Multinational	Severe pneumonia with sepsis	No specific organism
Rello et al.	291	Retrospective cohort study	Adults	USA	VAP	No specific organism
El-Solh et al.	294	Observational	Elderly	USA	Aspiration pneumonia	No specific organism

RCT, randomized controlled trial; HIV, human immunodeficiency virus; CAP, community-acquired pneumonia; VAP, ventilator-associated pneumonia; SARS, severe acute respiratory syndrome; SARS-CoV, SARS-associated coronavirus; P. carinii, Pneumocystis carinii; S. pneumoniae, Streptococcus pneumoniae.
Source: Author's own.

References

1. Black RE, Morris SS, Bryce J. Where and why are 10 million children dying every year? *Lancet* 2003; **361**: 2226–34.

2. Hoyert DL, Arias E, Smith BL, Murphy SL, Kochanek KD. Deaths: final data for 1999. *Natl Vital Stat Rep* 2001; **49**: 1–113.

3. Kaplan V, Angus DC, Griffin MF, Clermont G, Scott Watson RS, Linde-Zwirble WT. Hospitalized community-acquired pneumonia in the elderly: age- and sex-related patterns of care and outcome in the United States. *Am J Respir Crit Care Med* 2002; **165**: 766–72.

4. Schito AM, Schito GC, Debbia E, Russo G, Linares J, Cercenado E, Bouza E. Antibacterial resistance in *Streptococcus pneumoniae* and *Haemophilus influenzae* from Italy and Spain: data from the PROTEKT surveillance study, 1999–2000. *J Chemother* 2003; **15**: 226–34.

5. Drazen JM. Case clusters of the severe acute respiratory syndrome. *N Engl J Med* 2003; **348** (20): e6–7.

6. British Thoracic Society guidelines for the management of community acquired pneumonia in adults. *Thorax* 2001; **56**(Suppl 4): 1–64.

7. American Thoracic Society guidelines for the management of adults with community-acquired pneumonia. Diagnosis, assessment of severity, antimicrobial therapy, and prevention. *Am J Respir Crit Care Med* 2001; **163**: 1730–54.

8. American Thoracic Society. Hospital-acquired pneumonia in adults: diagnosis, assessment of severity, initial antimicrobial therapy, and preventative strategies. A consensus statement. *Am J Respir Crit Care Med* 1995; **153**: 1711–25.

9. Chastre J, Fagon JY. Ventilator-associated pneumonia. *Am J Respir Crit Care Med* 2002; **165**: 867–903.

18

Prophylaxis and vaccination against infection

Introduction

The effective and safe prevention of infection undoubtedly represents the ideal way forward for the field of pneumonia. This chapter will discuss a paper on whether secondary *Pneumocystis carinii* pneumonia prophylaxis is still required in the age of highly active antiretroviral therapy (HAART) in patients with human immuno-deficiency virus (HIV) infection. The second paper follows on the fungal theme by discussing the effect of environmental fungi on childhood respiratory illness, raising important questions on whether and how we should tackle potential fungal patho-gens. Thereafter emphasis turns to the effect of pneumococcal vaccination, first in young children (including HIV-positive children) and then in adults. Finally, the benefits of influenza vaccination in the elderly will be discussed.

Discontinuation of secondary prophylaxis for *Pneumocystis carinii* pneumonia in human immunodeficiency virus-infected patients: a randomized trial by the CIOP Study Group

Mussini C, Pezzotti P, Antinori A, *et al.* for the Changes in Opportunistic Prophylaxis Study Group. *Clin Infect Dis* 2003; **36**: 645–51

BACKGROUND. The introduction of HAART signalled a significant improvement in prognosis for HIV-infected patients. The improved immune function associated with HAART suggested that the requirement for (potentially toxic) prophylaxis against important opportunistic infections should be reviewed. From a pulmonary point of view *P. carinii* pneumonia continues to be a prominent pathogen in HIV-infected patients, leading to a traditional role for primary and secondary prophylaxis. This study therefore aimed to determine the long-term safety of discontinuing secondary prophylaxis for *P. carinii* pneumonia in patients established on HAART.

INTERPRETATION. Over a follow-up period averaging more than 2 years, two out of 77 patients who discontinued secondary prophylaxis had a further episode of *P. carinii* pneumonia and both responded well to conventional treatment. It appears that discontinuation of secondary prophylaxis for *P. carinii* pneumonia is generally safe in

HIV-positive individuals with a CD4+ T-lymphocyte count above 200 cells/μl. However, *P. carinii* pneumonia should remain high in the differential diagnosis of patients presenting with dyspnoea after discontinuation, even when the CD4 count exceeds 200 cells/μl.

Comment

This was an open-label, multicentre (41 Italian hospitals), randomized, controlled, subgroup trial set within a larger study simultaneously evaluating discontinuation of primary prophylaxis. Patients were included if they were HIV-positive adults with a confirmed history of previous *P. carinii* pneumonia for which they were receiving conventional secondary prophylaxis. Patients were also required to have had a CD4 count below 200 cells/μl at the time of commencing an effective HAART regimen and for the count to have risen subsequently to at least 200 cells/μl (a threshold below which *P. carinii* pneumonia is known to be significantly more likely) on two consecutive occasions 1 month apart in the run-up to enrolment. Eligible patients were randomized to continuation or discontinuation of secondary prophylaxis. The patients had regular clinical reviews and blood sampling. The primary end-point was confirmed or presumed *P. carinii* pneumonia, the presumptive diagnosis resting on a clear response to *P. carinii* pneumonia treatment in the absence of another identifiable microorganism.

The patients were relatively well matched at baseline ($n = 77$ in the discontinuation group and $n = 69$ in the control group), although the discontinuation group had a significantly higher CD4 count. The discontinuation group also had a relatively high proportion of patients who had acquired HIV through intravenous drug use and a relatively low proportion of patients acquiring HIV through heterosexual transmission. The median follow-up period was similar in both groups, approximating to 26 months or 150 person-years. During this time, no patients in the control group developed *P. carinii* pneumonia, as opposed to two (one confirmed and one presumed) cases in the discontinuation group (no significant difference). The two patients with *P. carinii* pneumonia had CD4 counts of 339 and 357 cells/μl respectively, and unremarkable viral loads. Both made a good response to treatment for *P. carinii* pneumonia. In addition, three patients (two in the discontinuation group) were withdrawn from the study because their CD4 counts fell below 200 cells/μl on two consecutive occasions.

This study supported findings from studies of shorter duration (generally around 1 year of follow-up) in which discontinuation of secondary prophylaxis was demonstrated to be safe |**1,2**|. A clear trend is therefore emerging for the safe discontinuation of secondary prophylaxis among patients with a CD4 count above 200 cells/μl. However, it is a pity that this study did not recruit more patients for longer, as there is very little evidence to support clinical decision making beyond 2 years without prophylaxis. It may also be relevant that the discontinuation group contained more intravenous drug users, as compliance with antiviral therapy may be lower in this group |**3**|. Similarly, the authors did not comment on smoking status, which has been shown to be associated with the development of *P. carinii* pneumonia |**4**|.

The overall conclusion would appear to be that considerably larger (and probably longer) trials will be required in order to answer definitively the questions of whether, when and for how long secondary prophylaxis can be discontinued. Despite this, the study by Mussini *et al.* adds sufficient weight to support discontinuation of potentially toxic secondary prophylaxis in patients with a CD4 count above 200 cells/μl so long as vigilant clinical follow-up is in place to pick up rare cases of relapse. Importantly, the study also reminds us that there is no clear threshold above which we can say *P. carinii* pneumonia will not recur and that the sick, breathless, HIV-positive patient may have *P. carinii* pneumonia even with CD4 counts well in excess of 200 cells/μl.

Fungal levels in the home and lower respiratory tract illnesses in the first year of life

Stark PC, Burge HA, Ryan LM, Milton DK, Gold DR. *Am J Respir Crit Care Med* 2003; **168**: 232–7

BACKGROUND. Childhood respiratory illness is associated with both household damp and mould. These associations strongly suggest a role for fungi in childhood respiratory illness. This study therefore set out to make a rigorous assessment of the interaction between fungi and lower respiratory tract infection specifically in infants.

INTERPRETATION. High domestic concentrations of fungi appear to be independently associated with an increased risk of lower respiratory tract illness in infants.

Comment

This study was set in the Boston area and made use of a large prospective birth cohort. Families in whom at least one parent had a history of allergy or asthma were screened and 505 children (499 households) aged approximately 2 months were followed until their first birthday. A single house visit collected detailed clinical and demographic data, but also involved vacuuming the 2 m^2 around the bed in which the child most often slept, with dust being filtered out for fungal culture. Airborne fungi were simultaneously assessed by placing plates 1–1.5 m above the area to be vacuumed. The main carer completed a telephone questionnaire every 2 months and the primary outcome variable was at least one description by that carer of a lower respiratory tract illness (pneumonia, croup, bronchitis or bronchiolitis) diagnosed by a doctor in the first year of life. Because fungi are ubiquitous, the authors considered a given fungus to be present in significant concentration (and therefore included in analysis) only if that concentration was above the 90th centile for the study and greater than 1 colony forming unit (CFU)/g (for dust) or greater than 1 CFU/m^3 (for air). Univariate analysis was performed in order to determine the clinical, demographic and socio-economic factors associated with lower respiratory tract illness, with subsequent multivariate analyses adjusted for the variables found to be significant. These included male sex, increasing number of siblings, water damage/

mould in the house (all positively associated with respiratory infection), winter birth and breast-feeding (protective of respiratory infection).

A wide variety of fungi were isolated in the bedrooms, as expected. However, a statistically increased risk of respiratory infection was associated with the presence of *Penicillium* in air (73% increased risk of infection) and *Zygomycetes* (96%), *Cladosporium* (52%) or *Alternaria* (51%) in dust. Interestingly, respiratory infection without wheeze was particularly associated with *Penicillium*, while infection with wheeze was strongly associated with *Zygomycetes* and *Alternaria*. When the presence of any significant fungal concentration in the household was entered into a multivariate analysis it was found to be the strongest independent predictor for respiratory infection and particularly for infection in the absence of wheeze (Table 18.1). Intriguingly, while the presence of mould/damp in the house was also associated with respiratory infection in infancy, there was no significant correlation between mould/damp and high fungal levels, implying that these may influence susceptibility to infection independently.

Inevitably, a number of questions crop up in a study such as this. The most important relates to the diagnostic criteria used. The trial did not attempt to demonstrate any indices of respiratory infection/inflammation at the time of illness. It is quite likely that the accuracy of the doctor's diagnosis was relatively low and there is no evidence that the investigators contacted the doctor for independent verification of his/her diagnosis and the grounds for it. The accuracy of a diagnosis of wheeze may have been particularly inaccurate as it was self-reported by the carer before or at the time of the doctor's diagnosis. These factors have the potential to influence the results significantly. On the other hand, it seems reasonable that carers/doctors would pick up episodes of breathlessness (irrespective of the cause). Thus, it seems plausible that episodes of breathlessness were accurately detected, but that a proportion of these were not caused by 'croup, pneumonia, bronchitis or bronchiolitis'.

Table 18.1 Final multivariate models

| Factor | Any LRI | | LRI without wheeze[1] | | LRI with wheeze | |
	RR	95% CI	RR	95% CI	RR	95% CI
Male child	1.64	1.21, 2.22	2.32	1.27, 4.26	1.54	1.04, 2.29
Water damage or mould/mildew	1.34	0.99, 1.82	–	–	1.35	0.90, 2.04
Born in winter	0.65	0.44, 0.97	0.84	0.44, 1.60	0.50	0.28, 0.91
Breast-fed ever	0.74	0.55, 0.98	0.54	0.31, 0.93	0.82	0.55, 1.21
Siblings	1.56	1.14, 2.15	1.51	0.85, 2.67	1.82	1.18, 2.79
High fungal levels	1.86	1.21, 2.88	3.88	1.43, 10.52	1.58	0.95, 2.64

LRI, lower respiratory illness; CI, confidence interval; RR, relative risk.
[1] Water damage or mould/mildew was not included in this model. It was not significant in a univariate model ($P = 0.15$), and the model with all six variables will not converge because of so few events.
Source: Stark *et al.* (2003).

The incidence of asthma in the study is not clear. In addition, the general applicability of the results is unclear, given that at least one parent had to have a history of allergy or asthma and that the cohort appears to have been relatively affluent. In addition, it is unclear whether factors such as season, temperature, the concentration of house dust mites in dust, the age of the home or location of the home may have influenced fungal concentrations and the morbidity. Furthermore, mortality of the respiratory illnesses are not described.

However, while the concerns about diagnostic criteria must be kept in mind, the association between fungi and lower respiratory tract illness in infancy is very striking in this study. The results are of major importance given that respiratory disease in infancy may predict for morbidity later in life. The apparent independence of fungal effects from visible mould in the house is also extremely interesting. The question ultimately is how and whether these findings should influence practice. Table 18.1 would appear to suggest that practical interventions for decreasing the risk of respiratory illness are limited to encouragement of breast-feeding and avoidance of damp/mould. The demonstration that fungi contribute independently (and strongly) poses more of a problem for intervention in that there are no easy prospective ways of identifying houses with fungi and, even if there were, it would be difficult, beyond the efficient removal of dust, to know how to limit fungi. As the authors stated, the challenge ahead is to work out the precise mechanisms by which fungi promote respiratory illness in infancy in the expectation that novel interventions will be suggested.

A trial of a nine-valent pneumococcal conjugate vaccine in children with and those without HIV infection
Klugman K, Madhi SA, Huebner RE, Kohberger R, Mbelle N, Pierce N. *N Engl J Med* 2003; **349**: 1341–8

BACKGROUND. Pneumonia is responsible for millions of deaths among children in developing countries and *Streptococcus pneumoniae* is a major cause of childhood pneumonia. Effective vaccination strategies against pneumococcal infection are therefore highly desirable, particularly for developing countries. Furthermore, antibiotic resistance to *S. pneumoniae* is increasing globally, reinforcing the need for effective vaccines. This prospective, double-blind, randomized, placebo-controlled study aimed to determine the effect of vaccination on the rates of invasive pneumococcal disease and radiographic pneumonia in children in Soweto, South Africa, which has a high prevalence of antibiotic resistance to *S. pneumoniae*. The vaccine comprised nine *S. pneumoniae* capsular sugar moieties conjugated to a diphtheria toxin mutant.

INTERPRETATION. This elegant and important study demonstrated a significant effect of a nine-valent pneumococcal vaccine in reducing first episodes of invasive pneumococcal disease and radiographic pneumonia in South African children. Invasive pneumococcal disease was also significantly reduced in the subgroup of children known to be HIV positive. Furthermore, the vaccine effectively reduced invasive pneumococcal disease attributable to antibiotic-resistant *S. pneumoniae*. The adverse effects included increased rates of viral pneumonia in the week after vaccination and a higher rate of bronchial hyper-reactivity.

Comment

The study enrolled children aged 4–14 weeks. Children were eligible if they had received bacille Calmette–Guérin (BCG) or polio vaccine at birth, but excluded if they were considered to have a progressive neurological disease, if they had a history of seizures or if they were likely to be moving from the Soweto area. Randomized children received vaccine or placebo on three occasions separated by at least 21 days, these being given concurrently with vaccines against hepatitis B, *Haemophilus influenzae* type b, diphtheria, pertussis and polio. No booster doses of trial vaccine were given subsequently. All children were tested for HIV by an enzyme-linked immunosorbent assay or polymerase chain reaction. The primary end-points were a first episode of invasive pneumococcal disease (as defined by positive blood cultures or cerebrospinal fluid cultures) or radiographic pneumonia presenting to the largest single hospital for children in the region. The secondary end-points included the rates of invasive pneumococcal disease and radiographic pneumonia specifically among HIV-positive children and the rate of antibiotic resistance among all children studied. The study enrolled for 32 months and follow-up continued until 15 HIV-negative children receiving all three doses of vaccine/placebo developed invasive pneumococcal disease (44 months from the start of the trial).

The vaccinated ($n = 19\,922$) and control ($n = 19\,914$) groups were well matched at baseline, with 37 057 children receiving all three trial doses. Vaccination conferred significant protection against invasive pneumococcal disease among HIV-negative and HIV-positive children (Table 18.2). This effect was associated with a reduction in antibiotic-resistant strains of *S. pneumoniae* (17 vaccinated children with invasive pneumococcal disease had a resistant strain, compared with 39 in the control group) ($P = 0.005$). In addition, 356 vaccinated children developed radiographic pneumonia compared with 428 control children ($P = 0.01$), the significance of this effect persisting for HIV-negative (but not HIV-positive) children. There were 13 fewer deaths in the vaccinated group, but this did not reach statistical significance. With regard to safety, vaccinated children were twice as likely to develop viral pneumonia (predominantly due to respiratory syncitial virus) in the 8 days after vaccination ($P = 0.03$) and to have bronchial hyper-reactivity ($P = 0.009$). There were also significantly more generalized seizures in vaccinated children, but the total rate of all seizures was similar in both groups.

It seems likely that many cases of invasive pneumococcal disease and/or pneumonia would have been missed by this study, assuming that a high proportion of the subjects may have moved away from the catchment area during the follow-up period, that some cases of pneumonia may have been managed in the community and that some children may have died before a diagnosis was established. Given that the study was double-blinded however, it is likely that the inclusion of such missing

Table 18.2 First episodes of invasive pneumococcal disease*

Variable	Vaccinated group	Control group	P-value	Vaccine efficacy (95% CI)
	no. of episodes			per cent
HIV-negative children				
Invasive pneumococcal disease	11	19	0.2	42 (–28 to 75)
Vaccine-serotype pneumococci	3	17	0.003	83 (39 to 97)
Non vaccine-serotype pneumococci	4	1	0.38	–300 (–19,599 to 60)
Vaccine-related serotype pneumococci	4	1	0.38	–300 (–10,599 to 60)
HIV-positive children				
Invasive pneumococcal disease	22	47	0.004	53 (21 to 73)
Vaccine-serotype pneumococci	9	26	0.006	65 (24 to 86)
Non vaccine-serotype pneumococci	9	8	1	–13 (–235 to 62)
Vaccine-related serotype pneumococci	6	16	0.05	63 (–1 to 88)
All children				
Invasive pneumococcal disease	33	66	0.001	50 (23 to 68)
Vaccine-serotype pneumococci	12	43	<0.001	72 (46 to 87)
Non vaccine-serotype pneumococci	13	9	0.52	–44 (–283 to 43)
Vaccine-related serotype pneumococci	10	17	0.25	41 (–36 to 75)

* Vaccine-serotype pneumococci were serotypes 1, 4, 5, 6B, 9V, 14, 18C, 19F and 23F. Vaccine-related pneumococci were serotypes 6A, 19A and 19B. CI, confidence interval; HIV, human immunodeficiency virus. For HIV-positive children and for all children, the sum of episodes involving vaccine, non-vaccine and vaccine-related serotypes exceeds the number of episodes of invasive pneumococcal disease because only the first episode of invasive disease was counted.
Source: Klugman *et al.* (2003).

cases would have further strengthened the observed protection of the vaccine. It is perhaps a pity that the study was stopped with a mean follow-up of 2.5 years and certainly the duration of efficacy of the vaccine cannot be inferred. It is also difficult to draw conclusions about cost-effectiveness for this vaccine and this may be important given that its greatest effect is to be expected in the world's poorest countries. A further interesting point about this study relates to the rate of invasive pneumococcal disease caused by serotypes distinct from or related to those in the vaccine. While virtually all cases of invasive pneumococcal disease in the HIV-negative controls were attributable to serotypes covered by the vaccine (Table 18.2), it is notable (and expected) that HIV-positive patients often had invasive pneumococcal disease caused by serotypes not covered by the vaccine. The implication is that the invasive pneumococcal disease rates in HIV-positive patients (but not HIV-negative patients) could be improved further by extending the vaccine valency. The other fascinating implication is that the vaccinated patients were more susceptible to specific serotypes not covered by the vaccine (Table 18.2), but the numbers are too small to draw firm conclusions on this subject.

Overall this trial represents an immensely important advance in our understanding of pneumococcal vaccination. The demonstration that this vaccine has efficacy in HIV-positive children has far-reaching implications. Furthermore, the reduction in the rate of pneumonia should not be underestimated, partly because pneumonia exerts such an unacceptable mortality among children |5| and partly because non-streptococcal organisms are likely to cause a high proportion of pneumonia in Sowetan children and so the vaccine probably had to exert a fairly profound effect on pneumococcal pneumonia to impact upon the rate of radiographic pneumonia. Further profound implications of the trial are that refinement of pneumococcal vaccines can improve efficacy in the future and that vaccination can have important beneficial effects as antibiotic resistance continues to spread at alarming rates.

Effectiveness of pneumococcal polysaccharide vaccine in older adults

Jackson LA, Neuzil KM, Yu O, *et al.*; Vaccine Safety Datalink. *N Engl J Med* 2003; **348**: 1747–55

BACKGROUND. The effectiveness of different formulations of pneumococcal vaccine remains a subject of considerable debate. In general, vaccination appears to protect elderly patients against pneumococcal bacteraemia, but conflicting data have emerged on the capacity for influencing the rates of community-acquired pneumonia. This large, retrospective, cohort study aimed to describe the effectiveness of the 23-valent pneumococcal polysaccharide vaccine against community-acquired pneumonia in an elderly population.

INTERPRETATION. The 23-valent pneumococcal polysaccharide vaccine was associated with a significant reduction in pneumococcal bacteraemia. However, it did not reduce the risk of community-acquired pneumonia or the risk of death from all causes. Indeed, in contrast, the data suggest a significant increase in community-acquired pneumonia requiring hospital admission among vaccinated subjects. Subgroup analysis, whilst harder to interpret, suggested that vaccination might have conferred small reductions in death among immunocompetent patients, without influencing the rates of community-acquired pneumonia.

Comment

This retrospective study ran from January 1998 to February 2001 and analysed data from 47 365 subjects in a health-managed organization in the north-west of the USA. Case records as well as databases pertaining to immunization status, laboratory results, X-rays and diagnosis were available. The primary outcome measurements were hospitalization for community-acquired pneumonia, outpatient community-acquired pneumonia and pneumococcal bacteraemia. The secondary outcomes included death from all causes. The authors assessed the risk of outcomes arising according to pneumococcal vaccination (subjects were assumed to have protective immunity 14 days after vaccination) using multivariate Cox proportional hazards models adjusted for a variety of confounding variables such as age, sex, cardiac disease, pulmonary disease, diabetes, cerebrovascular disease, immunosuppression, smoking and influenza vaccination.

In total 1428 patients were admitted with a diagnosis of community-acquired pneumonia (this excluded re-admissions), 3061 had an episode of outpatient community-acquired pneumonia and a total of 5690 patients died during the study period. Sixty-one patients had pneumococcal bacteraemia. The main results of the study are shown in Table 18.3, in which the results are expressed as hazards ratios (HRs) whereby a result >1 indicates that vaccinated subjects have an increased (and a result <1 a reduced) association with the outcome, e.g. an HR of 1.21 means the risk of that outcome was 21% more likely in subjects vaccinated with the 23-valent pneumococcal polysaccharide vaccine. The third row of the table is most important, indicating that vaccinated subjects were significantly less likely (by 44%) to have pneumococcal bacteraemia, but also suggesting they were 14% more likely to be hospitalized with community-acquired pneumonia! The fourth row is included because the study enrolled a relatively high proportion of subjects in whom no smoking data were available and so the model was revised to include only patients with clearly documented smoking status. With this adjustment the increased risk of community-acquired pneumonia in vaccinated patients was preserved, but no longer statistically significant, while a trend began to emerge for the vaccine protecting against death from all causes.

Interestingly, the authors extended these observations to a subgroup analysis on the basis of underlying immunocompromise (including cancer, immunosuppressive medication, chronic liver disease or chronic renal disease). Vaccination did not significantly influence any of the study outcomes among patients with immuno-compromise ($n = 9158$), whereas it was associated with significant reductions in pneumococcal bacteraemia and death in immuncompetent subjects. This trend persisted (and indeed was strengthened) in immunocompetent patients receiving influenza vaccination. Importantly, vaccination showed no significant influence on any of the outcomes among the subset of immunocompetent patients with chronic lung disease, though it should be noted that this group of patients was relatively small ($n = 3126$).

The study benefits greatly from the size of the population sampled. The obvious limitation of the study, as the authors discussed, is that it is retrospective and that misclassification bias cannot be controlled for. Thus, we cannot be sure that all pneumococcal vaccinations were accurately recorded (particularly in the first 2 years, which were before the vaccination database for the study was established), nor is it entirely clear that the 23-valent pneumococcal polysaccharide vaccine was the only vaccination available to the study population. Similarly, it is highly likely that cases of community-acquired pneumonia were missed and that there were several false-positive diagnoses

Table 18.3 Incidence and risk of pneumonia, pneumococcal bacteraemia and death from any cause in relation to pneumococcal-vaccination status*

Variable	Hospitalization for community-acquired pneumonia verified by medical record review	Outpatient pneumonia	Pneumococcal bacteraemia	Hospitalization with a discharge diagnosis code for pneumonia†	Death from any cause
Unadjusted rate per 1000 person-years					
Unvaccinated	10.4	23.2	0.68	18.8	50.1
Vaccinated	11.8	25.7	0.38	19.9	42.0
Age-adjusted hazard ratio for all subjects (95% CI)	1.21 (1.08–1.35)	1.14 (1.06–1.23)	0.58 (0.35–0.96)	1.12 (1.02–1.22)	0.88 (0.84–0.93)
*P*value	0.001	≤0.001	0.03	0.01	<0.001
Multivariate-adjusted hazard ratio for all subjects (95% CI)	1.14 (1.02–1.28)	1.04 (0.96–1.13)	0.56 (0.33–0.93)	1.06 (0.98–1.16)	0.96 (0.91–1.02)
*P*value	0.02	0.31	0.03	0.16	0.19
Multivariate-adjusted hazard ratio for subjects with smoking status data (95% CI)‡	1.11 (0.98–1.26)	1.02 (0.94–1.10)	0.53 (0.31–0.93)	1.05 (0.95–1.15)	0.94 (0.87–1.01)
*P*value	0.09	0.69	0.03	0.34	0.08

* The hazard ratios are for vaccinated subjects as compared with unvaccinated subjects. The multivariate hazard ratios were adjusted for age (65–74, 75–84, or more than 84 years); sex; nursing-home residence or non-residence; receipt or non-receipt of influenza vaccine; smoking status (currently smoking, not currently smoking, or no data); presence or absence of coronary artery disease, immunocompromised status, diabetes mellitus, chronic lung disease, and dementia or stroke; number of outpatient visits in the year before cohort entry (fewer than 6, 6–12, or more than 12); and any hospitalization for pneumonia in the year before study entry. CI, confidence interval.

† *International Classification of Diseases, 9th Revision, Clinical Modification* codes 480 through 487.0 denoted pneumonia.

‡ The analysis excludes 6343 subjects for whom no data on smoking were available.

Source: Jackson *et al.* (2003).

of community-acquired pneumonia, given that community-acquired pneumonia requiring hospitalization was dependent on discharge coding (traditionally notoriously inaccurate). Similarly, a diagnosis of outpatient community-acquired pneumonia was based only on the combination of a chest X-ray result and prescription of an antibiotic. Furthermore, the authors indicated that, of 2455 hospitalizations for pneumonia, only 1600 were considered to be community-acquired pneumonia, even after exclusion of re-admissions and nosocomial infections. The cause of pneumonia (other than community-acquired pneumonia) is not clearly explained for the remaining 855 patients and bias in case selection cannot be excluded. Finally, in the absence of extensive microbiological surveillance, it is inevitably impossible to say what proportion of community-acquired pneumonia was attributable to S. pneumoniae in this population. Clearly, if this were relatively low, then a protective effect against community-acquired pneumonia would be more difficult to detect.

Despite these concerns, which are inevitable for retrospective analyses of community-acquired pneumonia, this is an extremely valuable study, with fascinating results. It is certainly worrying that the 23-valent pneumococcal polysaccharide vaccine may increase community-acquired pneumonia in the elderly. No mechanism can be inferred, but it is tempting to speculate that vaccination may alter streptococcal rates in the nasopharynx, resulting in flora with an increased propensity for infecting the lower respiratory tract whenever the host is susceptible. Equally it is fascinating that, in the immunocompetent elderly subject, vaccination may reduce the risk of death in a way that has nothing to do with protection against pneumonia. This requires further study.

However, the pragmatic question is whether this should change our vaccination practice. Certainly the data support the use of vaccination to protect against pneumococcal bacteraemia. However, the study raises a variety of important questions. For example, should the immunocompromised elderly patient be vaccinated when there is no clear protection against bacteraemia, but a trend towards more death and community-acquired pneumonia? On the other hand, can we identify and target specific groups of patients in whom vaccination reduces death (e.g. immunocompetent subjects vaccinated against influenza) thus expanding considerably the clinical usefulness of the vaccine? Ultimately the authors make the important point that, while the 23-valent pneumococcal polysaccharide vaccine is clearly effective against pneumococcal bacteraemia, it now seems important to assess other vaccine preparations in the hope that they may reduce (rather than increase) the far commoner clinical manifestation of S. pneumoniae, non-bacteraemic community-acquired pneumonia. It seems certain therefore that the debate on pneumococcal vaccination will continue and important studies on the efficacy of alternative preparations are awaited with huge interest.

Influenza vaccination and reduction in hospitalizations for cardiac disease and stroke among the elderly

Nichol KL, Nordin J, Mullooly J, Lask R, Fillbrandt K, Iwane M. *N Engl J Med* 2003; **348**: 1322–32

BACKGROUND. Influenza epidemics are undoubtedly associated with higher rates of pneumonia and death, and influenza vaccination has been shown to reduce these complications among elderly patients. However, the effect of influenza vaccination on the incidence of heart disease and stroke has been less clear. This observational study of elderly subjects therefore aimed to determine the impact of influenza vaccination on death from all causes and on hospitalization associated with influenza/pneumonia, congestive heart failure, ischaemic heart disease or acute cerebrovascular disease.

INTERPRETATION. Influenza vaccination significantly reduced the risk of death among elderly subjects (approximately 50% reduced risk as compared with unvaccinated subjects). Similarly, vaccination significantly reduced the risk of congestive cardiac failure (approximately 20%), acute cerebrovascular disease (approximately 20%) and influenza/pneumonia (approximately 30%). This study argues strongly for widespread vaccination of patients aged 65 years and older.

Comment

This large, community-based, observational study pooled demographic and clinical data from three geographically distinct US managed-care organizations. The authors analysed two separate influenza seasons, these defined as the time between the first influenza isolate and 2 weeks after the last isolate in each separate region. Subjects had to be 65 years or older at the start of each study period (1 October 1998 or 1 October 1999) and had to have been enrolled for the full influenza season and the 12 months prior to it (the latter effectively used as a 'run-in' period in which to collect baseline data). The subjects' records were used to identify a wide variety of co-morbidities, number of hospitalizations and uptake of vaccination. Outcomes within the influenza seasons were defined as death from any cause or hospitalization associated with either 'influenza or pneumonia', congestive cardiac failure, ischaemic heart disease or acute cerebrovascular disease. The authors used multivariable logistic regression to compare outcomes in vaccinated and unvaccinated subjects, adjusting for confounding variables such as demographic factors and co-morbidities.

The results obtained were remarkably similar in each of the two consecutive influenza seasons. Vaccination conferred risk reductions of approximately 50% for death, while hospitalizations were reduced by 30% for 'pneumonia or influenza', 19% for 'cardiac disease' (congestive heart failure and/or ischaemic heart disease) and approximately 20% for acute cerebrovascular disease. It is worth noting that, in both influenza seasons, vaccination significantly reduced hospitalization due to congestive cardiac failure, but protection was only conferred against hospitalization for ischaemic heart disease in 1998–1999.

The authors estimated that, in the 1998–1999 influenza season, 95 subjects would have required influenza vaccination for one life to be saved. Interestingly, the protective effects of vaccination against death appeared to be preserved regardless of the age of the subjects and the presence or absence of significant co-morbidities. Together these data strongly suggest that the benefits of influenza vaccination extend well beyond the prevention of pulmonary complications and strengthen the argument for vaccinating elderly subjects without co-morbidities. They also provide further supportive evidence for an association between influenza and heart disease/cerebrovascular disease and hint that vaccination may benefit significant numbers of subjects younger than 65 years, though clearly this would require to be formally confirmed in prospective studies.

The strengths of this study lie in the large numbers enrolled, the ability to adjust for important and diverse confounding variables and the demonstration that the findings were reproducible both in consecutive influenza seasons and in geographically distinct regions of the USA. Furthermore, the baseline data period of 12 months before each influenza season allowed the authors to demonstrate that vaccinated patients comprised a group who were older and had significantly more risk factors for complications of influenza than did the unvaccinated patients. This not only implies that sicker, more elderly patients were appropriately 'targeted' with influenza vaccination, but makes it less likely that the study was biased towards detecting a protective effect of vaccination. For all these reasons, this study adds significantly to our understanding of influenza vaccination.

Despite the impressive design of the study however, a few cautions should be sounded. In particular (as the authors conceded) misclassification of patients may be an important factor in an observational study such as this. This applies not only to the specificity of the medical diagnoses in the study, but to the accuracy of the databases in recording the uptake of influenza vaccination. In this regard it is of some concern that incomplete data excluded subjects from the New Jersey, Pennsylvania and Connecticut areas for reasons that are not entirely explained. Secondly, the effects of smoking or of specific antithrombotic treatments do not appear to have been incorporated into the statistical models: vaccinated patients had a higher rate of detected cardiorespiratory disease and it is conceivable that this cohort may therefore have received more aggressive smoking cessation therapies (and/or antithrombotic treatments) than the unvaccinated patients. Any such effect might bias towards reduced vascular events in the vaccinated group. In addition, a retrospective observational study such as this makes it impossible to determine how many of the unvaccinated (or indeed the vaccinated) subjects had serologically confirmed influenza infection during the study periods and certainly further studies would be required to determine whether influenza has a direct causative association with vascular disease in susceptible individuals.

Overall however, this study provides compelling evidence to support vaccination of subjects aged 65 years or older and demands further study of vaccination in younger subjects.

References

1. Lopez Bernaldo De Quiros JC, Miro JM, Pena JM, Podzamczer D, Alberdi JC, Martinez E, Cosin J, Claramonte X, Gonzalez J, Domingo P, Casado JL, Ribera E for the Grupo de Estudio del SIDA 04/98. A randomized trial of the discontinuation of primary and secondary prophylaxis against *Pneumocystis carinii* pneumonia after highly active retroviral therapy in patients with HIV infection. *N Engl J Med* 2001; **344**: 159–67.

2. Koletar SL, Heald AE, Finkelstein D, Hafner R, Currier JS, McCutchan JA, Vallee M, Torriani FJ, Powderly WG, Fass RJ, Murphy RL; ACTG 888 Study Team. A prospective study of discontinuing primary and secondary *Pneumocystis carinii* prophylaxis after CD4 cell counts increase to $>200 \times 10^6$/l. *AIDS* 2001; **15**: 1509–15.

3. Laing R, Brettle R, Leen C, Hulks G. Features and outcome of *Pneumocystis carinii* pneumonia according to risk category for HIV infection. *Scand J Infect Dis* 1997; **29**: 57–61.

4. Miguez-Burbano MJ, Burbano X, Ashkin D, Pitchenik A, Allan R, Pineda L, Rodriguez N, Shor-Posner G. Impact of tobacco use on the development of opportunistic respiratory infections in HIV seropositive patients on antiretroviral therapy. *Addict Biol* 2003; **8**: 39–43.

5. Black RE, Morris SS, Bryce J. Where and why are 10 million children dying every year? *Lancet* 2003; **361**: 2226–34.

19

Viral infections and their treatment

Introduction

This chapter will focus solely on two infections. Following on from the previous chapter, the vexed question of whether antiviral therapies are effective in patients with influenza will be addressed. Thereafter attention will turn to the terrible severe acute respiratory syndrome (SARS) epidemic that began in China in late 2002. A seminal paper confirming the causative agent will be discussed, followed by a paper describing one of the first attempts to develop evidence for treatment efficacy in SARS.

Impact of oseltamivir treatment on influenza-related lower respiratory tract complications and hospitalizations
Kaiser L, Wat C, Mills T, Mahoney P, Ward P, Hayden F. *Arch Intern Med* 2003; **163**: 1667–72

BACKGROUND. Debate continues as to whether antiviral agents have a place in the management of acute influenza. Logical viral targets include neuraminidase, leading to the development of specific neuraminidase inhibitors such as oseltamivir carboxylate. This study pooled data from ten prospective, randomized, placebo-controlled trials of oseltamivir for influenza-like symptoms and determined the drug's effect on the frequency of lower respiratory tract complications requiring antibiotics.

INTERPRETATION. Within the limitations of the study, a trend appeared to emerge suggesting that oseltamivir is associated with a small reduction in lower respiratory tract complications of influenza requiring antibiotics.

Comment

This study amalgamated the results from ten randomized, double-blind, placebo-controlled, multicentre, phase III trials in which the design was conserved but the subjects' characteristics were variable (some trials confined to elderly subjects, some to younger adults and some restricted to adults with chronic obstructive pulmonary disease [COPD]). The commercial sponsorship of the study was acknowledged.

Recruited patients had a fever, at least one respiratory symptom and at least one constitutional symptom. If symptoms had been present for less than 36 h, patients were randomized to receive 150 mg of oseltamivir twice daily ($n = 2023$) or placebo ($n = 1541$). The mean age of the patients studied was approximately 43 years. The patients were evaluated over a 28-day period and the primary end-point was the presence of a lower respiratory tract complication requiring antibiotics. A 'lower respiratory tract infection' comprised bronchitis, lower respiratory tract infection or pneumonia as defined by the attending physician. Confirmation of influenza was defined as a positive isolation of influenza from nose and throat swabs and/or a four-fold rise in influenza antibody titres. By these criteria 68% of the patients had confirmed influenza. Just under 20% of all the patients had been vaccinated against influenza. Interestingly, a higher proportion of the patients receiving placebo were elderly and/or had cardiorespiratory disease.

Oseltamivir was associated with a significant reduction in lower respiratory tract complications requiring antibiotics among the patients with confirmed influenza (4.6 versus 10.3% in the placebo-treated patients). Interestingly, by far the common-est complication of influenza was bronchitis and, while oseltamivir seemed to reduce the incidence of this complication, the numbers were too small to demonstrate a significant reduction in influenza-associated pneumonia. The trend in oseltamivir reducing lower respiratory tract complications was maintained when the patients were stratified according to the presence or absence of significant risk factors for influenza.

Oseltamivir made no impact on the rate of lower respiratory tract complications among the patients with no laboratory confirmation of influenza, thereby implying an influenza-specific effect for the drug. Curiously, hospitalization was extremely rare in this study and, while a trend towards reduced hospitalization in oseltamivir-treated patients emerged, it is hard to draw definitive conclusions. Very little infor-mation was provided with regard to toxicity, but it would appear that oseltamivir was well tolerated.

This study undoubtedly benefited from the large numbers of patients recruited, the consistent protocol and the multinational, multicentre design. However, a number of potential limitations make it difficult to interpret the data. In particular, the validity of pooling studies that set out specifically to analyse patients with differ-ent characteristics (e.g. healthy younger adults and elderly patients with COPD) seems questionable. A further significant criticism is that no diagnostic standards were used in confirming 'lower respiratory tract complications' and it seems highly unlikely that antibiotics were clinically indicated for all of the complications identi-fied, particularly when the significant majority of these were 'bronchitis'. It would have been very interesting to have some idea of illness severity among the patients receiving antibiotics (e.g. the oxygen saturation of arterial blood [SaO_2]), but this was lacking. These potential problems are significantly compounded by the fact that the patients in the placebo group were older with significantly more risk factors for influenza. This not only questions the effectiveness of the randomization strategy, but biases towards an effect for oseltamivir.

Aside from these more important criticisms it could also be argued that, in an intention-to-treat study such as this, it is disappointing that the two groups of patients randomized were not directly compared, i.e. those with influenza-like illness randomized to either oseltamivir or placebo (instead subgroups were compared depending on whether influenza was confirmed in the laboratory). In 'real life' it is highly unlikely for laboratory results to be available within the time frame in which oseltamivir is considered effective. Furthermore, while the trial protocol aimed for patients with symptoms for less than 36 h to be recruited, it is frustrating that a number of the patients had symptoms for longer than this (one patient appeared to have had symptoms for 229.3 h!). Data interpretation is also made more difficult by the inclusion of a small number of patients already on antibiotics and by the fact that 20% of the patients were already vaccinated against influenza (the influence of vaccination on the data is not apparent).

For the reasons discussed the results of this study are extremely hard to interpret. On balance it seems plausible that oseltamivir reduces the incidence of influenza-associated bronchitis, but in the absence of widely available rapid diagnostic facilities for influenza and without knowing the morbidity caused by influenza-associated bronchitis, it is difficult to see a clear place for oseltamivir at the present time. From a practical point of view vaccination seems a more effective strategy, but it remains to be seen whether oseltamivir and other anti-influenza drugs have a place in susceptible patients who decline vaccination or in whom it is contraindicated.

Newly discovered coronavirus as the primary cause of severe acute respiratory syndrome

Kuiken T, Fouchier RAM, Schutten M, *et al. Lancet* 2003; **362**: 263–70

BACKGROUND. The international outbreak of SARS in late 2002 and early 2003 had an associated mortality of approximately 10%. The rapid dissemination of the disease from a distinct geographical locus in China immediately suggested an infective aetiology, prompting coordinated attempts at identifying the agent responsible. A number of candidate microorganisms were rapidly associated with SARS and prominent among these was SARS-associated coronavirus (SARS-CoV) |1,2|. This study aimed to establish whether SARS-CoV satisfied the criteria for a causative role in SARS.

INTERPRETATION. This landmark study provided persuasive evidence that SARS-CoV was the causative agent in a high proportion of (but not all) cases of SARS in the 2002–2003 outbreak.

Comment

This comprehensive study made use of clinical samples from 436 patients fulfilling the case criteria for SARS derived from twelve, well-defined cohorts in Southeast Asia and Western Europe. Evidence of infection with SARS-CoV was established for each patient's samples either by serological detection of antibody to SARS-CoV and/or by analysis of body fluids/secreta/tissue for detection of viral RNA and/or direct isolation of the virus in culture. Similar serological and/or reverse transcriptase polymerase chain reaction-based assays and/or isolation techniques were used for assaying samples from the same cohorts for another agent that was originally thought to be linked with SARS, the human metapneumovirus (hMPV), though in this case samples from only 335 patients were analysed. Evidence for SARS-CoV antibody and/or viral RNA was found in 75.5% of tested patients, while the corresponding figure for hMPV detection was 12.2%. Interestingly, more than 50% of the patients in ten of the twelve cohorts studied had evidence of infection with SARS-CoV, the remaining two cohorts with far lower rates of SARS-CoV infection being European (UK and France), while only one cohort (from Hong Kong) contained more than five patients with evidence of hMPV. It should be noted that no respiratory pathogen was consistently isolated in those cases negative for SARS-CoV. These human data seem extremely robust. The sensitivity and specificity of the serological tests are not discussed and no single virological assay was applied to all samples, but there is no clear reason to doubt the reproducibility of the tests. The human data suggest a strong association between SARS-CoV and SARS. However, there is also a tantalizing suggestion that other aetiologic agents may be responsible for SARS in specific cohorts.

The other part of the study involved inoculating four macaques with a clinical isolate of SARS-CoV. Each animal received intratracheal, intranasal and conjunctival inocula. Clinical samples were collected on days 0, 2, 4 and 6 and the animals were killed on day 6 for detailed post-mortem analysis. Importantly, three of the macaques developed evidence for diffuse alveolar damage, the histological pattern associated with human SARS (Fig. 19.1). In addition, virus shedding was detected from the respiratory tract of three of the animals from day 2 and electron microscopy of lung tissue showed particles morphologically indistinguishable from SARS-CoV. It is interesting that relatively few cells stained positively for SARS-CoV antigen using an immunohistochemical technique and that no serum antibody to SARS-CoV was detected in the animal studies. The former observation could represent a limitation of the (novel) assay. Alternatively, however, it may imply that the virus is cleared rapidly, but nevertheless sets in train the impetus for profound and ongoing inflammatory responses.

The most important aspect of this study is that it provided the final pieces of evidence for fulfilling the criteria establishing a causative role for a virus in an infective disease, as modified from Koch's postulates. Thus, we know that SARS-CoV can be isolated and purified from humans with SARS, it can subsequently be grown in human cells, it can imitate human disease closely in experimental models, it can be re-isolated after experimental infection and a specific immune response is elicited after experimental infection (the latter being proven in separate studies [3]). Taken together there is therefore now overwhelming evidence to implicate SARS-CoV as a cause of SARS. It remains likely that other as yet unidentified agents cause up to one-quarter of SARS cases. However, this study was one of a number of key reports providing very significant impetus to understanding more about SARS-CoV in the

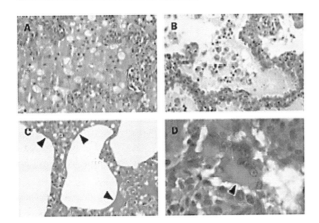

Fig. 19.1 Histological lesions in lungs from cynornolgus macaques infected with SARS-CoV. (A) Early changes of diffuse alveolar damage, characterized by disruption of alveolar walls and flooding of alveolar lumina with serosanguineous exudate admixed with neutrophils and alveolar macrophages. (B) More advanced changes of diffuse alveolar damage, characterized by thickened alveolar walls lined by type 2 pneumocytes, and mainly alveolar macrophages alvolar lumina. (C) Arrows show hyaline membranes on surfaces of alveoli. (D) A characteristic change is presence of syncytia (arrowhead), here in the lumen of bronchiole. All slides haematoxylin and eosin stained. Source: Kuiken *et al.* (2003).

hope that new treatments and vaccinations can be developed for this important disease.

High-dose pulse versus non-pulse corticosteroid regimens in severe acute respiratory syndrome

Ho JC, Ooi GC, Mok TY, *et al. Am J Respir Crit Care Med* 2003; **168**: 1449–56

BACKGROUND. The SARS epidemic in late 2002 and early 2003 posed significant therapeutic dilemmas in the absence of definitive data on the causative organism or the pathogenesis of the disease. Treatment was largely empirical, based on the principle that therapy should include antibiotics for severe community-acquired pneumonia (given that SARS presents in the same way), antiviral agents (as a viral aetiology was implied) and corticosteroids (as a florid inflammatory response is characteristic of SARS). In the absence of randomized, controlled trials there is no hard evidence to support these approaches, yet no convincing alternatives are available. Therefore, experience from the last SARS outbreak must be analysed critically in the hope of planning better treatment (and organizing important trials) in time for the next outbreak of the disease. This study therefore assessed the clinical and radiographic responses to different corticosteroid regimens used in centres of excellence during the Hong Kong outbreak.

INTERPRETATION. High-dose pulsed methylprednisolone was associated with significantly lower oxygen requirements and improved radiographic scores when compared with 'non-pulsed' steroid therapy. The early implementation of pulsed corticosteroids appears to be associated with a better outcome in SARS without evidence of significant adverse effects related to treatment.

Comment

This retrospective study was concerned with all 72 patients admitted to hospital in Hong Kong with probable SARS over a 40-day period from 9 March 2003. Serological and/or virological confirmation of SARS-CoV was subsequently available for 69 patients. All patients received standard antibiotics for severe community-acquired pneumonia, as well as a 10–14-day course of ribavirin. In addition, patients received corticosteroids based on two regimens, these comprising (1) 8–12 mg/kg/day hydrocortisone for 3–5 days (or 2–3 mg/kg/day methylprednisolone for 5 days) followed by 2 mg/kg/day prednislone, reducing as necessary ('non-pulse steroids' [non-PS]) and (2) 500 mg of methylprednisolone per day for 5 days (or 1 g per day for 3 days) then 50 mg of prednisolone twice daily reducing to 20–30 mg daily on day 21 ('pulse steroids' [PS]).

Steroids were generally started in response to clinical deterioration or lack of clinical improvement and increasing clinical suspicion of SARS (contact with the disease or laboratory findings such as lymphopenia or transaminitis). The patients had a daily clinical assessment, blood sampling and chest X-ray, the latter being scored on a serial basis by an experienced radiologist. Patients from either group who failed to respond or who deteriorated on steroids were given 'rescue' pulse methylprednisolone (500 mg daily for 3–5 days).

The mean age of the patients was 37 years and there was a low incidence of recorded co-morbidity. At baseline, patients in the PS group had a significantly lower SaO_2 than those in the non-PS group (95 versus 96%), but their baseline characteristics were otherwise very similar. Patients in the PS group were significantly less likely to require rescue pulse methylprednisolone (Fig. 19.2) or supplemental oxygen, had significantly better radiographic scores and were four times less likely to require admission to an intensive care unit. However, no clear differences in the rate of death or mechanical ventilation were noted when comparing the two groups. Interestingly, the cumulative dose of corticosteroid was similar in both groups, reflecting the high requirement for rescue methylprednisolone in the non-PS group. Furthermore, adverse effects were similar for both treatments with the exception that hyperglycaemia was significantly less likely in the PS group.

The authors readily conceded that interpretation of these data is limited by the retrospective nature of the study. It should also be noted that PS therapy was introduced on day 30 of the study period specifically because of anecdotal evidence suggesting its efficacy and, indeed, it became the routine treatment from that point onwards. The authors stated that treatment did not otherwise change from day 30, but it is conceivable that nursing and medical experience accumulated over the first 30 days of the outbreak improved patient care/outcome in the subsequent 10 days

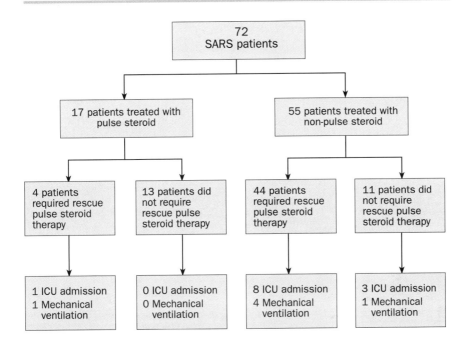

Fig. 19.2 Schematic diagram showing the study profile and major clinical outcomes for 72 patients with severe acute respiratory syndrome (SARS) receiving pulse steroid (methylprednisolone 500 mg daily) or lower-dosage non-pulse steroid therapy. ICU, intensive care unit.
Source: Ho *et al.* (2003).

and that there may have been an associated Hawthorne effect whereby introduction of a potentially more efficacious treatment for this severe disease may have subtly improved staff morale and performance. In addition, it would have been useful to know the change in the partial pressure of oxygen in arterial blood resulting from treatment (only the patients' SaO_2 values were recorded). Finally, it is not explained how three patients in the non-PS group ended up in intensive care (one died) without receiving rescue pulse methylprednisolone (see the right side of Fig. 19.2).

Despite these considerations, these data suggest that early intervention with PS appears to make a difference to the outcome in probable SARS. This is therefore an extremely valuable study, which is likely to have a significant impact upon the management of the next outbreak, at least until more is known about the pathogenesis of the disease and until prospective, randomized, clinical trials have demonstrated efficacy for alternative treatments.

References

1. Ksiazek TG, Erdman D, Goldsmith CS, Zaki SR, Peret T, Emery S, Tong S, Urbani C, Comer JA, Lim W, Rollin PE, Dowell SF, Ling AE, Humphrey CK, Shieh WJ, Guarner J, Paddock CD, Rota P, Fields B, De Risi J, Yang JY, Cox N, Hughes JM, leDuc JW, Bellini WJ, Anderson LJ and the SARS Working Group. A novel coronavirus associated with severe acute respiratory virus. *N Engl J Med* 2003; **348**: 1953–66.

2. Drosten C, Günther S, Preiser W, Van der Werf S, Brodt HR, Becker S, Rabenau H, Panning H, Kolesnikova L, Fouchier RA, Berger A, Burguière AM, Cinatl J, Eickmann M, Escriou N, Grywna K, Kramme S, Manuguerra JC, Müller S, Rickerts V, Stürmer M, Vieth S, Klenk HD, Osterhaus ADME, Schmitz H, Doerr HW. Identification of a novel coronavirus in patients with severe acute respiratory syndrome. *N Engl J Med* 2003; **348**: 1967–76.

3. Fouchier RA, Kuiken T, Schutten M, Van Amerongen G, Van Doornum GJ, Van den Hoogen BG, Peiris M, Lim W, Stohr K, Osterhaus ADME. Aetiology: Koch's postulates fulfilled for SARS virus. *Nature* 2003; **423**: 240.

20

Community-acquired pneumonia

Introduction

Community-acquired pneumonia is extremely common and continues to be associated with a high mortality [1,2]. While we now have useful guidelines for how to identify patients with life-threatening pneumonia, we require a much better understanding of how pneumonia develops and how to tailor our investigations and management. This chapter therefore begins by assessing genetic predisposition to pneumococcal disease, followed by papers dealing with the management of community-acquired pneumonia in a variety of settings (from outpatient childhood pneumonia in developing countries through to severe, life-threatening pneumonia in the intensive care unit [ICU]).

Pneumococcal septic shock is associated with the interleukin-10–1082 gene promoter polymorphism

Schaaf BM, Boehmke F, Esnaashari H, *et al. Am J Respir Crit Care Med* 2003; **168**: 476–80

Association of IL-10 polymorphism with severity of illness in community-acquired pneumonia

Gallagher PM, Lowe G, Fitzgerald T, *et al. Thorax* 2003; **58**: 154–6

BACKGROUND. The temporal balance between pro-inflammatory and anti-inflammatory cytokines during severe bacterial infection and sepsis is thought to be critical in determining outcomes. Thus, an excess of tumour necrosis factor-α (TNF-α) has been associated with adverse outcomes, but so has neutralization of this pro-inflammatory cytokine. Similarly, whilst interleukin-10 (IL-10) can protect against certain types of experimental infection, high concentrations can undoubtedly be associated with severe sepsis. The critical balance of cytokines promoting bacterial clearance has yet to be defined. This background has inevitably led to a hunt for polymorphisms in pro- and anti-inflammatory cytokine genes. These studies therefore characterized the frequency of a single nucleotide polymorphism (SNP) at position −1082 in the IL-10 promoter (IL-10−1082, which is associated with increased IL-10 secretion) and an SNP at position −308 in the TNF-α promoter (TNF-α−308) and assessed the influence of the polymorphisms on the severity of sepsis in microbiologically proven streptococcal disease (Schaaf *et al.*) or the severity of community-acquired pneumonia (Gallagher *et al.*).

INTERPRETATION. The IL-10−1082 G allele is associated with increased disease severity both in pneumococcal sepsis and in community-acquired pneumonia. These data have significant implications for understanding genetic susceptibility for pneumococcal disease and for designing novel therapeutic strategies.

Comment

These two studies are considered together because they provided the same important and novel general message, were remarkably similar in design principles and were published at approximately the same time.

Schaaf *et al.* prospectively recruited 69 patients with culture-proven pneumo-coccal disease (61 had pneumonia, five had meningitis and three had both pneumonia and meningitis, while 44 had bacteraemia and 24 had positive respiratory cultures) over a period of 3.5 years. Patients with immunocompromise were excluded. All patients were stratified by sepsis severity using validated definitions (non-sepsis, simple sepsis, severe sepsis and septic shock). The control group comprised 50 age- and sex-matched patients attending for elective orthopaedic surgery who were without systemic features of inflammation. In contrast Gallagher *et al.* recruited 93 patients with community-acquired pneumonia (aetiology not determined) and stratified these patients according to the severity of associated systemic inflammatory response syndrome. They included 90 controls drawn from medical outpatient departments. Both studies characterized IL-10−1082 and TNF-α−308 genotypes using standard molecular biology techniques (in addition, Schaaf *et al.* studied a polymorphism in the lymphotoxin-α gene and Gallagher *et al.* assessed the IL-6−174 promoter polymorphism: lymphotoxin-α and IL-6 are pro-inflammatory cytokines).

The allele frequency was similar among patients and controls in both studies. In the German study homozygosity for the IL-10−1082 G allele was significantly asso-ciated with septic shock. Furthermore, increasing severity of shock was significantly associated with increasing frequency of the G allele genotype (Table 20.1). This closely parallels the findings in the Irish study in which the frequency of the G allele was sig-nificantly associated with an increasing severity of systemic inflammatory response syndrome (Table 20.2). Gallagher *et al.* did not find an association between bacter-aemia and the IL-10 genotype, but the number of positive blood cultures was low in their study, which of course was not confined to patients with *Streptococcus pneu-moniae*. In neither study were pro-inflammatory cytokine polymorphisms associated with disease severity, although the frequency of the TNF-α−308 mutation in both studies was very low, such that an association cannot be rigorously excluded in these relatively small studies.

Interestingly, Schaaf *et al.* found that cells from patients with the IL-10 G allele genotype released significantly more IL-10 in response to lipopolysaccaride *in vitro*, yet patients with septic shock did not have significantly elevated levels of IL-10 in their serum. In contrast, the opposite was true for TNF-α, i.e. stimulated cells from patients with the IL-10 G allele genotype secreted unremarkable levels of TNF-α *in*

Table 20.1 Association between genotype interleukin-10–1082 GG and sepsis severity tested with the Cochrane-Armitage trend test

	Interleukin-10–1082				OR	95% CI	Corrected *P*
	AA/AG		GG				
	n	%	*n*	%			
Non-sepsis	16	30.19	2	12.50			
Sepsis	23	43.40	5	31.25	2.065	1.156–3.870	
Severe sepsis	8	15.09	2	12.50	4.264	1.337–14.977	
Septic shock	6	11.32	7	43.75	8.805	1.545–57.962	0.027

CI, confidence interval; OR, odds ratio.
IL-10 GG is associated with increasing sepsis severity, most prominent for septic shock. The *P*-value is corrected for testing multiple polymorphisms (times three).
Source: Schaaf *et al.* (2003).

Table 20.2 IL-10, TNF-α and IL-6 SNP distribution in patients with CAP grouped according to SIRS score

SNP	Illness severity group			
	Non-SIRS	SIRS 2	SIRS 3	SIRS 4
IL-10 GG*	5 (26%)	3 (18%)	12 (36%)	12 (50%)
IL-10 GA	7 (37%)	10 (59%)	12 (36%)	9 (38%)
IL-10 AA	7 (37%)	4 (24%)	9 (27%)	3 (13%)
IL-10 G allele**	17 (45%)	16 (47%)	36 (55%)	33 (69%)
TNF-α GG	10 (53%)	7 (41%)	20 (61%)	14 (58%)
TNF-α GA	9 (47%)	9 (53%)	11 (33%)	10 (42%)
TNF-α AA	0 (0)	1 (6%)	2 (6%)	0 (0)
TNF-α A allele	9 (24%)	11 (32%)	15 (23%)	10 (21%)
IL-6 GG	3 (16%)	6 (35%)	9 (27%)	7 (29%)
IL-6 GC	12 (63%)	8 (47%)	19 (58%)	11 (46%)
IL-6 CC	4 (21%)	3 (18%)	5 (15%)	6 (25%)
IL-6 G allele	18 (47%)	20 (59%)	37 (56%)	25 (52%)

SNP, single nucleotide polymorphism; CAP, community-acquired pneumonia; IL, interleukin; SIRS, systemic inflammatory response syndrome; TNF-α, tumour necrosis factor alpha.
* $P < 0.05$, non-parametric test for trend; ** $P = 0.02$, non-parametric test for trend.
Source: Gallagher *et al.* (2003).

vitro, yet this cytokine was significantly raised in the serum from patients with septic shock. This reinforces the concept that a complex interaction between apparently opposing cytokines may profoundly influence the outcome of streptococcal infection.

A few points should be considered in interpreting these data. First, the studies were small, with particularly low numbers when the patient groups were stratified by severity (in addition, the subsets of sepsis and systemic inflammatory response syndrome were slightly artificial manipulations of the severity continuum in these conditions). Sample size and difficulties in defining a very specific disease phenotype are the principal difficulties facing studies such as these. Nevertheless, the designs were robust enough to detect significance for the IL-10 polymorphism (the jury must remain out on the pro-inflammatory cytokines). Secondly, the controls might have been drawn instead from a healthy population and it cannot be assumed that patients with inflamed joints or attending medical outpatients are not predisposed to inflammation, but this is perhaps a pedantic point. Thirdly, it must be remembered that the G allele genotype was present in approximately 20% of the controls in both studies: as such it appears that nothing can be inferred about the susceptibility of carriers of the G allele to the acquisition of pneumococcus, but if a G allele individual does become infected with the organism, defence against severe disease appears to be impaired. Finally, the factors linking genotype to disease severity are likely to involve much more complex explanations than a single gene polymorphism and it is likely that interactions between a host of genes involved in innate (and adaptive) immunity require to be elucidated. This in turn will require further, larger studies.

Despite such inevitable considerations these studies are of great potential importance to understanding the biology of the host response to pneumococcus. While emphasizing the need for characterizing the interaction between cytokines more comprehensively in infected patients, they have other far-reaching implications, for example such findings may allow us to identify patients at high risk for severe pneumococcal sepsis.

Microbiological testing and outcome of patients with severe community-acquired pneumonia

Rello J, Bodi M, Mariscal D, *et al. Chest* 2003; **123**: 174–80

B A C K G R O U N D . The debate surrounding whether aggressive microbiological testing affects outcome in the ICU has largely been confined to the setting of ventilator-associated pneumonia |3|. Relatively little is known about the impact of microbiological assessment in the context of severe community-acquired pneumonia requiring admission to the ICU and this group therefore addressed this question retrospectively based on 7 years of clinical experience.

I N T E R P R E T A T I O N . Microbiological testing yielded a high rate of presumed aetiological pathogens in severe community-acquired pneumonia, frequently resulting in relevant and important changes in antibiotic therapy. While the aetiology of severe community-acquired pneumonia is likely to vary by location and season, in this study three organisms (*S. pneumoniae, Legionella pneumophila* and *Pseudomonas aeruginosa*) were associated with almost 60% of deaths in which positive microbiology was identified. These data strongly support the use of aggressive microbiological testing in severe community-acquired pneumonia.

Comment

This group has contributed enormously to the understanding of infection in the ICU and made use of their established, prospectively formulated database for describing the microbiology and outcomes in consecutive patients admitted to their ICU with severe community-acquired pneumonia from 1993 to 1999. A diagnosis of community-acquired pneumonia depended on a compatible chest X-ray and examination. The exclusion criteria included recent hospitalization or nursing home residence, immunosuppression associated with transplant, haematological malignancy or chemotherapy, and terminal disease complicated by pneumonia. A total of 210 patients were identified, of whom six were excluded on the grounds of clinical evidence of *Varicella zoster* pneumonia. Strict criteria for intubation and mechanical ventilation were met by 106 patients, with 81 of the remaining patients managed with non-invasive ventilation. All patients received empirical antibiotics on admission to hospital (presumed to be before ICU presentation in all/most cases). A wide variety of microbiological tests were employed, including tests for *L. pneumophila* and (in intubated and mechanically ventilated patients) bronchoscopic sampling with quantitative cultures. However, it should be noted that this was not an epidemiological surveillance study (i.e. not all patients had every microbiological test, indeed no single test was performed in all patients). Organisms were considered causative if they were isolated in blood, pleural fluid or bronchoscopic samples (using strict quantitative criteria), if serology showed a fourfold rise in titre or if there was any isolation of *Pneumocystis carinii, L. pneumophila* or *Mycobacterium tuberculosis* using standard tests. Organisms in tracheal aspirates were considered causative only if they were isolated within 1 h of intubation, while sputum isolates were considered as 'probable' pathogens.

The age range of the patients was wide with a mean of approximately 60 years and 80% of the patients were male. Microbiological tests led to identification of a pathogen in 117 patients with severe community-acquired pneumonia (57%). The yields were generally good for blood cultures (21% of those sampled), pleural fluid (22%) and bronchoalveolar lavage fluid (34%), particularly when it is considered that antibiotics had already been administered to patients. In total approximately 20 different organisms were identified, but 80% of the isolates were explained by *S. pneumoniae* ($n = 41$), *L. pneumophila* ($n = 23$), *Haemophilus influenzae* ($n = 11$), *P. carinii* ($n = 10$) and *P. aeruginosa* ($n = 8$). The microbiological yield was higher still in mechanically ventilated patients (69%), in whom testing was more frequent and more invasive. Empirical antibiotic management was altered on the basis of microbiology in 85 patients (i.e. 42% of all the patients and 73% of patients in whom microbiology was positive), usually resulting in simplification of treatment. However, in at least seven patients the introduction of antibiotics tailored to a newly isolated organism resulted in significant clinical improvement. The overall mortality in the study was 48 out of 204 (24%), this figure rising to 47 out of 106 (44%) among the mechanically ventilated patients. The predominant organisms associated with mortality were *S. pneumoniae*, *L. pneumophila* and *P. aeruginosa*. Mortality was not significantly different in those with (27%) and those without (20%) a microbiological diagnosis.

The authors pointed out that it is hard to extrapolate these data directly to other ICUs (local epidemiology, local resistance patterns and seasonal variations all have to be taken into account), but the general principles seem applicable. One or two findings in the trial are worthy of comment. First, each case in this study seems to be attributed to a single organism and this is perhaps surprising for severe community-acquired pneumonia, suggesting that some important organisms may have been missed. This theme is extended in that it is surprising that only one viral pneumonia, three atypical organisms other than *L. pneumophila*, and two anaerobic infections were identified. Furthermore, the timing of the positive samples relative to the time of ICU admission is not described. This may be relevant in that some of the organisms in the mechanically ventilated group are traditionally nosocomial and associated with antibiotic resistance (indeed 23 patients in the mechanically ventilated group had antibiotic-resistant organisms and 15 of these patients died). Therefore, the key question is whether these organisms were truly community acquired or hospital acquired. In this regard, the fact that the inclusion criteria contained acquisition of bacteria out of hospital and the fact that the time to death in ventilated patients was generally short (i.e. generally before acquisition of antibiotic-resistant, nosocomial pathogens) suggest that the majority of the fatal organisms were indeed community acquired. This has far-reaching implications. Indeed, the wide range of pathogens in this study suggests it is hard to select simple empirical therapy for covering the majority of important pathogens in severe community-acquired pneumonia requiring ICU admission (in distinct contrast to less severe pneumonia requiring admission to hospital). This in itself advocates increasingly aggressive microbiological testing for establishing the causative pathogen in severe community-acquired pneumonia.

The obvious final question is whether microbiological testing affects the outcome (and particularly mortality) in severe community-acquired pneumonia. There is certainly circumstantial evidence in this study to suggest that it does. The counter-argument would be that the mortality was slightly higher in the patients with a microbiological diagnosis in this study, but this ignores the fact that microbiology was more aggressively pursued in the sickest patients in the study. The inevitable conclusion is that prospective trials will be required in order to answer this question definitively. This brings us back to similarities with ventilator-associated pneumonia, in which the largest trial to date showed clear benefit for an invasive diagnostic strategy |4|. In the meantime this important study from Rello *et al.* strongly supports aggressive microbiological testing in patients with severe community-acquired pneumonia requiring admission to an ICU.

Clinical efficacy of 3 days versus 5 days of oral amoxicillin for treatment of childhood pneumonia: a multicentre double-blind trial

Pakistan Multicentre Amoxicillin Short Course Therapy Pneumonia Study Group. *Lancet* 2002; **360**: 835–41

BACKGROUND. The number of children under the age of 5 years who die each year is as shocking as it is depressing |5|. Poverty and inadequate healthcare systems contribute enormously to this problem. The unacceptable fact remains that a high proportion of these deaths are attributable to preventable or curable infection, often in the respiratory tract. Judicious use of simple, inexpensive, effective antibiotic regimens for pneumonia would represent a significant advance, particularly in developing countries. This study therefore aimed to compare the efficacy of 3 and 5-day courses of amoxicillin for the treatment of non-severe childhood pneumonia.

INTERPRETATION. A 3-day course of amoxicillin appears to be as effective as a 5-day course in the treatment of non-severe childhood pneumonia. However, each regimen was associated with a treatment failure rate of 20%. It remains possible that a high proportion of patients in this study did not have infection of the alveolar regions of the lung.

Comment

This was a large, randomized, double-blind, placebo-controlled, multicentre study. Children at least 2 months old but under 5 years of age were enrolled if they satisfied World Health Organization criteria for non-severe pneumonia, comprising cough and/or difficulty breathing in conjunction with a respiratory rate of 50 or more in children aged 2–11 months or 40 or more in children aged 12–59 months. The respiratory rate was assessed with the child quiet, eating or sleeping. Children were excluded if they had chronic illness, asthma, episodic wheeze or if they had received antibiotics in the previous 2 days. Parents were issued two treatment bottles, the first containing amoxicillin to be given orally for 3 days (15 mg/kg three times a day) and the second containing the same amoxicillin preparation or placebo, to be taken for a further 2 days. Children were assessed clinically on days 3, 5 and 14 and the majority of children (92%) had a chest X-ray. The primary outcome measurement was 'treatment failure' defined as a change in treatment for pneumonia in the first 5 days, lack of clinical improvement (as assessed by respiratory rate), progression of disease or death. The secondary outcome measurement was relapse, defined as evidence of pneumonia in the 6–14 days after recovery of initial tachypnoea. Two thousand children were randomized based on power calculations and over half of these were less than 1 year old. Only 14% of the children who were X-rayed had radiological evidence of pneumonia.

The rate of treatment failure was approximately 20% in each group and the rate of relapse approximately 1.3% in each group (no significant differences). Compliance (assessed by examining treatment bottles) was remarkably high and seems to have been greater than 90%: we are told that compliance in the 5-day group was significantly lower than for the first 3 days of amoxicillin in the 3-day group (but for some reason we are not told whether compliance was preserved in the subsequent 2 days when placebo was taken by the 3-day group). Logistic regression analysis suggested that non-compliance with treatment, age below 1 year, vomiting, a longer duration of illness and more severe tachypnoea were associated with treatment failure.

This study is important and has far-reaching implications, yet some potential concerns should be discussed. Most importantly, as the authors mentioned, there was no confirmation of the diagnosis of pneumonia, nor were extensive microbiological data available. That many of the children did not have infection in the distal, alveolar regions of the lung is suggested by the fact that only 14% of the chest X-rays were compatible with pneumonia and that the failure rates were high despite apparently excellent compliance. If one assumes that a moderate number of children had something other than infection of the lung parenchyma and that viruses or atypical organisms caused a proportion of bona fide pneumonias, then the study would naturally be biased towards no difference in efficacy between the 3- and 5-day courses of amoxicillin. Of course this is a central dichotomy in designing such studies: rigorous confirmation of bacterial pneumonia would be extremely difficult, time-consuming and expensive and would mean that pragmatic trials such as this would have to rely either on very small numbers, on many more centres or on greatly prolonged study periods. The other inevitable question, given the diagnostic and microbiological uncertainty, is whether the failure rate would have been any/much higher had placebo (with supportive care) been used throughout. It would be very difficult to make an ethical argument for a 5-day placebo limb in trials such as this and yet one of the arguments for the shorter course treatment is that antibiotic resistance should be less. Following this argument to its logical conclusion, one challenge ahead is to develop systems where bacterial pneumonia can be rapidly and accurately identified, such that short versus long courses of antibiotics can be compared in that population, while antibiotics can be specifically avoided in patients with no evidence for bacterial disease or predisposition.

The compliance and low dropout rates of this study were amazingly good. No specific data are provided, but the sceptic might argue that, in Pakistan's current healthcare system, such rates of compliance might be more likely among affluent, more educated families, raising concerns that the study may not be representative of the population in which morbidity and mortality from pneumonia is highest. In addition, it would have been interesting to know more about the formulation of the placebo: the vast majority of children had improved significantly by day 3 and it would seem intuitive that some parents would not start the second treatment bottle in the trial, again biasing towards equal efficacy of 3- and 5-day treatments. Finally, it is presumably a typographical error that 'all patients gave verbal, witnessed, informed consent' when most patients were under 1 year old!

Despite these considerations, many of which are inevitable in designing pragmatic trials of this nature, this is a most welcome addition to the literature suggesting that antibiotic courses can be shortened without losing efficacy. On the one hand, these data should encourage other developing countries to design trials assessing shorter courses of inexpensive, effective antibiotics for childhood pneumonia. On the other hand, the data reinforce the need for developing better yet simple systems with which to identify accurately when the breathless patient has bacterial pneumonia, non-bacterial pneumonia or a disease other than pneumonia.

Implementation of an evidence-based guideline to reduce duration of intravenous antibiotic therapy and length of stay for patients hospitalized with community-acquired pneumonia: a randomized controlled trial
Fine MJ, Stone RA, Lave JR, *et al. Am J Med* 2003; **115**: 343–51

BACKGROUND. The optimal duration of intravenous antibiotics and length of hospital stay for patients with community-acquired pneumonia remain controversial. Evidence exists to suggest that conversion of intravenous to oral antibiotics may lag some way behind clinical stability in community-acquired pneumonia |6| and the implication is that unnecessary intravenous antibiotic use is widespread, thus wasting resources and potentially promoting antibiotic resistance. This study aimed to determine whether introduction of an evidence-based guideline could promote earlier conversion of intravenous to oral antibiotics and earlier hospital discharge for stable patients with community-acquired pneumonia.

INTERPRETATION. The evidence-based guideline was associated with a trend towards earlier conversion to oral antibiotics, but this did not reach statistical significance. Introduction of the guideline was not associated with adverse effects and it appeared to be associated with a reduction in in-hospital medical complications.

Comment
Seven sites in the Pittsburgh region participated in this randomized, controlled trial. The guideline to be implemented in the active arm was based on existing literature and local expert opinion and is summarized in Table 20.3. Randomization in this trial was by physician groups, in other words teams of physicians treating community-acquired pneumonia were assigned to administer either the active arm of the trial only or the control arm of the trial only. The active arm of the trial consisted of an educational package for physicians, daily assessments of patient stability and a clear strategy with which to implement the guidelines shown in Table 20.3. Teams treating patients with community-acquired pneumonia in the control arm received only the educational package. Patients were eligible if they had a documented treatment plan for community-acquired pneumonia and a chest X-ray showing new alveolar infiltrates. A wide variety of exclusion criteria were employed, ensuring particularly that

Table 20.3 Medical practice guideline for conversion from intravenous to oral antibiotic therapy and hospital discharge

Step 1: Assess stability for conversion from intravenous to oral antibiotic therapy*

Recommend conversion when patient meets the following criteria:

(a) Ability to digest tablets, capsules, or liquids; and
(b) Stable vital signs for ≥24 hours:
  • Temperature ≤38.0°C (100.4°F)
  • Heart rate ≤100 beats per minute
  • Spontaneous respiratory rate ≤24 breaths per minute
  • Systolic blood pressure ≥90 mmHg (≥100 mmHg for patients diagnosed with hypertension) without vasopressor support

Step 2: Assess stability for hospital discharge*

Recommend discharge when patient meets the following criteria:

(a) Criteria for conversion to oral antibiotic therapy (in Step 1);
(b) Baseline mental status;
(c) No evidence of acute, serious co-morbidity, or laboratory abnormality that necessitates continued hospitalization†; and
(d) Adequate oxygenation on room air or ≤2 l of oxygen therapy (Pao_2 ≥60 mmHg; or pulse oximetry ≥92% for white patients; 94% for non-white patients). For patients with chronic hypoxaemia or chronic oxygen therapy, Pao_2 or pulse oximetry measurement must be at baseline.

* Criteria for antibiotic conversion and hospital discharge could be met simultaneously or sequentially. Stability for antibiotic conversion was required at or before the time of a discharge recommendation.
† Medical reasons for continued hospitalization included the following within the past 24 hours: transfer to a coronary care or intensive care unit, unstable angina, myocardial infarction, venous thromboembolism, worsening heart failure, atrial or ventricular arrhythmia with hypotension, cardiopulmonary arrest, gastrointestinal haemorrhage requiring blood transfusion, diarrhoea or vomiting with volume depletion, bowel obstruction or perforation, seizure, stroke or transient ischaemic attack, exacerbation of asthma or emphysema requiring parenteral corticosteroids, respiratory failure, pneumothorax, gross haemoptysis, acute renal failure, urinary retention requiring surgical intervention, or an operative procedure.
Pao_2, partial pressure of oxygen in arterial blood.
Source: Fine *et al.* (2003).

study patients were adults with no significant immunosuppression, nosocomial infection, active tuberculosis or cystic fibrosis. The primary outcomes were defined as the duration of intravenous antibiotics and length of hospital stay.

Interestingly, although 1660 patients were eligible during the 14-month study period, only 668 were randomized, largely because consent was withheld either by patients or physicians. The reasons for this unusually high failure to secure consent are not clear. A further 60 patients were withdrawn after enrolment leaving 283 patients in the intervention group and 325 in the control group. The groups were extremely well matched with mean age approximately 69 years and approximately 50% of the patients having pre-existing respiratory co-morbidity. Approximately half of the patients in each group had a Pneumonia Severity Index of class IV or V, representing relatively severe pneumonia.

Hazards ratio analysis suggested that patients in the intervention group had a shorter time to both conversion to oral antibiotics (HR 1.23) and discharge (HR 1.16), but neither of these observations was statistically significant ($P = 0.06$ and 0.11, respectively). When analysing a variety of secondary outcomes it was found that the rate of in-hospital medical complications was lower in the intervention group (55 versus 63%) ($P = 0.04$).

This study may have suffered from the fact that inpatient stays for a variety of medical conditions, including community-acquired pneumonia, were already falling between the planning of the study and its start date. This is disappointing, as carefully designed, randomized, controlled trials like this are badly required for assisting in the rationalization of treatment and discharge planning in community-acquired pneumonia. The authors readily highlighted potential weaknesses of the study including the fact that the physicians were not blinded (by necessity) and the possibility that local colleagues discussing their role in the intervention arm influenced the physicians administering the control arm. In addition, caution must be exercised in generalizing these data for several reasons. First, the remarkable number of eligible patients who were not enrolled were generally older and sicker than the patients who entered the study and stringent exclusion criteria were exercised in defining eligibility in the first place: therefore, the population studied was not strictly representative of patients admitted with community-acquired pneumonia in Pittsburgh. Furthermore, these data cannot be readily extrapolated to other healthcare systems such as the British National Health Service, where the use of intravenous antibiotics would likely be much lower in patients with community-acquired pneumonia of comparable severity and more patients would be cared for by respiratory specialists (who represented only approximately 8% of the physicians in this study).

One final limitation of the study relates to the unexpected finding that one-quarter of the patients in the intervention group were discharged before they reached stability as defined in the guidelines. This calls into question the level of adherence with the guidelines among the physicians in the intervention arm: while it appears that adherence was moderate to good, it is difficult to make a clear conclusion from the data presented.

So where does this study leave us? We are left in the frustrating situation where it seems logical to base therapeutic rationalization and discharge planning on stability indices, yet the evidence provides only a non-significant trend. On balance, however, at the present time, whilst we await future, larger trials, it seems reasonable to base discharge planning and conversion from intravenous antibiotics on stability guidelines, particularly when this study suggests it is eminently safe to do so.

Effectiveness of oral moxifloxacin in standard first-line therapy in community-acquired pneumonia

Torres A, Muir JF, Corris P, *et al. Eur Respir J* 2003; **21**: 135–43

BACKGROUND. Recent years have seen increasing interest in the potential use of fluoroquinolones as single-agent therapy for community-acquired pneumonia, particularly in light of the increasing spread of microbial resistance to penicillins and macrolides. This study therefore compared the clinical effectiveness of twice-daily oral moxifloxacin against that of standard therapy for community-acquired pneumonia using an imaginative design whereby the standard therapy could be given as oral amoxicillin alone (three times daily), oral clarithromycin alone (twice daily) or a combination of amoxicillin and clarithromycin whilst remaining a double-blind, controlled trial.

INTERPRETATION. Moxifloxacin and standard therapy were equally effective in the treatment of community-acquired pneumonia.

Comment

This phase IIIb study set out to encompass the analytical rigour of a randomized, multinational, double-blind, controlled trial, whilst preserving sufficient pragmatism to allow clinical flexibility such as would be found in 'real-life' medicine. In particular, the trial allowed clinicians to say whether they would have treated the index patient (had he/she not been in a trial) with amoxicillin (500 mg three times daily), clarithromycin (500 mg twice daily) or both. The patient was then randomized to moxifloxacin (400 mg twice daily) or the physician's choice of standard treatment in a double-blind fashion. Similarly, the physician controlled radiographic and microbiological decision making throughout, with the exception that a baseline chest X-ray consistent with pneumonia was one of the inclusion criteria.

Adult patients were enrolled if they satisfied the criteria for community-acquired pneumonia as defined by fever, leukocytosis, compatible symptoms or signs and the radiographic features described above. Exclusion criteria included pregnancy/lactation, allergy or severe reaction to quinolones, severe renal or hepatic disease, co-administration of drugs known to affect the cardiac output interval and hospitalization for more than 2 days. The patients were assessed clinically at days 3–5, days 7–10 ('test of cure') and days 28–35. In addition, the trial incorporated a symptom questionnaire and a well-validated quality of life tool. The primary end-point was defined as clinical response at days 7–10 in a per protocol (as opposed to intention-to-treat) analysis. A range of secondary outcomes were determined on an intention-to-treat basis. The trial incorporated 64 centres from 13 European countries. The authors stated that the study was commercially funded.

A number of the 563 patients randomized were withdrawn for a variety of reasons, leaving 477 patients in the intention-to-treat analysis and 446 in the per protocol analysis: 215 received moxifloxacin and 231 received standard care (37 amoxicillin alone, 57 clarithromycin alone and 137 amoxicillin and clarithromycin). The patients were well matched at baseline, with mean age approximately 50 years and over 50% of patients in Pneumonia Severity Index classes I and II (in keeping with the principle that the severity of illness should be broad but generally tailored towards pneumonia encountered in general practice).

The clinical success rates were extremely high (over 93% at days 7–10) in both arms of the study (Table 20.4), this trend extending across all severities of pneumonia. Similarly, the symptom and quality of life scores were almost identical. Adverse effects were similar in the two groups, but the authors found that 'adverse effects possibly related to therapy' were significantly less frequent in the moxifloxacin group. Curiously, however, the paper lists only five common side effects for each treatment, explaining 30 out of 55 and 40 out of 86 of these adverse effects for moxifloxacin and standard therapy, respectively: we are not told the nature of the remaining 25 and 46 adverse events, respectively. Furthermore, the trial may be biased towards finding more adverse effects for standard treatment because the exclusion criteria incorporated known adverse effects or allergy associated with moxifloxacin, but not standard care. The authors also described more side effects associated with amoxicillin alone than with amoxicillin and clarithromycin together, which is hard to explain. Moxifloxacin and standard treatment were associated with similar numbers of deaths (four and five, respectively) and withdrawals due to adverse events (25 and 23, respectively) and it seems likely that the undescribed adverse events were relatively minor.

This trial undoubtedly benefited from its innovative design and yet a couple of points require attention. First, the number of patients withdrawn after randomization is surprisingly high and includes 82 patients in whom 'essential data were missing or invalid', raising potential concerns over data collection. The withdrawal rate seems to relate to the criteria for intention to treat, which seem unusual in stipulating that clinical evaluation data at days 7–10 were required for inclusion in the

Table 20.4 Clinical success rates at test of cure (TOC) and follow-up (per-protocol [PP] and intention-to-treat [ITT] populations)

Clinical success	TOC#		Follow-up*	
	Moxifloxacin	**Standard treatment**	**Moxifloxacin**	**Standard treatment**
PP population				
Success	201/215 (93.5%)	217/231 (93.9%)	183/192 (95.3%)	207/221 (93.7%)
95% CI	−4.2–3.3		−2.2–5.2	
ITT population				
Success	218/233 (93.6%)	229/244 (93.9%)	196/208 (94.2%)	218/234 (93.2%)
95% CI	−3.9–3.3		−2.9–4.8	

CI, confidence interval
7–10 days post-therapy; * 28–35 days post-therapy.
Source: Torres *et al.* (2003).

statistical analysis. Secondly, while power calculations are described in detail, it is hard to conceive how moxifloxacin could have been shown to be more effective than standard care (which effected a 94% cure rate) without greatly increased recruitment. It is also slightly frustrating that the rates of amoxicillin- or clarithromycin-resistant *S. pneumoniae* in the study centres were not discussed. Some of the centres participating may have had unusually high rates of resistance, potentially introducing an advantage in favour of moxifloxacin.

However, this study unquestionably provides valuable information. Certainly moxifloxacin monotherapy appears to be as effective as standard treatment for community-acquired pneumonia and at least as well tolerated. Given that fluoroquinolones are currently much more expensive than standard treatment, moxifloxacin is most unlikely to displace standard treatment on the basis of results such as these (i.e. currently available treatment is effective, safe and cheap). However fluoroquinolones may find a specific niche in the setting of areas where antibiotic-resistant *S. pneumoniae* is particularly prevalent and future trials in this setting are awaited with interest.

Multicenter, double-blind, placebo-controlled study of the use of filgrastim in patients hospitalized with pneumonia and severe sepsis

Root RK, Lodato RF, Patrick W, *et al*. for the Pneumonia Sepsis Study Group.
Crit Care Med 2003; **31**: 367–73

BACKGROUND. Pneumonia is characterized by neutrophil accumulation in the alveolar space. In order to achieve resolution of pneumonia, neutrophils must be recruited appropriately to the lung, where they must effect phagocytosis and killing of bacteria then undergo apoptosis without extracellular release of toxic neutrophil products. In the design of new treatments for pneumonia it would be highly desirable to harness the beneficial effects of neutrophils while avoiding the undoubted potential of neutrophils for causing pulmonary damage. Granulocyte colony-stimulating factor (G-CSF) stimulates a florid neutrophil leukocytosis and has been used to good effect in experimental models of pneumonia and in human febrile neutropenia. This multicentre, randomized, double-blind, placebo-controlled trial aimed to determine whether filgrastim (recombinant human G-CSF) could influence mortality in patients with pneumonia and associated sepsis.

INTERPRETATION. Filgrastim had no effect on mortality among patients with established pneumonia and associated sepsis. It remains possible that earlier administration of filgrastim may have a place in the management of severe pneumonia, but further trials are clearly required.

Comment

This was a well-designed and rigorous trial involving 96 centres in three continents. Eligible patients had to be adults with clinical features and a chest X-ray consistent with community-acquired pneumonia or nosocomial pneumonia, as well as positive microbiology (sputum and/or blood cultures) and evidence of pneumonia-related severe sepsis as characterized by well-defined organ dysfunctions. Appropriate exclusion criteria were employed. All patients received intravenous antibiotics at the discretion of ICU physicians, but in addition were randomized to receive filgrastim (300 μg intravenously once a day) or placebo for 5 days or until their white cell count exceeded $75 \times 10^9/l$ or until antibiotics were discontinued, whichever came first. A variety of clinical and laboratory indices were followed. The primary outcome measurement was death from any cause by day 29. The secondary outcomes included organ dysfunction, a requirement for mechanical ventilation and the length of stay in ICU. Safety outcomes were also built in. The authors acknowledged the commercial sponsorship of the trial.

The trial ran for almost 4 years, with 701 patients randomized (348 in the filgrastim group), 80% of whom had community-acquired pneumonia. The two groups were extremely well matched at baseline, with mean age approximately 60 years, similar co-morbidities and Acute Physiology and Chronic Health Evaluation (APACHE) II scores of approximately 24. The commonest pathogen isolated was *S. pneumoniae*. The results were analysed on an intention-to-treat basis and 589 patients received the full 5-day course. No differences in mortality (Fig. 20.1), secondary outcomes or adverse effects were observed in the two groups.

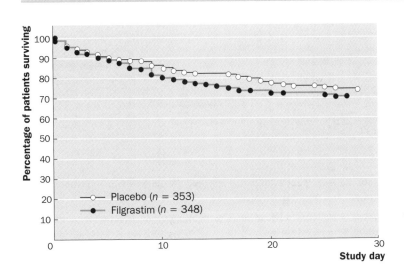

Fig. 20.1 Kaplan–Meier plot and log-rank test for time to death (expressed as percentage of patients surviving). Log-rank test, 1.262; $P = 0.261$.
Source: Root *et al.* (2003).

The strength of this trial lay in its rigorous insistence upon microbiological confirmation of bacterial pneumonia, its robust, multicentre design and its size. In fact, the trial may have suffered from advances in ICU care in the period between the design and the end of the study, as the authors made power calculations on the basis of a presumed mortality of 35% in the control group, whereas Fig. 20.1 shows that the actual mortality was only 25% in this group. Clearly this would make any effect of filgrastim harder to detect. Nevertheless, there is no hint of any effect of filgrastim on mortality. There is no doubt that filgrastim had biological efficacy as the median white cell count approximately doubled in the filgrastim group after 4 days, with no change in the placebo group. The authors speculated that the lack of effect on outcomes might relate to the fact that pneumonia and sepsis were already fully established at the time of administration of filgrastim. It certainly seems plausible that circulating neutrophils induced by filgrastim may have had difficulty accessing the appropriate regions of the lung owing to established ventilation–perfusion mismatch. Unfortunately, no bronchoscopic sampling was incorporated in this trial and therefore there are no data pertaining to neutrophil count, neutrophil products or bacterial counts in the lung. The authors hinted that G-CSF might be more efficacious if administered earlier in the course of infection (or even as a preventative measure in susceptible patients), at a time when neutrophils may have better access to their required site of action, which in turn may represent a less 'hostile' environment for efficient phagocytosis and apoptosis.

Ultimately, these data are in keeping with a recent Cochrane review [7], which concluded there is currently no place for G-CSF in the management of adult pneumonia, whilst acknowledging that earlier administration deserves further attention.

References

1. British Thoracic Society guidelines for the management of community acquired pneumonia in adults. *Thorax* 2001; **56**(Suppl 4): 1–64.

2. American Thoracic Society guidelines for the management of adults with community-acquired pneumonia. Diagnosis, assessment of severity, antimicrobial therapy, and prevention. *Am J Respir Crit Care Med* 2001; **163**: 1730–54.

3. Chastre J, Fagon JY. Ventilator-associated pneumonia. *Am J Respir Crit Care Med* 2002; **165**: 867–903.

4. Fagon JY, Chastre J, Wolff M, Gervais C, Parer-Aubas S, Stéphan F, Similowski T, Mercat A, Diehl JL, Sollet JP, Tenaillon A for the VAP Trial Group. Invasive and non-invasive strategies for management of suspected ventilator-associated pneumonia. *Ann Intern Med* 2000; **132**: 621–30.

5. Black RE, Morris SS, Bryce J. Where and why are 10 million children dying every year? *Lancet* 2003; **361**: 2226–34.

6. Halm EA, Fine MJ, Marrie TJ, Coley CM, Kapoor WN, Obrosky DS, Singer DE. Time to clinical stability in patients hospitalized with community-acquired pneumonia: implications for practice guidelines. *J Am Med Assoc* 1998; **279**: 1452–7.

7. Cheng A, Stephens D, Currie B. Granulocyte colony stimulating factor (G-CSF) as an adjunct to antibiotics in the treatment of pneumonia in adults. *Cochrane Database Syst Rev* 2003; **4**: CD004400.

21

Miscellaneous respiratory infections

Introduction

We all recognize that a small number of important pneumonias are relatively rare in practice, yet are associated with significant morbidity and mortality. The rarity of such infections means they are difficult to study and that experience in their management is often lacking. Such infections include ventilator-associated pneumonia, which is associated with considerable morbidity and mortality |1|, and aspiration pneumonia |2|. These are considered in turn.

Epidemiology and outcomes of ventilator-associated pneumonia in a large US database
Rello J, Ollendorf DA, Oster G, *et al.* for the VAP Outcomes Scientific Advisory Group. *Chest* 2002; **122**: 2115–21

BACKGROUND. Ventilator-associated pneumonia is associated with considerable morbidity, a high crude mortality rate and an enormous impact on healthcare resources. Considerable effort has been channelled into identifying risk factors in the hope of introducing effective preventive measures. Until recent years most studies on the epidemiology and outcomes associated with ventilator-associated pneumonia have been relatively small. This study took advantage of a large US database to identify risk factors for ventilator-associated pneumonia among patients admitted to an intensive care unit (ICU) and to determine the effect of ventilator-associated pneumonia on mortality, use of hospital resources and costs.

INTERPRETATION. Within the limitations of a retrospective design, this study identified male gender and trauma as risk factors for ventilator-associated pneumonia. The study could not identify excess attributable mortality for ventilator-associated pneumonia in the ICU, but patients with ventilator-associated pneumonia had significantly longer mechanical ventilation, ICU stay and hospital stay, in association with excess costs of over $40 000 per patient.

Comment

This retrospective, matched, cohort study took advantage of a large database that gathers admission information for all patients whose hospital is linked to the system. It is hard for the non-American reader to work out from the paper the geographical representation of the hospitals in the database or the relationship between the corporation running the database and the hospitals. Nevertheless, it appears that important information is collected in a way that allows key clinical events, investigations and costs to be followed temporally for each admission. The clear advantage of the database is that it allowed data for over 9000 individuals to be collated over only 18 months of study.

The database was used to identify all patients admitted to an ICU who were mechanically ventilated for at least 24 h, excluding those with evidence of pneumonia prior to mechanical ventilation. From the remaining cohort, patients with and without ventilator-associated pneumonia were identified, the diagnosis of ventilator-associated pneumonia requiring only evidence of hospital-acquired pneumonia occurring at least 24 h after mechanical ventilation. A variety of clinical and demographic details were collected and univariate analysis was used to identify the risk factors associated with ventilator-associated pneumonia. In the second part of the study, patients with ventilator-associated pneumonia (cases) were each matched to up to three controls on the basis of the duration of mechanical ventilation, illness severity at the time of admission, the reason for ICU admission (medical, surgical or trauma) and age. The purpose of this part of the study was to identify whether ventilator-associated pneumonia was specifically associated with excess mortality, length of stay (ICU or hospital) and hospital costs.

The database identified a total of 9080 patients admitted to an ICU who received mechanical ventilation for at least 24 h, 842 of whom (9.3%) satisfied the study criteria for ventilator-associated pneumonia. Patients with ventilator-associated pneumonia were on average significantly younger and more likely to be male, to have a diagnosis of coma/stupor and to be admitted because of trauma. Curiously, ventilator-associated pneumonia was also associated with a moderate level of illness severity, i.e. patients with low illness severity and very high illness severity appeared to be relatively protected from ventilator-associated pneumonia for reasons that are not clear. In the case–control study, 816 of the patients with ventilator-associated pneumonia were closely matched to 2243 controls. The in-hospital mortality was similar in the two groups at just over 30%. However, the duration of mechanical ventilation and length of both ICU- and hospital-stay were markedly and significantly increased in ventilator-associated pneumonia (Fig. 21.1), with an estimated excess cost per patient of $41 000.

The considerable strength of this study relates to its size and the comprehensive nature of the database employed. Certainly this is the largest study of its kind in relation to ventilator-associated pneumonia. In general it is reassuring that such a large study confirmed previous observations, including male gender and trauma as risk factors, and the identification of strikingly high attributable health costs, length

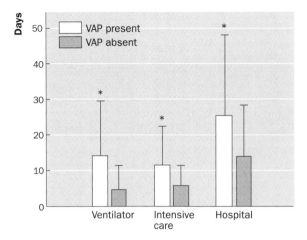

Fig. 21.1 Health and economic outcomes associated with VAP. Mean values and standard deviations are shown. VAP, ventilator associated pneumonia; SD, standard deviation.
*P <0.001 for all comparisons.
Source: Rello *et al.* (2002).

of stay and the duration of mechanical ventilation. However, the authors readily acknowledged the potential limitations of a retrospective study design. In particular, they made the important point that the database was unable retrospectively to retrieve data on a wide variety of risk factors demonstrated to be important in other studies of ventilator-associated pneumonia, in particular prior antibiotic use |3|. It may also be relevant that the cases and controls in the second part of the study were likely to be drawn from different hospitals.

A couple of other potentially very important points should be made in trying to interpret this study. First, allowing the case definition of ventilator-associated pneumonia to include infection acquired less than 48 h after intubation is controversial. Traditionally, studies of ventilator-associated pneumonia have only considered infections arising at least 48 h after intubation, though there are emerging reasons to believe that ventilator-specific lung infection can emerge before this |4|. Certainly it seems highly likely that some cases of 'incubating' nosocomial pneumonia (or even community-acquired pneumonia) acquired prior to mechanical ventilation contaminated the study group. Such organisms are likely to be much less virulent and antibiotic resistant than the pathogens traditionally associated with ventilator-associated pneumonia and therefore use of the 24-hour cut-off period may have profound implications, for mortality analysis in particular. Secondly, the actual diagnosis of ventilator-associated pneumonia must be called into question for a significant number of patients in this study, not just for the reasons described in the previous few sentences, but because strictly speaking the cohort had *suspected* ventilator-associated pneumonia and in this setting more detailed analyses have yielded alternative diagnoses to ventilator-associated pneumonia in over 50% of patients |5|. This raises again the thorny issue of whether microbiological confirmation is required for a diagnosis of ventilator-associated pneumonia and, if so, how it should be made. Although respiratory microbiology was obtained in 72% of the patients in this study, it is not clear in what proportion the distal airway was sampled (as opposed to relying on tracheal aspirates). Those in the 'invasive microbiological' camp would therefore contend that this study may have significantly overestimated true ventilator-associated pneumonia. Again this might explain the inability to detect a significant attributable mortality for ventilator-associated pneumonia.

Despite these considerations it is abundantly clear that ventilator-associated pneumonia as defined in this study is associated with significantly increased lengths of stay and costs. As described above, it is very comforting that this large study using a pragmatic definition of ventilator-associated pneumonia not only broadly supports the findings of studies using stricter definitions of ventilator-associated pneumonia but does so using large numbers of patients. Ultimately this important study achieves its aims in that, for ventilator-associated pneumonia as defined here, it reinforces understanding of the risk factors, emphasizes the healthcare implications of the disease and suggests end-points that might be targeted in important interventional studies aiming to reduce the incidence and burden of ventilator-associated pneumonia.

Microbiology of severe aspiration pneumonia in institutionalized elderly

El-Solh AA, Pietrantoni C, Bhat A, *et al. Am J Respir Crit Care Med* 2003; **167**: 1650–4

BACKGROUND. Traditional teaching contends that anaerobic organisms play a significant part in the pathogenesis of aspiration pneumonia. Although some evidence has emerged to challenge the importance of anaerobes in this setting |2|, the difficulties inherent in defining aspiration pneumonia have limited the number of studies addressing this issue. These investigators therefore aimed to establish the effects of microbial aetiology and prognostic factors on mortality in severe aspiration pneumonia acquired in long-term care facilities.

INTERPRETATION. This small study demonstrated that Gram-negative aerobic bacilli are the predominant pathogens isolated in aspiration pneumonia. Severe aspiration pneumonia carried a high mortality, which was not adversely influenced by isolation of anaerobic organisms. Indeed, nearly all patients with anaerobic isolates that were not covered by appropriate initial antibiotics showed features of improvement in the first 72 h. These data emphasize the need to cover Gram-negative pathogens when severe aspiration pneumonia is suspected. They similarly call into question the need to cover anaerobic organisms, although larger prospective, randomized trials will be required in order to address this issue comprehensively.

Comment

This study is to be admired for addressing such a difficult clinical problem. All residents of long-term care facilities aged 65 years or more admitted to the ICU in Buffalo, New York, with features of severe pneumonia were screened prospectively for features of aspiration pneumonia over a 34-month period. Patients were considered to have severe aspiration pneumonia if they had clinical and radiographic features compatible with pneumonia, required mechanical ventilation and had evidence of risk factors for oropharyngeal aspiration, defined as documented evidence of abnormal swallowing caused by neurological dysphagia, disruption of the oesophagogastric junction or anatomical abnormalities of the upper aerodigestive tract. The exclusion criteria incorporated clear evidence for immunosuppression and either hospitalization or antibiotics in the 30 days prior to admission. A variety of clinical and laboratory indices were assessed, including the APACHE II score, Activity of Daily Living score and a quantitative assessment of dentition. Microbiological analysis appears to have been comprehensive (though the handling and culture of anaerobic cultures are not discussed in great detail) and within 4 h protected bronchoalveolar lavage was performed for quantitative culture. In addition, the authors assessed whether initial antibiotic therapy, given before microbiology was available, was adequate (i.e. where isolated organisms proved to be sensitive) and/or effective (i.e. where the clinical situation remained stable for 72 h with a fall in fever and leukocytosis).

No consent was obtained for 43 of the 138 patients enrolled, leaving 95 for evaluation. Positive microbiology was obtained in 54 patients (57%), leading to the generation of three subgroups namely patients with anaerobes ($n = 11$), patients who had only aerobes isolated ($n = 43$) and patients with no microbiological confirmation of pneumonia ($n = 41$) (it is not clear how alternative diagnoses were pursued in the latter group). The three groups were generally well matched at presentation, although the group with no microbiological diagnosis had a trend towards more florid radiographic disease. Interestingly, dental disease (which is associated with aspiration pneumonia) was equally distributed among the three groups. Indeed, the only outcome differences in the study groups were a significantly greater length of ICU stay and mechanical ventilation in the group with no microbiological diagnosis and a significantly reduced functional status among patients with anaerobic organisms isolated. The mortality was similar in all three groups (33–41%).

The detailed microbiological profile is shown in Table 21.1. The striking features are that the microbiology bears no resemblance to the profile in community-acquired pneumonia, that Gram-negative aerobic bacilli are so well represented and that six of the eleven patients with anaerobes isolated had simultaneous isolation of a Gram-negative organism. Two of the eleven anaerobes were resistant to penicillin *in vitro* and another was resistant to both penicillin and metronidazole, but all eleven

Table 21.1 Microbial aetiology of pulmonary aspiration

	Aerobic group ($n = 43$)	Anaerobic group ($n = 11$)
Gram-positive aerobic cocci		
Streptococcus pneumoniae	5	–
Streptococcus spp.	6	–
Staphylococcus aureus	8	–
Gram-negative aerobic bacilli		
Haemophilus influenzae	2	–
Escherichia coli	11	2
Klebsiella pneumoniae	8	2
Serratia spp.	7	1
Proteus mirabilis	6	1
Enterobacter cloacae	1	–
Pseudomonas aeruginosa	2	–
Anaerobic		
Prevotella spp.	–	6
Fusobacterium spp.	–	3
Bacteroides spp.	–	1
Peptostreptococcus spp.	–	1

Source: El-Solh *et al.* (2003).

were sensitive to clindamycin. However, interestingly, while initial empirical anti-biotics did not cover seven of the eleven anaerobes, clinical effectiveness was still demonstrated for six of these seven patients, potentially suggesting that the anaer-obes were not making a significant contribution to morbidity. It is also interesting and reassuring that only two cases of methicillin-resistant *Staphylococcus aureus* were identified in this series.

These data provide a crucial addition to the understanding of severe aspiration pneumonia. However, certain methodological issues should be discussed. First, the number of patients with anaerobic infection was obviously small and definitive con-clusions on how best to treat anaerobic infection cannot be drawn (as the authors stated, this will require future prospective, randomized, clinical trials). Secondly, while the criteria for aspiration pneumonia are robust, there is still no way of know-ing whether these patients actually aspirated or whether their pneumonia was acquired without a direct contribution from aspiration. This problem is central to the design of large trials of aspiration pneumonia. Third and perhaps most import-antly, it seems strange that for bronchoalveolar lavage the quantitative culture threshold for pneumonia was taken to be 10^3 CFU/ml, when a cut off of 10^4 CFU/ml is the accepted norm for bronchoalveolar lavage (particularly when this group used a cut-off of 10^4 colony-forming units (CFU)/ml in a recent study of institutionalized elderly patients [6]). Unfortunately this seriously calls into question the specificity of the microbiological results. Finally, it would have been interesting if the authors had included a control group of patients from the same long-term care facilities presenting with severe pneumonia with no risk factors for aspiration pneumonia.

Whilst keeping the size of this study and the troublesome issue of the microbiological cut-off for bronchoalveolar lavage in mind, these data remain very important. The overwhelming messages would seem to be that Gram-negative aerobic bacilli should be covered in patients with suspected severe aspiration pneumonia and that this condition continues to carry a poor prognosis. Other implications are first that an aggressive microbiological approach would appear to be useful in this setting, and, secondly, that anaerobic cover is not as essential as previously thought. However, these two implications should be considered no more than assumptions in the absence of randomized trials for testing them formally.

References

1. Chastre J, Fagon JY. Ventilator-associated pneumonia. *Am J Respir Crit Care Med* 2002; **165**: 867–903.
2. Marik PE. Aspiration pneumonitis and aspiration pneumonia. *N Engl J Med* 2001; **344**: 665–71.
3. Rello J, Ausina V, Ricart M, Castella J, Prats G. Impact of previous antimicrobial therapy on the etiology and outcome of ventilator-associated pneumonia. *Chest* 1993; **104**: 1230–5.
4. Ewig S, Bauer T, Torres A. The pulmonary physician in critical care 4: nosocomial pneumonia. *Thorax* 2002; **57**: 366–71.
5. Meduri GU, Mauldin GL, Wunderink RG, Leeper KV, Jones CB, Tolley E, Mayhall G. Causes of fever and pulmonary densities in patients with clinical manifestations of ventilator-associated pneumonia. *Chest* 1994; **106**: 221–35.
6. El-Solh AA, Aquilina AT, Dhillon RS, Ramadan F, Nowak P, Davies P. Impact of invasive strategy on management of antimicrobial treatment failure in institutionalized older people with severe pneumonia. *Am J Respir Crit Care Med* 2002; **166**: 1038–43.

Overall conclusion

Significant advances have been made in respiratory infection in the past year and the papers discussed reflect a small proportion of these. In particular we now have much better information on the safety and efficacy of pneumococcal and influenza vaccines and we should now turn our attention to expanding the clinical utility of these. Last year also saw an impressive response from the scientific and medical community to the severe acute respiratory syndrome epidemic, with rapid identification of the causative virus. The next step is to develop effective treatments or, better still, vaccines. The field of community-acquired pneumonia research appears to have concentrated appropriately on the rationalization of investigations, the stratification of patients by illness severity and the design of better management plans. Important advances have been made in these areas. Finally, it is reassuring that rare but important infections such as ventilator-associated pneumonia are receiving increasing attention, with particular emphasis on the identification of risk factors in the hope that effective preventive strategies can be developed.

Part VI

Thoracic malignancy

Thoracic malignancy

R FERGUSSON

Introduction

Lung cancer is the most frequent cause of death from malignant disease in the Western world today. Globally more than a million new cases are diagnosed each year. The prognosis for these patients remains extremely poor with only 5–15% surviving 5 years. This figure has remained unchanged for the last two decades in the face of modest therapeutic advances in all treatment modalities. How can this dire situation be changed? There are three areas where urgent progress is needed.

Firstly, the vast majority of symptomatic patients have advanced stage disease at diagnosis. This narrows therapeutic options and makes cure and even prolonged survival unlikely. Patients who have their tumour picked up 'by chance' on an x-ray performed for an unrelated reason often have early stage disease which may be cured with radical treatment. There is little doubt that cancers arise from a single cell. This means that a tumour, which may have a doubling time of up to 6 months, must grow undetected for many years before becoming clinically apparent. These tantalising facts have led workers to pursue screening programmes to detect early lung cancer in asymptomatic smokers. The results of the early trials using chest x-rays and sputum cytology were negative and enthusiasm was quickly lost. In the last 5 years impressive detection of early stage disease using low-dose computed tomography (CT) scanning has emerged from the USA and Japan. Current trials will show whether this approach will improve survival and if other tools such as positron emission tomography (PET) scanning are useful in this context.

Secondly, for patients who are diagnosed conventionally, few effective treatments are available. Surgery is associated with the best survival but resection rates in most countries are below 20% due to unfavourable stage at presentation and the existence of significant smoking-related co-morbidity. Radical radiotherapy has similar problems and the real therapeutic need is for effective chemotherapy which may down-stage patients to make them suitable for a multi-modality approach. Specific molecular targeted therapies have also shown promise even in previously treated patients, and developments in this area are eagerly awaited.

Lastly, the most obvious avenue for progress in a tumour that is caused in the vast majority by cigarette smoking is disease prevention. Smoking rates in most Western countries have been declining recently and this is now being followed by a decrease in the incidence of lung cancer, especially in men. Interest has also been shown in using experimental 'chemo-protective' agents in high-risk groups, although early results have been disappointing. Unfortunately smoking rates in 'developing' countries are extremely high and lung cancer will continue to be a major killer for many years.

Malignant pleural mesothelioma is caused by occupational exposure to asbestos and is increasing dramatically in incidence in most Western countries. Like lung cancer it is preventable and perhaps even more resistant to standard treatments. Advances in its detection and management have appeared in the literature in the last few years.

22

Malignant pleural mesothelioma

Introduction

Pleural mesothelioma is a malignant tumour arising in the pleural surfaces and usually caused by asbestos exposure. The tumour is locally invasive and rapidly fatal with most sufferers dying within 1 year of diagnosis. The disease is rare in women and a history of occupational asbestos exposure usually 30 years previously is obtained in the vast majority of patients. This indicates that most are due to occupational rather than environmental exposure. The incidence of mesothelioma has risen dramatically around the world in the last two or three decades |**1**|. Epidemiological analysis has indicated that the worst affected cohorts in the UK were born in the late 1940s and that the peak incidence for mesothelioma in men will be reached around 2020 (Fig. 22.1) |**2**|, whereas data from North America suggest that this peak will be reached before 2020 as occupational exposure occurred at an earlier age in the USA.

For many years there has been great nihilism about the treatment of this tumour, with the median survival in patients treated with supportive care being approximately 6–9 months. Surgical resection is possible in a minority of highly selected patients, but survival in this group, which usually also receives multimodality treatment with radiotherapy and chemotherapy, is usually less than 15% at 5 years |**3**|. The early trials of chemotherapy were extremely disappointing with no significant prolongation of survival at the cost of much toxicity. The results of radiation therapy have also been poor, with great technical difficulties encountered in irradiating a disease that can spread locally across the whole pleural surface. Single-agent phase II chemotherapy trials with drugs such as cisplatin, doxorubicin and gemcitibine have shown little evidence of activity |**4**|. The combination of these agents has also proved disappointing. This nihilism about the treatment of mesothelioma, a condition for which the pathogenesis and biology are poorly understood, is understandable. The diagnosis is often made late in the disease and most patients do not receive specific anticancer therapy. However, the increasing incidence of the condition has led to some recent attempts to improve this dire situation. One of the first advances was an agreement to develop an internationally accepted staging system based on the tumour and nodes metastases system |**5**|. This has allowed more rational clinical trial designs with standardization of the treatment responses. The recent increase in incidence in the condition has also been accompanied by a surge of reports in the

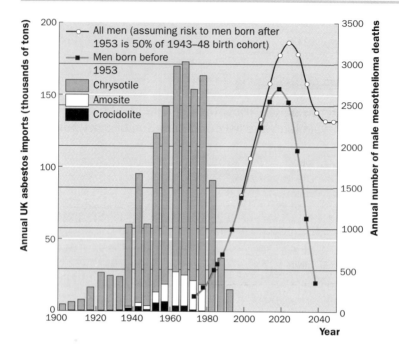

Fig. 22.1 Predicted mesothelioma deaths in British men and UK asbestos imports. Source: [**2**].

literature concerning all aspects of the disease. Some of the important advances in 2002–2003 are summarized below.

Aetiology

In the first half of the twentieth century malignant pleural mesothelioma was very rare and of unknown aetiology. Clusters of patients from asbestos mining areas in Africa first hinted that this was an occupational disease. Subsequent studies confirmed the strong association between mesothelioma and exposure to crocidolite. A number of unresolved questions concerning the causation of mesothelioma remain. One is that there would appear to be a long latent period between exposure to asbestos and the development of mesothelioma. This is certainly more than 20 years and often in the region of 50 years. The reason for this is not known. It is also not clear why only a small proportion of men exposed to asbestos actually develop mesothelioma. Whilst there is undoubtedly a dose–response effect there would appear to be a requirement of host susceptibility before the tumour develops. There has recently been interest in whether exposure to contaminated polio vaccination in the 1950s may have an important place in the development of this tumour. Two papers (one from the USA and one from Denmark) looking at this possibility have appeared in the last year.

Trends in US pleural mesothelioma incidence rates following simian virus 40 contamination of early poliovirus vaccines

Strickler HD, Goedert JJ, Devesa SS, Lahey J, Fraumeni JF, Rosenberg PS.
J Natl Cancer Inst 2003; **95**(i): 35–45

BACKGROUND. Vaccines produced 40 years ago against the poliovirus were contaminated with a monkey virus (simian virus 40) that causes tumours in rodents. Simian virus 40 DNA sequences have been found in some human cancers, particularly pleural mesothelioma. Could accidental exposure to this virus during vaccination in childhood predispose an individual to contracting mesothelioma in later life?

INTERPRETATION. This study was performed using data from the Surveillance, Epidemiology and End-result Programme for estimating the incidence rates of mesothelioma from 1975 to 1997. The poliovirus vaccination prevalence during the period of simian virus 40 contamination was determined for each birth cohort from published survey data. The trends in mesothelioma incidence were then compared with the trends in relevant exposure. The age-standardized pleural mesothelioma incidence rates increased in males from 0.79 per 10^5 person-years in 1975 to a peak of 1.69 per 10^5 person-years in 1992. The group with the greatest increase in rates (75 years of age or older) were least likely to have been immunized against poliovirus. In the age groups most heavily exposed to simian virus 40-contaminated vaccine the incidence rate of mesothelioma remained stable or decreased from 1975 through to 1997. Similar trends were seen amongst females.

Comment

This study concluded that there was no connection between contamination of poliovirus vaccines in the 1950s and 1960s and the increasing incidence of mesothelioma. The data concerning mesothelioma were taken from the Surveillance, Epidemiology and End-result Programme database, which comprises a representative sample of approximately 10% of the US population. The study was limited by the fact that the absolute number of mesothelioma cases in the USA is small and decreasing. Secondly, individual exposure data were not available and, thirdly, the fact that trends in incidence derived from surveillance data will reflect the impact of all risk factors rather than a single effect also limited the study.

Cancer incidence in Denmark following exposure to poliovirus vaccine contained with simian virus 40

Engels EA, Katki HA, Nielsen NM, *et al. J Natl Cancer Inst* 2003; **95**(7): 532–9

B A C K G R O U N D . Early poliovirus vaccines were contaminated with simian virus 40 as these vaccines were produced in infected monkey kidney tissue. Simian virus 40 has been shown to cause malignancy in rodents including mesothelioma. Denmark had a particularly high rate of poliovirus vaccination in the 1950s. These viruses were contaminated with simian virus 40. Has this led to an increased incidence of mesothelioma?

I N T E R P R E T A T I O N . Between 1955 and 1956 the vast majority of Danish children and young adults received poliovirus vaccine. In some cohorts, e.g. 7–14 years, 99% of children were vaccinated. This high level of vaccination continued into the early 1960s. This virus was widely contaminated with simian virus 40. This study looked at any association between simian virus 40 contamination and cancer risk by examining the cancer incidence in Danish cohorts with varying exposure to simian virus 40-contaminated vaccine. The cancer incidence was examined in children who were 0–4 years of age before, during and after the period of vaccine contamination. After 69.5 million person-years of follow-up individuals exposed to simian virus 40-contaminated vaccine as infants or children had a lower overall cancer risk than unexposed individuals born after the vaccine was cleared of simian virus 40 contamination (age-adjusted relative risk [RR] = 0.86 and 95% confidence interval [CI] = 0.81–0.91 for infants and age-adjusted RR = 0.79 and 95% CI = 0.75–0.84 for children) (P <0.001 for both).

Comment

These data back up the larger series from North America and show that exposure to simian virus 40-contaminated poliovirus vaccine in Denmark was not associated with an increased cancer incidence and specifically an increased incidence of mesothelioma.

One problem in all these studies has been the fact that it is not known whether simian virus 40 infects humans or whether it is transmitted amongst asymptomatic individuals after vaccination. The strength of this study was the availability of high-quality data on cancer incidence in a small country. These clinical studies therefore conflict with laboratory data reporting the presence of simian virus 40 DNA sequences in human tumours. The authors of this study raised the possibility that the finding of simian virus 40 DNA in human tumours may be a laboratory artefact.

The link between exposure to simian virus 40 and mesothelioma appears fairly tenuous. However, could there be a link between this virus and survival in patients who do develop mesothelioma?

Expression of p21 in SV40 large T antigen-positive human pleural mesothelioma: relationship with survival

Baldi A, Groeger AM, Esposito V, *et al. Thorax* 2002; **57**(4): 353–6

BACKGROUND. Although the vast majority of patients developing mesothelioma have had occupational exposure to asbestos the mechanism of carcinogenesis is unknown. Approximately 20% of patients do not have a clear history of asbestos exposure and it is known that probably only 10% of workers with high levels of asbestos exposure develop the tumour. Approximately 10 years ago it was found that the antigen simian virus 40 large T had a role in the pathogenesis of mesothelioma with simian virus 40 large T sequences found in a significant percentage of cases. It was also found that p53 mutations are extremely rare in mesothelioma patients and it has been postulated that simian virus 40 large T is able to bind to p53. It is therefore thought that p53 is the most important target of simian virus 40 oncoproteins in mesothelioma. The ability of simian virus 40 oncoproteins to inactivate p53 suppressor proteins has been proposed as an important step in the pathogenesis of mesothelioma.

INTERPRETATION. In this study the authors examined tissue from 29 patients with malignant mesothelioma (16 epithelial, six sarcomatous and seven mixed). These patients had been treated over a 13-year period. Survival data were available. The expression of a cell cycle inhibitor p21, a downstream target of p53, was measured immunohistochemically in these tissue specimens. All 29 had already been characterized for the presence of simian virus 40 large T sequences. There was no correlation between p21 expression and histological type. However, there was a significant positive relationship between p21 expression level and the patient's overall survival (Table 22.1). Patients with less than 10% p21 expression ($n = 15$) had a median survival of only 5 months compared with 12 months in 14 patients with greater than 10% p21 expression ($P \leq 0.001$).

Table 22.1 Correlation between p21 and histology with survival in patients with mesothelioma

Variable	No. of patients	Median survival (months)	Standard error	P-value
p21 expression				<0.001
<10%	15	5.00	0.76	
>10%	14	12.00	1.87	
Histology				0.577
Epithelial	16	10.00	0.99	
Sarcomatoid	6	5.00	2.45	
Mixed	7	8.00	2.62	

Source: Baldi *et al.* (2002).

Comment

By measuring the expression of a downstream target of p53 the authors produced further evidence that this mechanism is important not only in the carcinogenesis of these tumours, but also in their prognosis. They concluded that the expression of p21 can be a useful prognostic marker and may even represent a new target for molecular approaches to treatment. This study provided useful information in the understanding of simian virus 40 large T in the pathogenesis of mesothelioma.

Diagnosis and staging

The diagnosis of malignant pleural mesothelioma is usually made from material taken at pleural biopsy. The tumour demonstrates a wide range of histological appearances, the main varieties being epithelial, sarcomatous and mixed patterns.

Histological examination of pleural biopsies in this disease is made difficult by the pleomorphic nature of mesothelioma. This is a particular problem for the pathologist when small samples are available. The main problems are of a differentiation between mesothelioma and secondary adenocarcinoma of the pleura, usually of pulmonary origin, and the separation of benign from malignant pleural disease.

Differentiation of mesothelioma from adenocarcinoma

Patients commonly present with a unilateral pleural effusion that contains undifferentiated malignant cells. Often there is a difficult diagnostic dilemma as to whether this is a primary mesothelioma of the pleura or pleural metastases from other tumours either in the lung or in other solid organs. The tumour type in this situation is usually adenocarcinoma. Whilst radiological evidence of a mass lesion would be in favour of mesothelioma diffuse pleural involvement with adenocarcinoma is common and, on the other hand, patients with mesothelioma may have a 'normal' looking pleura on computed tomography (CT) scanning. Since therapeutic options differ greatly between mesothelioma and adenocarcinoma there have been numerous attempts to try and facilitate the distinction between these two tumours using pathological markers. A single marker specific for mesothelioma has yet to be identified and the immunohistochemical diagnosis of mesothelioma is often based on the use of a battery of markers that may be either positive or negative. Unfortunately, a large number of antibodies that react with mesothelioma frequently cross-react with adenocarcinoma. Controversy therefore exists regarding the value of some of these markers as well as which combination is the most useful in distinguishing between epithelioid mesothelioma and pulmonary adenocarcinoma.

The immunohistochemical diagnosis of mesothelioma. A comparative study of epithelioid mesothelioma and lung adenocarcinoma

Ordonex NG. *Am J Surg Pathol* 2003; **27**(8): 1031–51

BACKGROUND. Numerous histochemical markers that could potentially facilitate the distinction between epithelioid pleural mesothelioma and pulmonary adenocarcinoma have recently become available. Whilst some are strongly positive in each diagnosis many react with both tumours. It is not known which are the best for discriminating between these malignancies.

INTERPRETATION. Sixty epithelioid mesotheliomas and 50 peripheral lung adenocarcinomas were investigated for the expression of 19 immunohistochemical markers. All cases were diagnosed using World Health Organization criteria. To evaluate the specificity of antibody, known positive and negative tissues were used as controls. The grading of the immunostaining was performed on a sliding scale of + to ++++ according to the percentage of reactive cells (+ = 1–25% and ++++ = 76–100%) The results of the immunohistochemical staining for the two tumour types are shown in Table 22.2. All mesotheliomas reacted for calretinin, cytokeratin 5/6 and mesothelin. In the adenocarcinomas 100% were positive for MOC-31, Ber-EP4 and EMA. It was concluded that calretinin, cytokeratin 5/6 and WT1 were the best positive markers and CEA, MOC-31, Ber-EP4, BG-8 and B72.3 were the best negative markers for mesothelioma. The author recommended a panel of four markers (two positive and two negative) for use in diagnosis. The best combination appeared to be calretinin and cytokeratin 5/6 (or WT1) for positive markers and CEA and MOC-31 for negative markers.

Comment

The recommendation that a panel of four markers (two positive and two negative) should be used seems reasonable. Obviously the choice of markers developed depends upon the availability in a given laboratory. One potential problem is the expression of some of the markers in non-pulmonary adenocarcinoma. For example, whilst WT1 is absent in lung adenocarcinomas it is strongly expressed in serous carcinomas of the ovary. Conversely, CEA is less common in ovarian cancer, but is often expressed in lung adenocarcinoma. This study provided a useful reference point by which histopathologists can base the differential diagnosis between mesothelioma of the epithelioid type and adenocarcinoma.

Imaging in pleural mesothelioma

Patients with pleural mesothelioma usually present with a pleural effusion. The pleura may appear thickened with a characteristic lobulated outline. These features may be demonstrated more clearly by a CT scan. In the small proportion of patients undergoing surgery CT scanning is mandatory and the international staging system for mesothelioma is based on the appearance at CT scan.

Table 22.2 Immunohistochemical results

Marker	Epithelial mesotheliomas						Pulmonary adenocarcinomas					
	(n = 60) + cases (%)	Grade of reactivity					(n = 50) + cases (%)	Grade of reactivity				
		Trace	1+	2+	3+	4+		Trace	1+	2+	3+	4+
Calretinin	60 (100)	0	0	0	15	45	4 (8)	2	2	0	0	0
Cytokeratin 5/6	60 (100)	2	3	7	16	32	1 (2)	0	1	0	0	0
WT1	56 (93)	0	4	9	16	27	0 (0)	0	0	0	0	0
Thrombomodulin	46 (77)	0	10	16	16	3	7 (14)	2	5	0	0	0
Mesothelin	60 (100)	0	11	4	17	28	19 (38)	0	8	5	5	1
N-cadherin	44 (73)	1	5	13	14	11	15 (30)	2	4	3	6	0
HBME-1	51 (85)	0	7	11	14	28	34 (68)	0	4	5	9	16
CD44S	44 (73)	0	7	4	11	17	24 (48)	0	14	7	2	1
MOC-31	5 (8)	5	3	0	0	0	50 (100)	0	3	7	19	21
E-cadherin	24 (40)	2	14	5	2	3	44 (88)	0	9	8	20	7
BG-8 (Lewis^y)	4 (7)	0	2	0	0	0	48 (96)	1	6	7	15	21
TTF-1	0 (0)	2	0	0	0	0	37 (74)	0	4	10	15	8
CEA	0 (0)	0	0	0	0	0	44 (88)	0	3	12	17	16
B72.3 (Tag-72)	0 (0)	0	0	0	0	0	42 (84)	0	7	12	15	8
Leu-M1 (CD15)	0 (0)	0	0	0	0	0	36 (72)	0	4	9	13	7
Ber-EP4	11 (18)	2	9	0	0	0	50 (100)	0	0	0	13	37
CA19-9	0 (0)	0	0	0	0	0	24 (48)	0	6	10	6	2
EMA	56 (93)	0	7	9	19	21	50 (100)	0	3	12	10	25
Vimentin	33 (55)	1	28	4	0	0	19 (38)	1	16	2	0	0

CEA, carcinoembryonic antigen; TTF, thyroid transcription factor; EMA, epithelial membrane antigen.
Source: Ordonex et al. (2003).

The value of chest computed tomography and cervical mediastinoscopy in the pre-operative assessment of patients with malignant pleural mesothelioma

Schouwink JH, Schultze Kool L, Rutgers EJ. *Ann Thorac Surg* 2003;
75: 1715–19

BACKGROUND. Multimodality therapy including surgery, radiotherapy and chemotherapy has been postulated to improve survival in patients with mesothelioma. Selection of the patients most likely to benefit from this aggressive treatment is important, as accurate staging of this disease is difficult. CT scanning is commonly used and cervical mediastinoscopy is also established as a method for assessing mediastinal lymph node involvement. The relative usefulness of these two assessments is unknown.

INTERPRETATION. This was a retrospective study comparing mediastinoscopy and CT scanning for diagnostic accuracy in detecting mediastinal lymph node metastases in patients with mesothelioma being screened for potential operability. Forty-three patients were assessed over a 3-year period in the Netherlands Cancer Institute. Thirty-nine per cent had enlarged lymph nodes (more than 10 mm) on CT scanning. The sensitivity, specificity and diagnostic accuracy of CT scanning were 60, 71 and 67% and those of mediastinoscopy were 80, 100 and 93%, respectively (Table 22.3).

Comment

This study highlighted the importance of mediastinoscopy as a pre-operative assessment tool in patients being considered for resection for mesothelioma. As a procedure it would appear to be more accurate than CT and should reduce the number of futile thoracotomies. The enthusiasm of the authors for mediastinoscopy ignored some of the shortcomings of the procedure. Twenty-one per cent of the patients were found to have N2 disease (mediastinal node involvement) that was not diagnosed by

Table 22.3 Sensitivity, specificity, positive predictive value, negative predictive value and accuracy of CT and CM

	CT	CM
Sensitivity	60%	80%
Specificity	71%	100%
Positive predictive value	53%	100%
Negative predictive value	77%	90%
Accuracy	67%	93%

CM, cervical mediastinoscopy; CT, computed tomographic scan.
Source: Schouwink *et al.* (2003).

mediastinoscopy either because the lymph nodes were missed or were inaccessible. The precise importance of N2 disease in this condition has not been established. It may be that histological type is more important and that a patient with epithelial histology with N2 disease may have a better outlook than patients with mixed histology and no lymph node involvement. Caution should therefore be exercised in basing a therapeutic decision on a single test.

Positron emission tomography scanning in mesothelioma

Positron emission tomography (PET) scanning is playing an increasingly important role in the assessment of all malignant diseases. Tumour tissue takes up labelled glucose more avidly than normal tissues and PET scanning is establishing a role in distinguishing benign from malignant involvement. Reports are now appearing in the literature of PET scanning in mesothelioma.

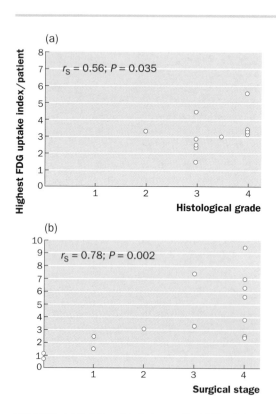

Fig. 22.2 (a) Relationship between the FDG uptake index and the histological grade. (b) Correlation between the highest FDG uptake index per patient and surgical stage. FDG, fluorodeoxyglucose.
Source: Gerbaudo *et al.* (2003).

Metabolic significance of the pattern, intensity and kinetics of ^{18}F-FDG uptake in malignant pleural mesothelioma

Gerbaudo VH, Britz-Cunningham S, Sugarbaker DJ, Treves ST. *Thorax* 2003; **58**(12): 1077–82

BACKGROUND. Few reports have appeared in the literature addressing the use of ^{18}F-fluorodeoxyglucose and PET scanning in the assessment of malignant pleural mesothelioma. It is not known whether the uptake of ^{18}F-fluorodeoxyglucose relates to tumour aggressiveness and whether PET scanning can be used as a prognostic indicator.

INTERPRETATION. Sixteen patients with pleural disease on CT scanning underwent PET imaging by comparing the lesion to background ratio. ^{18}F-Fluorodeoxyglucose uptake was quantified and its uptake over time (malignant metabolic potential index) was correlated with surgical stage and histological grade. Twelve patients had histologically proven mesotheliomas. A number of interesting findings were reported. The intensity of the ^{18}F-fluorodeoxyglucose uptake was a better marker of disease aggressiveness than the histological grade of the tumour. However, there was a good correlation with the surgical stage (Fig. 22.2). Metastatic and recurrent diseases were more ^{18}F-fluorodeoxyglucose avid than primary lesions. The increment in ^{18}F-fluorodeoxyglucose uptake over time was a good estimate of aggression as defined by surgical stage (Fig. 22.3).

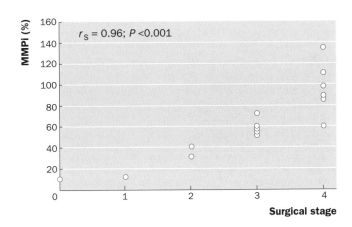

Fig. 22.3 Increment of FDG uptake as a function of time (MMPi) and surgical stage. MMPi, malignant metabolic potential indices.
Source: Gerbaudo *et al.* (2003).

Comment

This was a small pilot study, but it produced interesting results. Larger studies of higher statistical power are required in order to confirm or refute the exact place of PET scanning as a prognostic indicator. This study did not look at the sensitivity and specificity of PET scanning in mesothelioma, but suggested that this technique may be useful once the diagnosis is confirmed histologically.

Positron emission tomography defines metastatic disease but not locoregional disease in patients with malignant pleural mesothelioma

Flores RM, Akhurst T, Gonen M, Larson SM, Rusch VW. *J Thorac Cardiovasc Surg* 2003; **126**(1): 11–16

BACKGROUND. Accurate staging of malignant pleural mesothelioma is difficult. The tumour commonly infiltrates locally along tissue planes and, although CT and magnetic resonance imaging (MRI) are used for staging mesothelioma, they often fail to detect tumour invasion of the chest wall and diaphragm as well as the presence of mediastinal nodal metastases. This is extremely important if surgical resection is being considered. It is not clear whether fluorodeoxyglucose PET scanning has a major role to play in the pre-operative staging of mesothelioma. Only a small series has appeared in the literature thus far.

INTERPRETATION. This was a single-centre series of PET scanning prior to surgery in mesothelioma reported from the Memorial Sloan-Kettering Cancer Centre in New York. A blinded review of PET scans as a staging tool was correlated with surgical and pathological findings. This allowed determination of the sensitivity and specificity for both the tumour and nodal status. Sixty-three patients were included in the study over a 2-year period. The PET scans were positive in all but one patient. The sensitivity of PET for accurately detecting tumour and nodal statuses was extremely poor (19 and 11%, respectively). Uptake of isotope by the tumour was not related to histology. The sensitivity and specificity of PET in predicting the tumour and nodal status are shown in Tables 22.4 and 22.5. The authors showed a weak association between increased uptake in the primary tumour and nodal disease. PET correctly identified six patients who had extrathoracic disease (supraclavicular N3 or M1).

Comment

The results of this study are disappointing though perhaps not surprising. PET scanning very commonly underestimated locoregional tumour and nodal status, but was reasonably good at identifying extrathoracic disease. The correlation between the uptake of isotope and N2 disease was interesting but predictable. It is known that the uptake of fluorodeoxyglucose is related to the mitotic rate and it is also known that tumours with such characteristics commonly have nodal disease at presentation. PET scanning would seem to have little benefit in assessing the local respectability of

Table 22.4 PET assessment of T status compared with surgical and pathologic staging of T status

		T status by PET		
		T0–T3	T4	Total no. patients
Surgical/pathologic T status	T0–T3	29	3	32
	T4	17	4	21
Total no. patients		46	7	53

PET, positron emission tomography; T, tumour.
Source: Flores *et al.* (2003).

Table 22.5 PET assessment of N status compared with the pathological N status

		N status by PET		
		N0 and N1	N2	Total no. patients
Pathologic N status	N0 and N1	19	3	22
	N2	8	1	9
Total no. patients		27	4	31

N, nodal.
Source: Flores *et al.* (2003).

mesothelioma, but may be useful in identifying patients who have unresectable disease due to more distant spread that has been missed on standard clinical assessment and CT scanning.

Treatment of mesothelioma

The results of treatment for pleural mesothelioma are extremely poor. At present there is no accepted curative therapy. There are reports of good survival from radical surgery for limited disease and from multimodality treatment including radiotherapy and chemotherapy [6].

It is likely that advances in survival will be achieved through multimodality therapy. In the last year there have been numerous reports in the literature of various combinations of different forms of therapy. Many of these have been given with radical surgery.

Radiotherapy

Although pleural mesothelioma is not particularly sensitive to radiotherapy this treatment modality has been used as both a radical treatment after surgery and for preventing tumour seeding at biopsy sites.

Hemithoracic radiation after extrapleural pneumonectomy for malignant pleural mesothelioma

Yajnik S, Rosenzweig KE, Mychalczak B, *et al*. *Int J Radiat Oncol Biol Phys* 2003; **56**(5): 1319–26

BACKGROUND. Few patients with pleural mesothelioma are suitable for radical therapy. Results suggest that patients who can be treated by resection with other treatment modalities such as radiotherapy and chemotherapy are a highly selected group, but have better survival. Local recurrence, however, is the most common form of relapse. Extrapleural pneumonectomy is a more radical form of surgery than pleurectomy and decortication. It is not known how to combine this with other modalities of therapy and whether this will reduce the incidence of local relapse.

INTERPRETATION. This paper summarized the experience of extrapleural pneumonectomy followed by high-dose hemithorax radiation therapy at the Memorial Sloan-Kettering Cancer Centre. Thirty-five patients with malignant pleural mesothelioma were treated in this way between 1990 and 2001. Extrapleural pneumonectomy was defined as resection of the entire pleura, lung and diaphragm with or without resection of the ipsilateral half of the pericardium. The radiation therapy target volume involved the entire hemithorax including the thoracotomy and chest tube incision sites. The total dose of radiotherapy delivered was 54 Gy in 30 fractions. This was a retrospective review of case records. Twenty-six of the 35 patients had epithelioid histology, four had stage I disease, eleven has stage II disease, 19 had stage III disease and one had stage IV disease. Radiation therapy appeared reasonably well tolerated, with the most common toxicity being nausea and vomiting (22 of the 35 with grade I and II toxicity). Grade I and II lung, skin and oesophageal toxicity was seen in more than 50% of the patients. Radiotherapy was delivered 3–6 weeks after surgery. Of the 33 patients available for follow-up 26 had died, two were alive with recurrent disease at the time of publication and only five patients were alive and free from disease with a median follow-up of 55 months. Two of these five had persistent pain over their surgical incision site leaving three with no major complaints.

Comments

This radical surgical and radiation therapy can only be administered to a small percentage of patients with malignant pleural mesothelioma. It is worth noting that this tertiary referral centre was only able to recruit approximately three patients per year to the regime. Local control was good but the overall survival was poor. The toxicity in what must have been a fit group of patients was acceptable. The authors highlighted the need for anatomically reconstructing the diaphragm in order to allow optimal post-operative radiotherapy. This involved placing of the radiotherapy field low enough to include the tenth intercostal space where the diaphragm is inserted. If the radiation field is planned without consideration for post-operative elevation of the hemidiaphragm then it is likely that disease will be left in the paravertebral gutter and will not receive treatment. This may explain why other series have found poor local control with aggressive therapy. The standard field of radiotherapy in this series had an inferior border at L2. Only two of their 35 patients had chest wall failures.

Treatment of intervention sites of malignant pleural mesothelioma with radiotherapy: a Dutch–Belgian survey

De Ruysscher D, Slotman B. *Radiother Oncol* 2003; **68**: 299–302

BACKGROUND. Tumour cell seeding at the biopsy site is common in patients with malignant pleural mesothelioma. The incidence of needle track subcutaneous metastases has been reported to be in the region of 20–50%. These metastases may be painful and once established are difficult to treat with either surgery, radiotherapy or chemotherapy. Two small, randomized trials of prophylactic radiotherapy to intervention sites have shown some evidence of benefit. A large phase III trial has not yet been performed in order to establish whether prophylactic local radiotherapy is of benefit. It is also not known how common the practice of prophylactic radiotherapy is.

INTERPRETATION. This small study reported a survey of radiotherapy practice of malignant mesothelioma in The Netherlands and Belgium. Questionnaires were sent to all radiotherapy departments in these two countries. Clinicians were asked whether patients with mesothelioma were offered prophylactic radiotherapy to intervention sites on a routine basis, which schedules were used and how many patients received this treatment annually. The clinicians were also asked whether they would be willing to participate in a phase III, randomized trial of this therapy. Further questions about the current practice of radiotherapy to symptomatic recurrences at intervention sites were also asked. All Dutch radiotherapists responded to the questionnaire and 65% of Belgian departments responded. This gave an overall response of 38 out of 47 centres (81%). Prophylactic radiotherapy to intervention sites was offered as routine practice in 84% of the centres. A wide variety of different hypofractionated schedules were used. Most centres treated less than ten patients per year. Just less than half the centres responding were interested in participating in a randomized trial. All centres offered radiotherapy to intervention site recurrences. Once again a wide variety of schedules was used.

Comment

This study suggested that the vast majority of radiotherapists in The Netherlands and Belgium believe that prophylactic and symptomatic radiotherapy to intervention sites is effective in patients with pleural mesothelioma. There are two randomized trials in the literature looking at this issue. Both were fairly small (40 and twelve patients). The larger study |**7**| supported the use of prophylactic radiotherapy whereas the smaller trial showed no such benefit |**8**|. A large, prospective, randomized trial looking at this treatment intervention is required. However, the relatively low incidence of mesothelioma and the fact that prophylactic radiotherapy is already considered standard treatment may make it difficult to recruit patients to such a study.

Chemotherapy

The failure of surgery and radiotherapy to have a major impact on survival in patients with mesothelioma has led to interest in systemic chemotherapy in this disease. Unlike surgery this form of treatment could possibly be available to the vast majority of patients with the disease. Reasonable studies are now appearing concerning the efficacy of chemotherapy in this disease.

Multicentre phase II study of gemcitabine and cisplatin in malignant pleural mesothelioma
Van Haarst JMW, Baas P, Manegold Ch, *et al. Br J Cancer* 2002;
86: 342–5

BACKGROUND. Malignant pleural mesothelioma is generally accepted to be a chemotherapy-resistant malignancy. Reports of chemotherapy trials have largely been in small groups of patients from single institutions often using single agents in heavily pre-treated patients. Larger studies are required in order to evaluate the efficacy of combinations of active drugs in this condition.

INTERPRETATION. This was a study from four cancer centres in The Netherlands and Germany. Thirty-two patients were enrolled into the study over an 8-month period. All had histologically proven mesothelioma and had not received prior chemotherapy. A dose of 1250 mg/m^2 gemcitabine was given on days 1 and 8 and a dose of 80 mg/m^2 cisplatin on day 1 in a three-week cycle to a maximum of six cycles. Responses and toxicity were evaluated using established criteria. Twenty-five patients had evaluable disease. Four partial responses were observed (16%). No unexpected toxicity occurred, with most patients having low-grade leucopenia, nausea, vomiting and fatigue. The median survival from diagnosis was 14.6 months and from the start of treatment 9.4 months. The median time to progression was 6.1 months. Quality of life data were available in approximately three-quarters of the evaluable patients. Chemotherapy was associated with less pain ($P \leq 0.05$). Unfortunately the compliance to quality of life scoring at further follow-up was <50% and reliable estimates beyond two cycles of treatment were impossible to make. The authors concluded that the trial excludes a response rate of >30% with 90% power in patients with mesothelioma from this chemotherapy regimen.

Comment

This regime appears to have manageable toxicity, but rather poor response rates. The dose of gemcitabine given was slightly lower than in other studies. The quality of life data were difficult to assess, as they were only really available at the start of the trial. However, it is an important measurement in what, for most clinicians, would be palliative treatment. It would appear, however, that gemcitabine and cisplatin cannot be recommended as stardard therapy in mesothelioma.

Gemcitabine combined with carboplatin in patients with malignant pleural mesothelioma. A multicentre phase II study

Favaretto AG, Aversa SML, Paccagnella A, *et al. Cancer* 2003; **97**: 2791–8

BACKGROUND. As yet there is no commonly accepted chemotherapy regimen for the management of patients with malignant pleural mesothelioma. Many different single-agent regimens have been studied. The response rates are generally lower than 20% and there is little data regarding survival or symptom control. The two classes of drugs that have been most favoured in this condition are the platinum analogues and the antimetabolites. This study looked at a two-drug combination (carboplatin and gemcitabine) in a group of patients with mesothelioma. There is little data in the literature about the activity of gemcitabine in this disease.

INTERPRETATION. This was a multicentre study performed in eight cancer centres in northeast Italy. The investigators enrolled 50 patients into the trial over a 4-year period. Most patients had an European Cooperative Oncology Group (ECOG) performance status of 1 or 0 and 56% had stage I or II disease. Three-quarters had epithelioid histology and around the same number had no previous treatment. Patients were treated with carboplatin with an area under the curve (AUC) 5 dose on day 1 with 1000 $\mu g/m^2$ gemcitabine on days 1, 8 and 15. The cycle was repeated every 4 weeks. Eight-two per cent of the planned dose of gemcitabine was delivered. The delivered dose intensity for carboplatin was 80 mg/m^2/week. Almost half of the day 15 gemcitabine was omitted. There were no complete responses. Twenty-six per cent of the patients had a partial response, the median duration of which was 55 weeks (range 13–113 weeks). Forty-six per cent of the patients had improvement in breathlessness with 40% gaining weight and 26% having less pain. Toxicity was predominantly haematological (grade III or IV) leucopenia and thrombocytopenia seen in 11 and 14% of patients, respectively. Life-threatening sepsis or haemorrhage was not seen. The median overall survival was 66 weeks with 1, 2 and 3 years' survival being 53, 30 and 20%, respectively. Patients with epithelial histology had a median survival of 90 weeks versus 42 weeks for non-epithelial type disease ($P = 0.03$).

Comment

This was a non-randomized, phase II trial looking at the ability of mesothelioma patients to take a novel combination of drugs known to have activity as single agents. The treatment had an acceptable toxicity profile and reasonable response rates. The authors concluded that gemcitabine/carboplatin for four cycles was a 'valid' option for the treatment of mesothelioma, but that there was much room for improvement.

It was suggested that an adjustment in schedule from 4 to 3 weeks might optimize the activity of the combination.

Pemetrexed (alimta)

In the past antifolates have had only a minor role in the treatment of most cancers, with methotrexate being the most widely used agent. Pemetrexed is a new anti-metabolite that has shown evidence of activity in pre-clinical cancer systems including mesothelioma. Publications about its clinical activity are now appearing. These have involved both phase II and III studies. More is known about the mechanism of action of the drug and other related compounds such as raltitrexed are being tested in mesothelioma patients.

Phase II study of Pemetrexed with and without folic acid and vitamin B$_{12}$ as front-line therapy in malignant pleural mesothelioma
Scagliotti GV, Shin D-M, Kindler HL, *et al. J Clin Oncol* 2003; **21**(8): 1556–61

BACKGROUND. Mesothelioma is notoriously chemoresistant. Numerous cytotoxic drugs either as single agents or as combinations have been evaluated in phase II trials with disappointing results. Single-agent studies have reported survival rates of between 7 and 9 months with response rates of 0–15%. Pemetrexed is a new antifolate with broad antitumour activity. Laboratory studies have shown that it attacks multiple enzyme targets, particularly dihydrofolate reductase, thymidylate synthetase and glycinamide transferase. This contrasts with other antifolates that have been shown to inhibit single enzymes. This study was designed for determining the efficacy of Pemetrexed as a single agent in patients with mesothelioma.

INTERPRETATION. Patients were included in the study if they had a histologically proven diagnosis of pleural mesothelioma and were not candidates for curative surgery. The patients were required to have measurable disease on CT or MRI scanning, a performance status of >70% on the Karnofsky scale and no previous chemotherapy. Prior radiotherapy was permitted. Sixty-four patients were enrolled into the study and were given 500 mg/m^2 Pemetrexed intravenously every 3 weeks. Two-thirds of the patients received vitamin supplementation with folate and vitamin B$_{12}$ and 21 patients did not. Overall the response rate was nine out of the 64 patients (14.1%). Seven of the nine responders were vitamin supplemented. The median overall survival for supplemented patients was 13 months (8 months for non-supplemented patients). Patients receiving vitamins completed more cycles of therapy (six versus two) and had a lower incidence of neutropenia.

Comment

This study showed that Pemetrexed has moderate antitumour activity in patients who have not received prior chemotherapy. The effect of vitamin supplementation is interesting. It allowed a higher dose of the active agent to be given, which presumably was the reason for the better response rates and survival in this group. There was no apparent adverse effect of vitamin supplementation on the drug's antitumour activity. This drug will have to be examined in a phase III setting in mesothelioma patients.

Phase III study of Pemetrexed in combination with cisplatin versus cisplatin alone in patients with malignant pleural mesothelioma

Vogelzang NJ, Rusthoven JJ, Symanowski J, *et al*. *J Clin Oncol* 2003; **21**(14): 2636–44

BACKGROUND. No standard treatment exists for patients with malignant pleural mesothelioma. The median survival is usually between 6 and 9 months for untreated patients. Pemetrexed is a novel mutlitargeted antifolate drug that has shown single-agent activity in phase II trials of patients with mesothelioma. This was a randomized, multicentre, international, phase III trial in patients with pleural mesothelioma.

INTERPRETATION. Four hundred and seventy-two patients with malignant pleural mesothelioma were recruited to the study between 1998 and 2002. All were not eligible for curative surgery and none had previous chemotherapy. The patients were randomly assigned to two treatment arms. One received 500 mg/m^2 Pemetrexed and 75 mg/m^2 cisplatin on day 1 or 75 mg/m^2 cisplatin alone on day 1. Both treatment regimens were given intravenously every 21 days. Four hundred and fifty-six patients were eventually randomized: 226 received Pemetrexed and cisplatin, 222 received cisplatin alone and eight did not receive either therapy. The median survival in the two-drug (Pemetrexed/cisplatin) arm was 12.1 months against 9.3 months in the control (cisplatin alone) arm ($P = 0.02$). The hazard ratio for death for patients in the Pemetrexed arm was 0.77 versus the control arm. The response rates were 41.3% in the Pemetrexed/cisplatin arm versus 16.7% in the cisplatin alone arm. A quarter of the way through the trial (117 patients) folic acid and vitamin B$_{12}$ were added to reduce toxicity after four drug-related deaths from febrile neutropenia were noted. These deaths were linked to increased homocystine levels. Vitamin supplementation reduced the toxicity of the chemotherapy in both arms. The overall survival in the treatment arm for patients receiving vitamin supplementation was 13.3 months compared with 10 months for the control arm ($P = 0.051$).

Comment

This was the first randomized study to show significant prolongation of survival and lengthening of time to disease progression with a 'new' treatment in this condition. The authors concluded that the combination of Pemetrexed and cisplatin with folic acid and vitamin B$_{12}$ should be considered the 'standard front-line therapy' for patients with malignant pleural mesothelioma. A number of criticisms of the trial

have been made. The inclusion of a control arm that had toxic chemotherapy is controversial. Some reviewers have felt that the inclusion of an active cytotoxic agent
nullifies the idea of the control arm, which should not include any form of either
active or toxic therapy. It may be that some of the improvements in the treatment
arm were exaggerated by a worsening of patients in the comparative control arm. The
survival difference was extremely borderline ($P = 0.051$ in patients receiving vitamin
therapy) and it would seem premature to label this as standard therapy. More trials
including the large UK-based MS01 trial which has a no treatment control arm are
urgently required.

A novel folate transport activity in human mesothelioma cell lines with high affinity and specificity for the new-generation antifolate, Pemetrexed

Wang Y, Zhao R, Chattopadhyay S, Goldman ID. *Cancer Res* 2002;
62: 6434–7

BACKGROUND. Much interest has been shown in a new generation of antifolate drugs
that have activity against mesothelioma in early clinical trials. Pemetrexed is the drug
that has shown most activity. It is dependent upon its metabolism to polyglutamate
derivatives. The compound is a potent inhibitor of thymidylate synthetase as well as
other enzymes involved in the metabolism of folates. A reduced folate carrier transports
Pemetrexed into malignant cells with similar transport kinetics to methotrexate.
Evidence of enhanced transport into cancer cells may explain the impressive results of
this drug in mesothelioma patients compared with other antimetabolites.

INTERPRETATION. This group from New York studied the influx of Pemetrexed and
methotrexate in human mesothelioma cell lines. Using the NCI-H28 line they were able to
demonstrate the presence of a novel high-affinity transport activity that appeared to be
highly specific for Pemetrexed. The substrate specificity pattern was quite different from
that of the reduced folate carrier and folate receptors. Interestingly, there was an apparent
relatively low affinity for other antifolate inhibitors of dihydrofolate reductase such as
methotrexate and aminopterin (Fig. 22.4).

Comment

The demonstration of a high-affinity folate transport mechanism for enhancing the
entry of Pemetrexed into mesothelioma cell lines is unique. This striking transport
advantage for Pemetrexed over several other antifolate thymidylate synthetase and
dihydrofolate reductase inhibitors would appear to play a role in the efficacy of
Pemetrexed in this disease. The high-affinity transporter functions most efficiently at
very low drug concentrations. This should be particularly effective in maintaining
high intracellular Pemetrexed levels in mesothelioma cells for long intervals beyond
the intravenous administration of a single dose when extracellular drug concentrations are in the nanomolar range. This should prolong the duration over which the

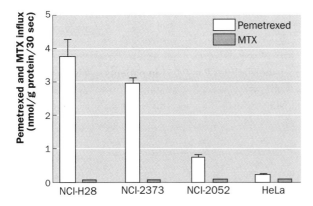

Fig. 22.4 A comparison of the initial rates of MTX and Pemetrexed uptake (over a period of 30 s) in three mesothelioma cell lines and HeLa cells. The extracellular concentration of drugs was 50 nm. The data are the average of three experiments. MTX, methotrexate. Source: Wang *et al.* (2002).

drug inhibits its target sites. This mechanism may also allow the design of newer, more specific drugs with activity in mesothelioma.

Combination of raltitrexed and oxaliplatin is an active regimen in malignant mesothelioma: results of a phase II study

Fizazi K, Doubre H, Le Chevalier T, *et al. J Clin Oncol* 2003; **21**(2): 349–54

BACKGROUND. Malignant melanoma is notoriously refractory to chemotherapy. No standard therapy is currently agreed for a condition in which surgery and radiotherapy do not increase survival. A number of compounds that inhibit folate metabolism are appearing and have been shown to have activity in this disease in pre-clinical models. Trials looking at these two therapies either alone or in combination with more established anticancer drugs are appearing in the literature.

INTERPRETATION. This was an open-label, phase II study evaluating the activity of raltitrexed (Tomudex) and oxaliplatin as a combination therapy in patients with malignant mesothelioma of the pleura. Seventy patients were enrolled in the trial, with median age 60 years. Fifteen had been pre-treated with chemotherapy and 55 were chemotherapy naïve. Two-thirds of the patients had advanced disease. The patients received 3 mg/m^2 raltitrexed followed by 130 mg/m^2 oxaliplatin in 3-weekly cycles. Fourteen patients (20%) had a partial response with 32 patients (46%) having stable disease. Approximately one-third of the patients had a symptomatic response in terms of shortness of breath and pain. The mean survival in patients who had not been treated previously was 31 weeks (95% CI = 23–40 weeks) from the start of treatment compared with 44 weeks (95% CI = 24–40 weeks) in pre-treated patients. The overall 1-year survival was 26% (22% in chemotherapy-naïve patients). The haematological toxicity was mild. The most common adverse events were asthenia, nausea and vomiting. There was no alopecia. No treatment-related deaths were seen.

Comment

This was an outpatient regimen of a new antifolate compound with a platinum-based drug. The regimen was given on an outpatient basis and had an acceptable tolerability profile. Responses that were encouraging were seen. The European Organisation for Research and Treatment of Cancer has set up a phase III randomized trial of cisplatin with and without raltitrexed. It is to be hoped that combined treatment modalities may deliver superior results to current treatments in this disease and folate analogues appear promising. It is interesting that in this trial patients were not given vitamin supplementation, which may have further ameliorated the small amounts of toxicity seen.

Immunotherapy and chemotherapy

Two interesting papers appeared in 2002 looking at immunotherapy and chemotherapy in malignant mesothelioma. The first was a systematic review of the literature and the second looked at the feasibility of giving a vaccine therapy in combination with chemotherapy.

Activity of chemotherapy and immunotherapy on malignant mesothelioma: a systematic review of the literature with meta-analysis

Berghmans T, Paesmans M, Lalami Y, *et al. Lung Cancer* 2002; **38**(2): 111–21

BACKGROUND. The exact role for chemotherapy in unresectable malignant pleural mesothelioma is as yet unclear. A number of reports of chemotherapy from phase I and II trials have appeared in the literature over the years. Most studies are small and a single agent or combination of agents has not emerged as being an 'accepted' chemotherapeutic regimen. A systematic review of the literature with meta-analysis may be helpful in trying to clarify this situation.

INTERPRETATION. The authors searched the English, French and Dutch literature between 1965 and 2001 using standard electronic databases looking for prospective, single or randomized, phase II or III trials concerning the treatment of malignant mesothelioma of the pleura. Trials with a minimum of 14 patients were included. Abstracts were excluded from the analysis. A team of seven doctors and one biostatistician

Table 22.6 Response rates according to treatment groups

	R/E patients	Response rate (%)	95% CI
Group 1	127/547	23.2	19.7–26.8
Group 2	24/213	11.3	7.0–15.5
Group 3	43/151	28.5	21.3–35.7
Group 4	164/1409	11.6	10.0–13.3

Group 1, trials testing cisplatin but not doxorubicin; Group 2, trials testing doxorubicin but not cisplatin; Group 3, trials testing cisplatin and doxorubicin; Group 4, trials without cisplatin and doxorubicin. R/E, number of patients responding to the allowed treatment between the number of evaluable patients according to ELCWP criteria. $P < 0.001$.
Source: Berghmans *et al.* (2002).

evaluated each trial. Trial quality was assessed according to a set protocol assessing internal and external validity measurements. The scores for each trial were therefore aggregated for the ten categories studied: each category received a maximal theoretical value of 10 points giving a total maximal theoretical score for each trial of 100 points. Eighty-three articles published between 1983 and 2001 met the selection criteria. Of these 80 were single-arm, phase II trials and three were randomized, phase II trials. The trials were separated into four groups according to treatment regimen. Group 1 ($n = 20$) included trials testing cisplatin, group 2 ($n = 8$) was composed of trials investigating doxorubicin without cisplatin and group 3 looked at cisplatin/doxorubicin combinations ($n = 6$). Group 4 comprised the remaining 54 trials, which had regimens without cisplatin or doxorubicin. The combination of cisplatin and doxorubicin had the highest response rate (28.5%) ($P < 0.01$). Cisplatin was the most active single agent (Table 22.6).

Comment

The authors based their conclusion that cisplatin and doxorubicin is the most active combination and cisplatin the most active single agent on their response rates. Data concerning survival and toxicity were inadequately reported in more than half the studies and could not be used as end-points. This is disappointing in view of the fact that the vast majority of patients are symptomatic and the aim of treatment is usually palliation. The authors concluded that the role of chemotherapy in malignant mesothelioma needs to be assessed in randomized, phase III trials and felt that the best available chemotherapy regimen to compare with new treatments would be cisplatin and doxorubicin. The first phase III trials are now appearing, e.g. Vogalzang *et al.* and indeed they did use cisplatin alone as a 'control arm'. It is strange that cisplatin which has the best single agent activity should be used as a control arm.

Clinical and immunological assessment of *Mycobacterium vaccae* (SRL172) with chemotherapy in patients with malignant mesothelioma

Mendes R, O'Brien MER, Mitra A, *et al. Br J Cancer* 2002; **86**: 336–41

B ACKGROUND. Many published studies have shown a poor response to chemotherapy in malignant mesothelioma. New treatments are required. There is little in the literature about immunotherapy for patients with mesothelioma. *Mycobacterium vaccae* is a fast growing virulent mycobacterium that is thought to have non-specific immunomodulating properties. One of the attractions of its use in mesothelioma is that it can easily be injected into the tumour. However, little is known about the potential toxicity of this form of therapy.

I NTERPRETATION. The objective of this small study was to determine the toxicity of both intratumoural and intradermal *M. vaccae* (SRL172) injections given prior to and with chemotherapy. Sixteen patients were included in this study. Thirteen had a pleural effusion and ten had epithelial histology. All had stage IV disease. The patients received chemotherapy (mitomycin C, vinblastin and cisplatin) on a 3-weekly basis for up to six courses. Incremental doses of intrapleural SRL172 injections were given 3 weekly prior to chemotherapy and escalated in tenfold incremental doses throughout the trial. The patients were also given intradermal SRL172. There was no dose-limited toxicity seen although there was greater toxicity at the higher dose and the main side effects were nausea, vomiting, constipation and hair loss. Two patients had flu-like symptoms and one required admission. Nine out of the 16 patients (56%) reported symptomatic benefit from the treatment. Ten out of 14 patients with pain were helped and seven out of nine patients with cough described improvement. Six of the 16 patients (37.5%) had a partial response. The median overall survival was 10.5 months (disease-free progression 8 months). There was a significant increase in the percentage of natural killer cell activation and a decrease in the percentage of CT3 plus T lymphocytes after treatment.

Comment

This study was performed in a group of patients with advanced disease. This trial showed that immunotherapy can be given safely into tumour deposits with acceptable toxicity. This trial also established a dose for this therapy and phase II trials are now required for this new form of treatment.

Hyperthermia

The resistance of mesothelioma to standard therapies has led researchers to look at other forms of treatment in an attempt to improve survival. This recently reported study looked at the effect of combining chemotherapy with whole-body hyperthermia.

Ifosfamide, carboplatin and etoposide combined with 41.8°C whole-body hyperthermia for malignant pleural mesothelioma

Bakhshandeh A, Bruns I, Traynor A, *et al. Lung Cancer* 2003; **39**: 339–45

BACKGROUND. Combined modality therapy using surgery (curative or debulking), adjuvant radiotherapy and chemotherapy has had little impact on survival in patients with malignant pleural mesothelioma. New treatment strategies are required in this disease. Hyperthermia has been shown to have an antitumour effect in laboratory models of cancer and in patients with other malignancies. It is thought that neoplastic cells are more sensitive to hyperthermia than normal cells due to inhibition of DNA repair enzymes, the induction of apotosis and inhibition of angiogenesis. However, there are few reports in the literature of hyperthermia alone or in combination with chemotherapy.

INTERPRETATION. Twenty-seven patients with histologically proven mesothelioma were enrolled into this German study over a 2-year period. Patients were treated with cycles of therapy every 28 days. Treatment involved ifosfamide, carboplatin and etoposide chemotherapy given in standard doses with granulocyte colony-stimulating factor and MESNA protection as standard. Whole-body hyperthermic treatment was defined as raising the patient's systemic temperature to 41.8°C for at least 60 min. A typical hyperthermia treatment session lasted 4 h with 1.3 h to reach the target temperature, 1 h at 41.8°C and a cooling phase of 1 h. The patients were sedated during this time. Hyperthermia was achieved using the 'aquatherm' system. The patients were evaluated after a minimum of two cycles of treatment. The majority of the patients had epithelial histology. Twenty-five of the 27 patients were evaluable for response. The overall response rate was 20% (all partial responses). One-quarter of the patients had progressive disease. The survival from the start of treatment for all patients was 76.6 weeks with that for progression-free survival being 29.6 weeks. The 1-year overall survival was 68% with 20% alive after 2 years. All patients were evaluable for toxicity. Grade 3–4 neutropenia and thrombocytopenia was seen in 74 and 33% of the treatment cycles, respectively. There was one septic death.

Comment

Hyperthermia has not yet been accepted as a standard anticancer treatment. This trial showed that it is possible to give fairly intensive chemotherapy on the same day as hyperthermia. What is unclear is whether this multimodality form of therapy actually improves survival. Obviously this was an uncontrolled study in a group of patients with good prognostic indicators and no prior treatment. There is a need for a randomized, phase III trial perhaps comparing chemotherapy and hyperthermia with chemotherapy alone in order to ascertain whether hyperthermia adds anything apart from toxicity to standard chemotherapy.

Prognosis

Stage, histological subtype and other prognostic factors such as haematological abnormalities are established as useful prognostic indicators in mesothelioma. The selection of patients who may respond well to therapy is needed as most treatments offer significant toxicity with little chance of prolonged survival. More refined methods for predicting prognosis are therefore needed.

Using gene expression ratios to predict outcome among patients with mesothelioma
Gordon GJ, Jensen RV, Hsiao L-L, *et al. J Natl Cancer Inst* 2003;
95(8): 598–605

BACKGROUND. The outcome of treatment in patients with mesothelioma is strongly related to histological subtypes. Patients with epithelial subtype show a survival benefit for a variety of treatments including multimodality therapy. Tumours can be profiled according to gene expression using oligonucleotide microassays. As yet these tools have not had a substantial impact on clinical management.

INTERPRETATION. The authors used surgical specimens from 60 patients undergoing extrapleural pneumonectomy for mesothelioma in Boston. This group had a long history of aggressive multimodality treatment. Seventeen samples were used for constructing an outcome predictor model on the basis of linked clinical data. The remaining 29 samples were used for a reverse transcriptase polymerase chain reaction analysis for validating the model. Genes were identified from the two outcome groups to form prognostic expression ratios. Four genes were found that were most statistically significantly over-expressed in each outcome group (favourable and poor). These were used to classify the 17 samples used for training the model with respect to group membership. Using this technique it was possible to predict treatment-related patient outcomes independent of histological subtype (Fig. 22.5).

Comment

This was an extremely complex study where genes that appeared to predict survival more accurately than current best prognostic indicators such as histological subtype and tumour stage were identified. The authors claimed that this technique could identify patients who are unlikely to respond to conventional treatment modalities thus sparing them from radical surgery. One weakness of the study is that it was performed in patients who had undergone surgery and it is known that these are a highly selected group of mesothelioma patients.

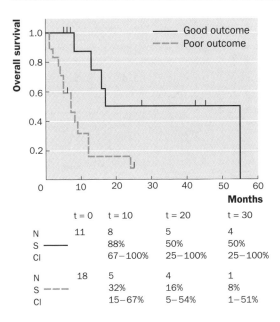

	t = 0	t = 10	t = 20	t = 30
N	11	8	5	4
S ———		88%	50%	50%
CI		67–100%	25–100%	25–100%
N	18	5	4	1
S ----		32%	16%	8%
CI		15–67%	5–54%	1–51%

Fig. 22.5 Independent validation of the four-gene expression ratio model. Overall survival in the test set of samples for good-outcome (median survival = 36 months) and poor-outcome (median survival = 7 months) groups as defined by the four-gene expression ratio model that used only reverse transcription–polymerase chain reaction for data acquisition. N and S indicate the number of patients at risk and the Kaplan–Meier estimate of overall survival, respectively, at the indicated time points. CI, 95% confidence interval for the Kaplan–Meier survival estimate. $P = 0.0035$. Source: Gordon *et al.* (2003).

Mesothelioma management guidelines

Mesothelioma is increasing in incidence in most Westernized countries. It is proving extremely difficult to manage, but small steps involving new chemotherapeutic agents are being taken. Reports summarizing standard patterns of care have appeared in the literature recently.

Statement on malignant mesothelioma in the United Kingdom

British Thoracic Society (BTS) Standards of Care Committee. *Thorax* 2001; **56**: 250–65

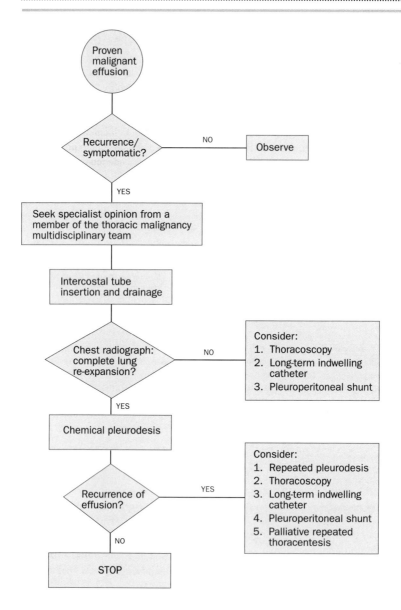

Fig. 22.6 Algorithm for the management of malignant pleural effusions.
Source: Antures *et al.* (2003).

BTS guidelines for the management of malignant pleural effusion

Antures G, Neville E, Duffy J, Ali N on behalf of the BTS Pleural Disease Group, a subgroup of the BTS Standards of Care Committee. *Thorax* 2003; **58**(Suppl 2): ii29–38

BACKGROUND. Although malignant mesothelioma is increasing in incidence, few centres have managed enough patients to acquire comprehensive clinical experience. The literature is full of non-randomized trials of the condition and evidence-based guidelines by which clinicians may base their practice do not exist.

INTERPRETATION. The BTS Standards of Care Committee has recently produced two important documents concerning the management of malignant pleural disease. Although the first statement was published in 2001 and is, therefore, outwith the scope of this chapter, it does however represent an important landmark in the mesothelioma literature and deserves mention. Although not strictly evidence based the committee attempted to review all the important evidence concerning many aspects of mesothelioma comprehensively. The statement is offered for guidance and is not an attempt to dictate management. Several important areas are covered, including epidemiology, prognosis, diagnosis, staging and treatment, while general management and palliative care are also covered. Key points are clearly stated at the end of each chapter and there are important sections concerning the claiming of benefit and compensation.

The BTS guidelines for the management of malignant pleural effusion comprises one section of a supplement of *Thorax* published in May 2003 devoted to the management of pleural disease in general (i.e. the subjects also covered include investigation of unilateral pleural effusion, management of pleural infection, spontaneous pneumothorax and guidelines for insertion of chest drains). The section on malignant pleural effusions covers both mesothelioma and patients with metastatic disease from other primaries. The guidelines produced are evidence based although the vast majority of recommendations carry a low (B or C) level of evidence. A useful algorithm for the management of malignant pleural effusions is included (Fig. 22.6).

Comment

These two papers provide useful guidelines for clinicians involved in the management of patients with mesothelioma. As with all guidelines they rapidly become outdated as new evidence appears in the literature. This is particularly true of new treatment modalities that have been reported since 2001. Most clinicians see only a handful of patients with mesothelioma and will find these guidelines extremely useful.

References

1. Peto J, Decarli A, La Vecchia C, Negri E. The European mesothelioma epidemic. *Br J Cancer* 1999; **79**(3/4): 666–72.

2. Peto J, Hodgson JT, Matthews FE, Jones JR. Continuing increase in mesothelioma mortality in Britain. *Lancet* 1995; **345**: 535–9.

3. Rusch VW, Venkatraman ES. Important prognostic factors in patients with malignant pleural mesothelioma, managed surgically. *Ann Thorac Surg* 1999; **68**: 1799–804.

4. Ryan CW, Herndon J, Vogelzang NJ. A review of chemotherapy trials for malignant mesothelioma. *Chest* 1998; **113**(Suppl 1): 66S–73.

5. Union International Coutre le Cancer. *TNM Classification of Malignant Tumours*. 6th edn. New York: Wiley-Liss, 2002.

6. Sugarbaker DJ, Flores RM, Jaklitseh MT, *et al.* Resection margins, extrapleural nodal status and cell type determine post-operative long-term survival in trimodality therapy of malignant pleural mesothelioma: results in 183 patients. *J Thorac Cardiovasc Surg* 1999; **117**: 54–63.

7. Boutin C, Rey F, Viallat JR. Prevention of malignant seeding after invasive diagnostic procedures in patients with pleural mesothelioma. A randomised trial of local radiotherapy. *Chest* 1995; **108**: 754–8.

8. O'Rourke N, Paul J, Hill J. Radiotherapy to mesothelioma drain sites may not be worthwhile – interim report of a randomised study. *Lung Cancer* 2000; **29**(Suppl 1): 168.

23

Lung cancer

Introduction

Lung cancer continues to be the leading cause of cancer deaths worldwide with an estimated 1.1 million people dying of the condition in 2000. This figure includes over one-third of a million deaths in Europe and an estimated 150 000 in the USA. Survival from lung cancer remains poor with most countries reporting 5-year survival rates of between 6 and 12%. Whilst it is accepted that cigarette smoking causes the vast majority of lung cancer cases, there is still much to learn about its causation, how best to pick up patients early and also how to increase survival with different treatment modalities.

In 2004 thousands of reports of research into lung cancer have appeared in the literature. This chapter covers a few selected papers addressing issues in the aetiology, screening, staging and treatment of lung cancer patients.

Aetiology

It is estimated that between 80 and 90% of patients with lung cancer have contracted the disease from tobacco smoking. Non-smokers who inhale other people's tobacco smoke (passive smokers) are also at increased risk of lung cancer. Women who have never smoked but have been exposed to environmental tobacco smoke from their spouses have a relative increased risk of 1.29 (95% confidence interval [CI] = 1.17–1.43) of developing lung cancer compared with unexposed women who have never smoked |1|. Other risk factors for the development of lung cancer include occupational or environmental exposure to various carcinogens as well as a small genetic predisposition. Little longitudinal data exist in the literature concerning the effects of air pollution on the development of lung cancer.

Lung cancer and air pollution: a 27 year follow-up of 16 209 Norwegian mean
Nafstad P, Hameim LL, Oftedal B, *et al. Thorax* 2003; **58**: 1071–6

BACKGROUND. Although the pathogenesis of lung cancer is clearly linked to cigarette smoking it has been known for many years that environmental exposure to carcinogens

is also important. The differences in lung cancer risk between urban and rural
populations cannot be fully explained by differences in cigarette smoke exposure. Is
there an association between urban air pollution and lung cancer?

INTERPRETATION. Sixteen thousand two hundred and nine out of a total of 25 915 Oslo
men aged between 40 and 50 years agreed to participate in a population-based, follow-up
study of cardiovascular diseases in 1972. Participation included a questionnaire
concerning occupation, education and smoking habits. These men were followed for the
next 27 years to 1998. Their data at presentation were linked to the average yearly air
pollution levels at their home address and to data from the Norwegian Cancer Register and
the Norwegian Death Register. Survival analyses were performed and the association
between exposure to air pollution and the incidence of lung cancer were examined. Four
hundred and eighteen men developed lung cancer in the follow-up period. The adjusted risk
ratio for developing lung cancer was 1.08 (95% CI = 1.02–1.15) for a 10 $\mu g/m^3$ increase
in nitrogen oxide exposure. These figures were controlled for age, smoking habits and
length of education. The figures for a similar increase in sulphur dioxide were 1.01 (95%
CI = 0.94–1.08).

Comment

This study had a number of advantages over previously published work. The follow-
up was over a long time period and the study population lived in one city. A reasonable number of lung cancers occurred during the study period. One of the weaknesses
of the study was that information on cigarette smoking was only taken at the beginning of the follow-up period and the possibility exists that changes in tobacco use
over the ensuing 27 years of follow-up may have had an influence on the development of lung cancer. The authors concluded that their study provides strong
evidence that exposure to pollutants (particularly nitrogen dioxide) is associated
with an increased risk of lung cancer. However, the effect seen with pollution was
extremely small compared with that of cigarette smoking.

Screening

For many years workers have been interested in screening the population for lung
cancer. The hope was that tumours could be picked up at an early stage and treated
more effectively. In the 1960s and 1970s the results of five randomized, clinical trials
performed predominantly in the USA with hundreds of thousands of patients suggested that neither chest x-rays nor sputum cytology were beneficial screening tools.
Neither appeared to prolong the life expectancy of an individual with the disease. In
the last 5 years attention has turned to the use of low-dose computed tomography
(CT) scanning for the early detection of lung cancer and encouraging early results
have been obtained. It is not known whether this strategy prolongs survival |2|. In the
last year reports have appeared on the use of positron emission tomography (PET)
scanning along with CT scanning as a screening tool. Interest has also been expressed
in the financial implications for a mass screening programme as commercial CT

systems are appearing on the market. Finally, a fascinating report about the possible advantage of CT screening in helping with smoking cessation has appeared.

Early lung cancer detection with spiral CT and positron emission tomography in heavy smokers: 2-year results
Pastorino U, Bellomi M, Landoni C, *et al. Lancet* 2003; **362**: 593–7

BACKGROUND. In the last 3 years low-dose spiral CT scanning of the chest has been shown to detect early stage lung cancer effectively in high-risk individuals. Unfortunately, many of the studies were complicated by the detection of a large percentage of benign nodules. Could the combining of repeated annual low-dose spiral CT and the selective use of PET be an efficient way of picking up lung cancers in a cohort of high-risk individuals?

INTERPRETATION. This study recruited volunteers through a media campaign in Milan, Italy. Subjects were eligible if they were current or former smokers and aged 50 years or older with no history of malignant disease. The patients also had to be fit enough to undergo thoracic surgery. All subjects underwent baseline and annual single-slice spiral CT scans. Nodules <5 mm or those containing calcium were deemed as non-suspicious. Larger and non-calcified nodules were rescanned and those showing positive enhancement went on to undergo a PET scan. Suspicious lesions were biopsied. One thousand and thirty-five smokers were enrolled in the study. Ninety-six per cent of the participants had undergone a first repeat (year 2) scan at the time of publication. Eleven lung cancers were detected on

Table 23.1 Results of low-dose spiral CT

	Baseline (*n* = 1035)	Year 2 (*n* = 996)	Total
Patients with nodules	199 (19%)*	99 (10%)†	298
1 nodule only	145	80	225
2 nodules	32	14	46
≥3 nodules	22	5	27
Total number of nodules	284	127‡	411
Nodules <6 mm	238	197	345
Nodules >5 mm	47 (4.4%)	20 (2.0%)	66
Non-nodular lesions	15 (1.4%)	14 (1.4%)	29
Thin-section CT	61 (5.9%)	34 (3.4%)	95
Contrast-enhanced CT	29 (2.8%)	7 (7.0%)	36
Median (IQR) time to diagnosis (days)§	121 (52–156)	45 (34–80)	
Lung cancers	11 (1.1%)	11 (1.1%)	22

* Proportion of low-dose CT (column %). † Patients with newly appeared or additional nodules.
‡ Total number of new or additional nodules. § Period elapsed from initial low-dose CT and final diagnosis.
CT, computerized tomography; IQR, interquartile range.
Source: Pastorino *et al.* (2003).

Table 23.2 Results of PET

	Baseline (n = 29)	Year 2 (n = 13)	Total (n = 42)
Results (standardised uptake value)			
True positive	8 (10.3)*	10 (4.9)	18
True negative	17	1	18
False positive	3 (3.9)	1 (4.9)	4
False negative	1†	1‡	2
Accuracy	86%	85%	
Positive stage 1 (<2 cm)	3 of 4 (2.0)	9 of 10 (4.0)	12
Positive stage II–III	5 of 5 (13.4)	0	5

*Average standardized uptake value. †8 mm well-differentiated adenocarcinoma.
‡11 mm adenocarcinoma with bronchoalveolar component.
Source: Pastorino *et al.* (2003).

the baseline scan and eleven out of 29 PET scans were positive with one false negative. In the follow-up year eleven new lung cancers were detected (six of these were actually seen on the baseline CT scan). Ten of 13 subsequent PET scans were true positives with one false positive, one false negative and one true negative. Twenty-one of the 22 patients had complete resection of their tumour, 17 of which were stage I (Tables 23.1 and 23.2).

Comment

Although the authors concluded that CT scanning combined with the selective use of PET can effectively detect early lung cancer, it is worrying that of the eleven tumours picked up in the second year more than half had been identified in the previous scan. The study once again highlighted the difficulty of using low-dose CT scanning in population-based studies. As with the American studies there were high levels of false-positive scans. PET scanning did not seem to add greatly to the diagnostic accuracy of the algorithm. It is possible, however, that these tumours were picked up slightly quicker than just using further interval CT scans. Once again it is not known whether this approach results in prolonged survival and we still await the results of ongoing randomized trials of CT scanning as a screening tool.

Lung cancer screening with helical computed tomography in older adult smokers: a decision and cost-effectiveness analysis

Mahadevua PJ, Fleisher LA, Frick KD, Eng J, Goodman SN, Powe NR. *J Am Med Assoc* 2003; **289**: 313–22

BACKGROUND. Clinicians are becoming more interested in screening for lung cancer with low-dose CT scanning. It is not known whether this improves survival in the absence of controlled studies. Little is known about the potential economic and safety consequences of a widely disseminated lung cancer screening programme.

INTERPRETATION. The authors performed a decision and cost-effective analysis of a hypothetical study population of 100 000 60-year-old heavy smokers. They postulated that all were eligible for lung resection surgery and that males comprised 55% of the cohort. These data mirror participants in the screening trials reported in the literature. The authors allowed for different levels of smoking cessation. The model assumed annual screening from aged 60 years to aged 80 years with follow-up potentially until aged 100 years. The authors used the best available data on outcomes, the cost of diagnosis and treatment. Over the 20 years of screening the authors postulated that in this population there would be 550 fewer lung cancer deaths but 1186 false-positive invasive tests performed. The cost of this screening for current, ceasing and former smokers varied from $116 300 to $2 322 700 per quality-adjusted life year (QALY) gained. Using the most favourable parameters the most cost-effective outcome for current smokers was still $42 500 per QALY.

Comment

This was an extremely complex model looking at an older lung cancer population. The results of this study would suggest that the current programmes for lung cancer screening are not cost-effective. This is an extremely pertinent result at a time when screening programmes are becoming commercially available to clinicians and members of the population. This study was also performed before it is known whether lung cancer screening is actually effective in detecting and curing early lung cancer.

Change in smoking status after spiral chest computed tomography scan screening

Cox LS, Clark MM, Jett JR, *et al*. *Cancer* 2003; **98**(11): 2495–501

BACKGROUND. Most smokers are keen to cease the habit, but smoking cessation rates are disappointingly low (the national cessation rate mean is 5–7% in the USA). Is the population who have undergone screening for lung cancer with spiral CT more likely to cease smoking at the time of their scan?

INTERPRETATION. This study from the Mayo Clinic looked at 901 current smokers and 574 former smokers participating in a low-dose spiral chest CT scan screening study for the early detection of lung cancer. All volunteers had smoked a pack or more a day for over 20 years. The self-reported point prevalence smoking abstinence 1 year after screening was assessed and correlated with different variables such as tomography result, pulmonary function and previous smoking history. Of the current smokers at baseline 14% reported smoking abstinence at follow-up at 1 year. Older age and poorer lung function were associated with smoking cessation. Ninety per cent of former smokers reported continuing abstinence at follow-up. A longer duration of smoking abstinence at baseline was found to be predictive of continuing abstinence in this group. The authors concluded that the smoking abstinence rate was higher than one would expect and that screening may be an ideal place for providing a smoking cessation message to this kind of individual. Interestingly, the results of screening had no effect on the cessation rate.

Comment

This link between lung cancer screening and accelerated rates of smoking cessation are interesting and provide evidence that this may be a valuable 'teachable moment' for a reduction in high-risk behaviour. One potential confounder of this conclusion is that this population of smokers and ex-smokers came forward themselves for screening and might therefore represent a selected population. Presumably their interest in lung cancer screening would make them more susceptible to smoking cessation interventions. It should also be noted that no active smoking cessation was targeted at the time of screening. Further research is needed in order to evaluate the potential of lung cancer screening as an opportunity for providing effective smoking cessation intervention such as nicotine replacement therapy.

Staging

Accurate staging of patients with non-small cell lung cancer is vital in determining the small proportion of patients with an operable lesion and to limit futile thoracotomies. However, it is also important not to deny curative treatment to patients who on initial testing may have apparently irresectable disease. Current staging is often based on the results of CT scanning where tissue confirmation is required before an accurate decision about surgery can be made. The same can be said for PET scanning, which is becoming more widely available to clinicians. Endoscopic ultrasound is emerging as a useful diagnostic tool in the pre-operative assessment of lung cancer patients. Its great benefit is that it can provide tissue proof of inoperability in a single staging test. Its weakness is that it cannot accurately stage all parts of the mediastinum. There are few data in the literature comparing these different staging techniques. An algorithm for staging patients with lung cancer is urgently needed, but requires careful comparisons of the strengths and weaknesses of each test.

Endoscopic ultrasound, positron emission tomography and computerized tomography for lung cancer

Fritscher-Ravens A, Davidson BL, Hauber H-P, *et al. Am J Respir Crit Care Med* 2003; **168**: 1293–7

BACKGROUND. CT has an established place in the staging of lung cancer patients, but is not particularly accurate. PET scanning and endoscopic ultrasound are becoming more available to lung cancer clinicians, but their precise place in the staging of potentially operable patients has not been established. These new tests are expensive. What is the most cost-effective way of assessing patients pre-operatively?

INTERPRETATION. In this study from Germany the authors compared CT scanning, PET scanning and endoscopic ultrasound with fine-needle aspiration for identifying inoperable patients in 79 consecutive patients with suspected or proven lung cancer. Each test was interpreted blinded with respect to the other tests. An economic analysis was performed to look at the cost-effectiveness of each test alone and in combination. Thirty-nine of the 79 patients were found to be inoperable by the test. A further patient's inoperability was missed by all three tests. The sensitivity of CT scanning was 43%, while PET and endoscopic ultrasound were more sensitive (68 and 63%, respectively). The negative predictive values of PET and endoscopic ultrasound were also similar (64 and 68%). Since it confirmed a histological diagnosis endoscopic ultrasound had a superior specificity (100 versus 72% for PET). Table 23.3 shows the cost in US dollars for each of the staging tests and their combinations. The authors assumed a false-negative rate of 10% for mediastinoscopy (Table 23.3). PET scanning appeared to be more expensive than all other tests. Adding endoscopic ultrasound to CT scanning did not increase the number of patients who were incorrectly thought to be inoperable, but reduced the proportion of surgical candidates with inoperable disease by over 50%.

Comment

These authors, who have published widely in the field of endoscopic ultrasound, came down heavily in favour of endoscopic ultrasound as the better test after an initial CT scan compared with PET scanning. The basis for this conclusion is that endoscopic ultrasound has a higher specificity than PET at considerably less cost. One disadvantage of endoscopic ultrasound is that it cannot identify extrathoracic metastases where PET is more useful. Once again the high frequency of false-positive scans in the mediastinum that necessitated tissue confirmation was a major weakness

Table 23.3 Cost and consequences of different staging strategies in 100 consecutive patients

Staging	Cost (US dollars)	False negatives*	False positives†
CT	$549	32	4
CT + PET	$2799 (PET $2250)	6	31
CT + EUS-FNA	$1695 (EUS-FNA $1146)	14	4
CT + mediastinoscopy	$2642 (outpatient mediastinoscopy $2093)	10	4

CT, computerized tomography; EUS, endoscopic ultrasound; FNA, fine-needle aspiration; PET, positron emission tomography.
Assumptions: (1) Biopsy costs incurred to exclude false positives not included in the table. (2) All EUS has FNA and associated cytopathology costs (in fact, if EUS is negative for lymphadenopathy, FNA is not done). (3) Thoracotomy (DRG 75) cost is for lobectomy. Chest wall resection would add $350, pneumonectomy would add $450, etc. (4) Unnecessary thoracotomies assume no further work-up before surgery. (5) The 10% false-negative rate for CT + mediastinoscopy is taken from the literature.
* Unnecessary thoracotomies at the rate of $22 536 each.
† Possibly surgically curable patients denied surgery unless tissue confirmation sought.
Source: Fritscher-Ravens *et al.* (2003).

of PET scanning. The authors suggested caution in the size of the study and high-lighted the fact that conventional mediastinal node sampling did not form part of their study. A larger study in different healthcare settings is clearly required before the exact place of endoscopic ultrasound versus PET is determined.

Staging of non-small cell lung cancer with integrated positron emission tomography and computed tomography
Lardinois D, Weder W, Hany TF, *et al. N Engl J Med* 2003; **348**(25): 2500–7

BACKGROUND. CT scanning of the thorax and upper abdomen is the standard pre-operative assessment tool in non-small cell lung cancer. However, it cannot differentiate between benign and malignant tissues. PET scanning has some theoretical advantages, but the false-positive rates are high and the accuracy of location of abnormal areas is poor. Can an integrated PET–CT scan improve results?

INTERPRETATION. This study from the University Hospital of Zurich assessed 50 patients with proven or suspected non-small cell lung cancer. All patients underwent conventional staging with contrast-enhanced CT and whole-body PET scanning. These scans were performed in an integrated fashion using a single PET/CT scanner. Shifting the examination table by 60 cm moved the patient from the CT to the PET gantry. The acquisition time for PET was 4 min per table position and 24 min in total. The patients had to hold their breath for 22 s during the CT imaging. PET image data sets were reconstructed with use of the CT data. Co-registered images were displayed for final viewing. Histological confirmation was performed at resection with total mediastinal lymph node dissection. Eight patients were excluded from surgery because of extrathoracic metastases. One patient was found to have a lymphoma. Images were prospectively analysed by two independent review boards that had no knowledge of the patients' clinical data. The first board assigned a tumour and nodes metastases stage on CT images alone and then interpreted the PET images with the knowledge of the CT findings. It was thought this was standard practice. The second review board assigned a tumour and nodes metastases stage using the integrated CT/PET images. The diagnostic accuracy of integrated PET/CT with CT alone, PET alone and visual correlation of PET and CT images is shown in Table 23.4. Integrated PET/CT provided additional information in 20 out of 49 patients (41%) beyond that provided by conventional correlation of PET and CT. Integrated PET/CT had a better diagnostic accuracy in assessing tumour and node staging. The authors concluded that integrated PET/CT scanning was a significant advance on the conventional single modalities alone.

Comment

This was a novel way of combining CT scanning and PET scanning. However, integrated PET/CT scanning did not provide any further help in detecting micro-scopic lymph node metastases. The authors agreed that histological confirmation (in this case with mediastinoscopy) was still required in order to confirm a patient's operability. The main drawback of PET scanning is the poor quality of the anatomical

Table 23.4 Comparison of the diagnostic accuracy of integrated PET–CT with CT alone, PET alone, and visual correlation of PET and CT images*

Variable	*P*-value
Tumour stage (*n* = 40)	
PET–CT vs CT alone	0.001†
PET–CT vs PET alone	<0.001†
PET–CT vs visual correlation of PET and CT	0.013†
Node stage (*n* = 37)	
PET–CT vs CT alone	0.12
PET–CT vs PET alone	0.013†
PET–CT vs visual correlation of PET and CT	0.021

* The paired sign test was used to calculate *P*-values. Stages assigned on the basis of CT alone, PET alone, and PET and CT were assessed by Review Board A, and stages assigned on the basis of integrated PET–CT were assessed by Review Board B.
† The *P*-value was significant after Bonferroni's correction.
PET, positron emission tomography; CT, computerized tomography.
Source: Lardinois *et al.* (2003).

information, which often does not allow precise assessment of the tumour and nodal stages. This weakness was not overcome by the integrated approach. One advantage of integrated PET/CT scanning is the faster acquisition time, which decreased the duration of the examination for patients.

Treatment

Survival from lung cancer has shown no dramatic change over the last few decades. The vast majority of patients still present with advanced disease and are treated with palliative intent. The best results are still obtained with surgery. Newer chemotherapeutic agents such as IRESSA are appearing and their place in the management of lung cancer patients is becoming established. In this section reports appearing in 2004 concerning advances in lung cancer treatment using these modalities are presented.

Surgery

Successful surgery is unfortunately only available to a small proportion of lung cancer patients. The results in stage 1a and stage 1b disease are encouraging with the 5-year survival being approximately 75% for those with non-small cell histology. The role of adjuvant therapy in this group of surgically treated patients is unclear.

Bestatin is a naturally occurring immunostimulator and inhibits aminopeptidase, inhibition of which increases tumour cell invasion and tumour angiogenesis. Bestatin has some antitumour activity *in vitro* and *in vivo*. However, there are few published studies of its effect in patients. A small, randomized, clinical trial of bestatin as a post-operative adjuvant treatment in patients with non-small cell lung cancer gave inconclusive results |3|. In 2003 a larger placebo-controlled trial of bestatin as post-operative adjuvant treatment was published.

Randomized, double-blind, placebo-controlled trial of bestatin in patients with resected stage I squamous-cell lung carcinoma

Ichinose Y, Genka K, Koike T, *et al.*; NK421 Lung Cancer Surgery Group.
J Natl Cancer Inst 2003; **95**: 605–10

BACKGROUND. Bestatin has immunostimulant and antitumour activity. It is a well-tolerated oral treatment. Could it have a place as a post-operative adjuvant treatment in patients with completely resected stage I squamous carcinoma?

INTERPRETATION. This was a large, randomized trial performed in 80 institutions in Japan. Four hundred and two patients were enrolled into the trial over an 8-year period. Two hundred and two were randomly allocated bestatin (30 mg daily by mouth) and 198 patients were treated with placebo. There were no significant differences between the two groups at the start of the study. The researchers assessed whether bestatin treatment was associated with any improvement in the overall and 5-year cancer-free survival. Safety data were also collected. The median follow-up for the surviving patients was 76 months (range 58–92 months). The overall 5-year survival was 81% in the bestatin group and 74% in the placebo group. The 7% difference was significant ($P = 0.033$). The 5-year cancer-free survival was 71% in the bestatin group and 62% in the placebo group ($P = 0.017$). Few adverse events were observed in either group although anorexia was seen more commonly with bestatin, with 15% having some reports of anorexia compared with 7% in the placebo group. In total, 97.6% of the projected dose of bestatin and 96.3% of the projected dose of placebo were administered. The overall survival in each group is shown in Fig. 23.1.

Comment

The fact that patients in the group treated with bestatin had significantly better survival than those taking placebo is interesting. There are few publications of similar trials examining adjuvant therapy post-operatively in the literature. A trial |4| reviewed in the *Year in Respiratory Medicine 2003* concluded that the retinoid isotretinoin did not influence survival or the development of secondary primary cancers. Although the aim of the bestatin study was not to look at the development of secondary tumours there was an apparent reduction in second primary cancers in the treated group (19 versus 30). This did not reach statistical significance. Bestatin is not currently available worldwide and data are still being collected concerning the safety of the drug. Clearly further work is required in order to determine whether it has a place in the post-operative management of good prognosis surgical patients.

The two common reasons why patients are considered unsuitable for surgery are either spread of cancer outwith the lung or a poor cardiorespiratory reserve due to other smoking-related co-morbidities. Surgeons in the past were keen on limited

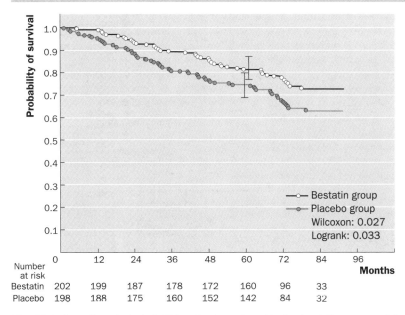

Fig. 23.1 Overall survival of all 400 patients assigned to the bestatin group and the placebo (control) group. Error bars = 95% confidence intervals; $P = 0.027$ (Wilcoxon test) and $P = 0.033$ (log-rank test). All statistical tests were two-sided.
Source: Ichinose *et al.* (2003).

resection for lung cancer, but abandoned this procedure in favour of lobectomy in patients with limited disease as this was thought to be a better curative operation. Is there a place for limited resection in the subgroup of patients who have apparently small peripheral tumours but are poor operative risks?

Intentional limited pulmonary resection for peripheral T1 N0 M0 small-sized lung cancer

Koike T, Yamato Y, Yoshiya K, Shimoyama T, Suzuki R. *J Thorac Cardiovasc Surg* 2003; **125**: 924–8

BACKGROUND. Limited pulmonary resection is rarely practised as a curative operation in patients with lung cancer after reports that recurrence was more common than in patients undergoing lobectomy. Segmentectomy and wedge resection have a low peri-operative mortality and morbidity. Is there a place for limited pulmonary resection for small peripheral cancers?

INTERPRETATION. This was a small, single-centre study from Japan. The authors reported their results of intentional limited resection and compared them with standard lobectomy. Patients were eligible for the study if they had a clinical stage Ia peripheral lung cancer (T1 N0 M0) with a maximum diameter of 2 cm or less on plain chest X-ray or CT scan. All patients had non-small cell histology and had to be fit enough for lobectomy. Two hundred and sixty-eight candidates satisfied these criteria, 80 of whom gave their consent for limited resection Seventy-six of these 80 patients underwent limited resection. Patients were included in the analysis if their pathological staging post-operatively was still stage 1a. Limited resections were performed in 74 patients and lobectomy in 159. Segmentectomy was performed in 60 of the 74 limited resection patients with the remaining 14 receiving a wedge resection. The patients' lymph nodes were sampled at the time of surgery. Follow-up was performed for 5 years post-operatively with annual CT scans. The 3- and 5-year survival rates were 97 and 90.1% in the lobectomy group and 94 and 89.1% in the limited resection group, respectively. This difference was not significant. Recurrence was detected in five of the limited resection group and in nine of the lobectomy group. Survival in the two groups was virtually identical ($P = 0.93$ for both the total survival and disease-free survival).

Comment

Limited resection has generally been performed in patients with poor cardiorespiratory reserve with compromised lung function. However, it has not been widely accepted as a reasonable operation after the results of a randomized trial showing a higher post-operative mortality and increased incidence of recurrence compared with lobectomy |5|. However, this study was not a randomized trial but a retrospective analysis of patients who consented to undergo limited resection. No difference in survival was seen compared with patients with lobectomy and local recurrence was not an issue. The authors suggested that a larger randomized trial is required. With the introduction of mass screening it is likely that more patients with stage 1a tumours will require surgery. It would be useful therefore to have more data in order to resolve the question of whether limited resection has any part to play in these patients, particularly in those with poor respiratory function.

Radio-frequency ablation

Radiotherapy is an established treatment for the management of lung cancer patients. This may be given in an attempt to cure the patient with radical doses or more commonly as a palliative measure in symptomatic patients with extensive disease. Radio-frequency ablation is a new form of treatment that has not been tried in lung cancer patients because of the difficulty in applying a thermal energy probe to a lesion in the lung. Temperatures of up to 100°C are created by ionic agitation resulting in necrosis and tissue destruction in the vicinity of the probe.

Radio-frequency ablation of pulmonary malignant tumours in non-surgical candidates
Herrera LJ, Fernando HC, Perry Y, *et al. J Thorac Cardiovasc Surg* 2003; **125**: 929–37

BACKGROUND. Radio-frequency ablation uses a thermal energy delivery system that applies an alternating current delivered through a needle electrode placed directly into the tumour. It has been used extensively in the treatment of liver tumours in patients who are not candidates for resection. Does it have a place in the treatment of malignant pulmonary disease?

INTERPRETATION. This was a retrospective review of 18 patients with lung tumours treated with radio-frequency ablation from the University of Pittsburgh. None of these patients were candidates for complete resection either because of patient refusal or a poor cardiorespiratory reserve. All patients had disease localized to the lungs although the vast majority had secondary tumours (72%). Five patients had non-small cell lung cancer. The vast majority of patients had received prior chemotherapy and radiotherapy or previous surgery. Thirty-three tumour nodules were treated in 18 patients. The tumours were approached by either mini-thoracotomy or by the CT guided route. The needle electrode was placed within the tumour and radio-frequency ablation performed. Pneumothorax and pleural effusion were common complications (Table 23.5). The response rates to radio-frequency ablation were fairly impressive (55% having complete or partial response, 33% stable disease and 17% progression). The response rates were better for smaller lesions (<5 cm). Unfortunately, half the patients with pulmonary metastases developed new lesions within the chest.

Table 23.5 Complications after radio-frequency abblation

Complication	n	%
Pleural effusion	9	50
Thoracocentesis	2	11
Pneumothorax (CT-guided group)	7	53.8
Delayed pneumothorax	1	5
Pneumonitis or pneumonia	4	22
Transient acute respiratory failure	1	5
Massive haemoptysis	1	5

CT, computerized tomography.
Source: Herrera et al. (2003).

Comment

This is a difficult group of patients who have a short life expectancy and progressive symptoms. This is a fairly invasive treatment that may involve a thoracotomy. This report was helpful in describing a new technique, but larger groups of patients are required before it will be known how effective a palliative treatment this is. Significant toxicity was observed in this small group of patients, but the response rates were fairly high. This is not a group where prolonged survival would be expected. More reports of this new form of treatment are awaited.

IRESSA

For the vast majority of patients with lung cancer, surgical resection is not a therapeutic option. This is because they either have advanced disease or their co-morbidity makes them unfit for surgery. Chemotherapy, if effective, would be the treatment of choice for most patients. This is certainly the case with small cell lung cancer, but the results of chemotherapy for non-small cell lung cancer have been less promising. Newer, more active drugs are urgently required.

Epidermal growth factor (EGF) receptor belongs to a family of four closely related cell surface receptors that are important in the regulation of cell growth and division. EGF receptor is expressed in a variety of tumours with increased levels being associated with advanced disease and poor prognosis. IRESSA is an orally active EGF receptor tyrosine kinase inhibitor. It blocks the proliferation, invasion, angiogenesis, apoptosis and metastases stimulated by EGF receptor. Further information outlining its efficacy, mode of action and safety in lung cancer has appeared in the last year.

The efficacy of gefitinib, an inhibitor of the epidermal growth factor receptor tyrosine kinase, in symptomatic patients with non-small cell lung cancer: a randomized trial

Kris MG, Natale RB, Herbst RS, *et al. J Am Med Assoc* 2003; **290**(16): 2149–58

BACKGROUND. IRESSA (ZD 1839) or gefitinib, blocks the EGF receptor tyrosine kinase and has shown positive results in phase I studies in non-small cell lung cancer. What is its effect on symptom control and response rates in pre-treated patients and what is the correct dose to use?

INTERPRETATION. This was a double-blind, randomized, phase II trial conducted in 30 US centres with 221 patients being enrolled into the study over a 6-month period. All patients had either stage IIIb or IV non-small cell lung cancer and had received prior chemotherapy regimens. The patients were randomized to receive either 250 mg or 500 mg of IRESSA over a 28-day treatment cycle. Symptoms were assessed using the Functional Assessment of Cancer Therapy – Lung (FACT-L) instrument. Radiographic responses were assessed using chest radiographs in a standard way. Two hundred and sixteen patients received IRESSA as randomized (102 received 250 mg). The patients receiving this lower dose were more likely to have an improvement in symptoms (43% of patients) (95% CI = 33–53%) compared with the dose of 500 mg where 35% (95% CI = 26–45%) showed symptomatic improvement. This improvement was seen in three-quarters of the patients within 3 weeks of starting treatment. The radiographic response rates were fairly low, seen in 12% of the group on 250 mg and 9% of the larger dose group. The vast majority of patients having a radiographic response also had a symptomatic response (Fig. 23.2). The 1-year survival (25% in the whole trial) was not influenced by the dose of treatment received. The larger dose of 500 mg was associated with more diarrhoea (75 versus 57%) (*P* = 0.006) and acniform rash (75 versus 62%) (*P* = 0.04) than in the group on a dose of 250 mg.

Comment

This trial was performed in a group of patients with advanced non-small cell lung cancer who had received a considerable amount of prior chemotherapy (at least two

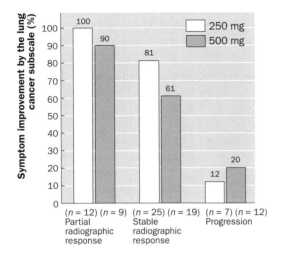

Fig. 23.2 Correlation between the symptom improvement rate and the best radiographic response rate following gefitinib administration. Measure of association (Goodman and Kruskal gamma coefficient) for 250 mg dose, 0.95; for 500 mg dose, 0.78; P <0.001 for both. Source: Kris *et al.* (2003).

different regimens). The symptomatic response to treatment was therefore encouraging as this was, by definition, palliative treatment. The lower dose (250 mg) gave better symptomatic and radiographic responses and was associated with lower adverse events. The results of this trial would support the use of this drug in patients who have received standard chemotherapeutic agents. As this treatment is given orally and is reasonably well tolerated, it is likely to establish a place as a maintenance therapy (rather like tamoxifen in breast cancer) rather than a first-line cytotoxic drug.

Epidermal growth factor receptor in non-small cell lung carcinoma: correlation between gene copy number and protein expression and impact on prognosis

Hirsch FR, Varrella-Garcia M, Bunn PA Jr, *et al. J Clin Oncol* 2003; **21**(20): 3798–807

BACKGROUND. It is known that EGF receptor is frequently over-expressed in non-small cell lung cancers. Much interest has been shown in EGF receptor inhibitors as new treatments for these patients. The molecular basis for this over-expression is poorly understood and it is not known whether this is an important prognostic indicator.

INTERPRETATION. The EGF receptor gene copy number and protein status was assessed in a group of 183 non-small cell lung cancer patients. Eighty-nine of the group had squamous cell histology. The remainder had either adenocarcinoma or undifferentiated non-small cell tumours. Immunohistochemistry was used for assessing protein expression and represented on a scale (0–400). This represented the staining intensity (0–4) × the percentage of positive cells seen. Gene copy numbers were identified by fluorescent *in situ* hybridization. EGF receptor protein over-expression was seen in 62% of the 183 patients and the score was greater than 300 in 37%. Patients with squamous cell histology were more likely to over-express EGF receptor protein compared with the non-squamous cell group (82 versus 44%) ($P \leq 0.001$). The small group of patients with bronchoalveolar cell carcinoma had a similar EGF receptor over-expression. The gene copy number correlated closely with protein expression ($r = 0.4$; $P < 0.001$). Disomy (40%) and trisomy (38%) for the EGF receptor gene was the prevalent pattern on *in situ* hybridization. Interestingly, EGF receptor over-expression or a high gene copy number was not significantly correlated with prognosis.

Comment

This study confirmed previous reports of over-expression of EGF receptor protein in non-small cell lung cancer. This is particularly true in squamous cell histology. Although a high gene copy number per cell showed a trend towards a poor prognosis, this effect was not statistically significant. Further studies are required in order to identify whether evaluation of the EGF receptor gene and EGF receptor protein status has any clinical use in terms of determining which patients may respond to EGF receptor inhibitors and whether measurements of these proteins have any prognostic significance. This study suggested that patients with squamous histology are more likely to respond to EGF receptor inhibitors.

Severe acute interstitial pneumonia and gefitinib
Inoue A, Saijo Y, Maemondo M, *et al. Lancet* 2003; **361**: 137–9

BACKGROUND. Gefitinib (IRESSA) has been shown to be an effective and emerging treatment for patients with advanced non-small lung cancer. This drug appears well tolerated, but reports have appeared from the Far East of possible more worrying side effects.

INTERPRETATION. Two reports of randomized, phase II trials of IRESSA (IRESSA Dose Evaluation in Advanced Lung cancer [IDEAL] I and IDEAL II) have shown promising results for its use as a second- or third-line chemotherapeutic agent. In IDEAL I two of the 102 Japanese patients developed interstitial pneumonia. Up to November 2002, 17 500 patients with non-small cell lung cancer had been given this drug in Japan. Two hundred and ninety-one patients had suspected interstitial pneumonia or acute lung injury associated with the drug with 81 deaths. However, detailed information was not available. This study reports on the 18 patients from a single centre (Tohoku University, Tokyo, Japan) who had received IRESSA. Four patients developed severe acute interstitial pneumonia. The diagnosis of interstitial pneumonia was made on characteristic CT appearances with ground glass opacities distributed diffusely. These patients had elevation of a serum marker (KL-6) that is raised in pulmonary injury and fibrosis. All four patients were treated with steroids and oxygen and two of the four responded to this. The other two died from progressive respiratory failure. Autopsies in these patients showed diffuse alveolar damage with features of acute respiratory distress syndrome. No evidence of lymphangitis carcinomatosis, pulmonary embolism or haemorrhage was seen. The authors appeared to exclude infection as a cause of this problem. Obviously these patients also received other chemotherapeutic agents and radiotherapy. One patient had underlying pulmonary fibrosis. None of the patients were current smokers although all had smoked previously. In one patient treatment with IRESSA had been completed for 83 days and stopped 1 month before the patient developed acute interstitial pneumonia.

Comment

The incidence of interstitial pneumonia in this small series of patients was extremely high. This level of pneumonitis has not been reported from other centres although the incidence of this complication in Japan runs at approximately 1.7%. It is not clear why these patients are more likely to develop this extremely serious complication compared with those of other ethnic origins. One problem in interpreting the significance of this report is the fact that acute respiratory distress syndrome has been reported in patients with cancer, particularly those receiving cytotoxic chemotherapy and high-dose irradiation. More reports concerning the safety of IRESSA and particularly this specific abnormality are eagerly awaited.

Lung cancer guidelines

Lung cancer continues to be a major health problem in both the Western and developing worlds. It is closely related to cigarette smoking and will, therefore, be a particular problem in the emerging nations where smoking is far more common than in 'civilized' societies where smoking rates in most groups are declining. The management of lung cancer will therefore continue to be a major health problem for decades to come. Whilst guidelines concerning many aspects of lung cancer have appeared over the years, an important landmark occurred in 2003 with the publication of comprehensive lung cancer guidelines by the American Academy of Chest Physicians.

Diagnosis and management of lung cancer. ACCP evidence-based guidelines

American Academy of Chest Physicians. *Chest* 2003; **123**(Suppl 1): 1–338

Background. Evidence-based guidelines for lung cancer do exist, but often do not cover all parts of the patient's management. They rapidly become outdated as new advances appear in the management of the condition.

Interpretation. This important series of articles was published as a supplement in *Chest.* At over 300 pages long it is hardly a pocket guide, but is a comprehensive summary of the current evidence for various aspects of lung cancer management. The methodology of this work is carefully set out using standard graded recommendations. Each recommendation was estimated in terms of benefit for lung cancer patients. This ranged from recommendations where implementation could not be justified on current evidence to those whose implementation would be associated with improvements in important health outcomes and where the benefits would substantially outweigh harm. Each recommendation was also based in terms of quality of evidence. The quality of evidence was rated as good, fair and poor. Thus, a recommendation based on good evidence with substantial benefit was graded as A and one based on a poor quality of evidence with no or negative benefit was labelled as I.

Comment

This system was used for assessing various features of lung cancer management throughout the guidelines. All areas, including prevention, screening, patient evaluation, diagnosis and staging, treatment of all tumour stages and types with all treatment modalities, follow-up and surveillance and palliative care were covered. As a reference text this provides an excellent overview of the evidence base for current lung cancer management practices. It is hoped that this will be updated at regular intervals in the future.

References

1. Taylor R, Cumming R, Woodward A, Black M. Passive smoking and lung cancer: a cumulative meta-analysis. *Aust NZ J Public Health* 2001; **25**: 203–11.
2. Swensen SJ, Jett JR, Sloan JA, Midthun DE, Hartman TE, Sykes AM, Aughenbaugh GL, Zink FE, Hillman SL, Noetzel GR, Marks RS, Clayton AC, Pairolero PC. Screening for lung cancer with low dose spiral computed tomography. *Am J Respir Crit Care Med* 2002; **165**: 508–13.
3. Yasumitsu T, Ohshima S, Nakano N, Kotake Y, Tominaga S. Bestatin in resected lung cancer a randomised clinical trial. *Acta Oncologica* 1990; **29**: 827–31.
4. Lippman SM, Lee JJ, Karp DD, Vokes EE, Benner SE, Goodman GE, Khuri FR, Marks R, Winn RJ, Fry W, Graziano SL, Gandara DR, Okawara G, Woodhouse CL, Williams B, Perez C, Kim HW, Lotan R, Roth JA, Hong WK. Randomized phase III intergroup trial of isotretinoin to prevent second primary tumors in stage I non-small-cell lung cancer. *J Natl Cancer Inst* 2001; **93**: 605–18.
5. Ginsberg RJ, Rubinstein LV for the Lung Cancer Study Group. Randomized trial of lobectomy versus limited resection for T, N0 non-small cell lung cancer. *Ann Thorac Surg* 1995; **60**: 615–23.

Part VII

Obstructive sleep
apnoea/hypopnoea syndrome

Obstructive sleep apnoea/hypopnoea syndrome

T MACKAY

Introduction

The obstructive sleep apnoea/hypopnoea syndrome was clinically recognized more than 30 years ago [1], but awareness of this condition outside the field of sleep medicine has been slow to develop. The obstructive sleep apnoea/hypopnoea syndrome can be defined as the co-existence of excessive daytime sleepiness with irregular breathing at night. It forms part of a spectrum of sleep-disordered breathing ranging from simple snoring at one end to profound nocturnal hypoventilation and respiratory failure at the far end of the spectrum. It is historically based upon the recognition of repetitive episodes of partial or complete upper airway obstruction during sleep leading to recurrent episodes of hypoxia and the production of impairment of sleep architecture with a reduction in the amount of slow wave sleep and an increase in sleep fragmentation [2]. These repeated episodes of airway obstruction are usually terminated by an arousal from sleep, which results in sleep fragmentation, the generation of unrefreshing sleep and subsequent excessive daytime sleepiness. The Wisconsin Sleep Cohort Study [3] defined obstructive sleep apnoea syndrome as the association of excessive daytime sleepiness with an apnoea/hypopnoea index of more than five events per hour slept. An apnoea is defined as complete cessation of airflow for at least 10 s and a hypopnoea is defined as a 50% reduction in airflow for at least 10 s, terminating in arousal or associated with an oxygen desaturation of at least 3%.

References

1. Guilleminault C, Tilkien A, Dement WC. Sleep apnoea/hypopnoea syndromes. *Ann Ref Med* 1976; 27: 465–84.

2. Kryger MH, Roth T, Dement UC. *Principles and Practice of Sleep Medicine.* Philadelphia: WB Saunders, 1989.

3. Young T, Palta M, Dempsey J, Sketred J, Weber S, Bader S. The occurrence of sleep disordered breathing among middle aged adults. *N Engl J Med* 1993; **328**: 1230–5.

24

Epidemiology

Introduction

Obstructive sleep apnoea is a significant public health problem and there is a large and increasing demand for sleep service facilities in many countries due to both the high prevalence of the condition and growing public awareness of sleep disorders in general. A conservative estimate of the prevalence of obstructive sleep apnoea in middle-aged men (30–65 years) is in the range 0.3–4%, with most studies giving a prevalence of 1–2% which is a similar prevalence to type I diabetes and approximately double that of severe asthma |1–3|.

The prevalence of obstructive sleep apnoea in middle-aged women is probably approximately half of that in males at around 0.5–1% |4|. However, there is increasing debate about which sleep study indices we should actually be measuring in order to predict the severity of obstructive sleep apnoea and subsequent outcome in response to treatment |5|.

However, there is no doubt that no matter how we measure sleep fragmentation at night there is evidence from methodologically sound cohort studies that undiagnosed obstructive sleep apnoea, with or without symptoms, is associated with significant consequences including an increased likelihood of daytime sleepiness, impairment of cognitive functioning, impairment of mood and personality changes |6|, hypertension |5|, cardiovascular disease and stroke |5|. Untreated sleep apnoea is also associated with a reduction in the quality of life |6| and there are also adverse effects on relationships between spouses and partners |6|. One of the most dangerous aspects of increased daytime sleepiness resulting from impaired concentration is an increased risk of road traffic accidents |7–10|. There is objective evidence for a 1.3- to twelvefold increase in accident rates amongst patients with untreated sleep apnoea |10|. Sleepiness at the wheel is estimated is to cause approximately 20% of road traffic accidents on major highways and these accidents often occur at high speed without any attempt at avoidance actions and they are therefore associated with serious injuries and a high mortality rate |9,10|.

The reduction of risk factors for obstructive sleep apnoea/hypopnoea syndrome through public health measures is vital. Potentially modifiable risk factors include obesity |11|, alcohol |12|, smoking |13| and post-menopausal oestrogen depletion |14|. The identification and treatment of obstructive sleep apnoea cases is one of the most important challenges faced by clinicians practising respiratory medicine.

Familial predisposition and co-segregation analysis of adult obstructive sleep apnoea and the sudden infant death syndrome

Gislason T, Johannson JH, Haraldsson A, *et al. Am J Respir Crit Care Med* 2002; **116**: 833–8

BACKGROUND. There have been several reports of a familial aggregation of patients with obstructive sleep apnoea |15|. Redline |16| reported that there was a twofold risk of obstructive sleep apnoea in first-degree relatives of 47 subjects with laboratory-proven sleep apnoea compared to control subjects and that the probability of sleep-disordered breathing increased progressively with increasing numbers of affected relatives. There may be an oligogenic inheritance of obstructive sleep apnoea in Caucasians |17|. It has also been observed that there is a resemblance between obstructive sleep apnoea and sudden infant death syndrome (SIDS) |18,19|. A familial association between obstructive sleep apnoea and SIDS has been reported, with allergy, narrow upper airways and a decreased hypoxic ventilatory response all being suggested as possible contributory factors. However, none of the previously reported studies have been population based. With this in mind this study, which was undertaken in Iceland, where there is a relatively homogeneous population base |20|, aimed to determine whether adult sleep apnoea and SIDS were familial diseases and whether or not sleep apnoea cases congregated with SIDS cases.

INTERPRETATION. Hospital-based lists of all Icelandic patients who were diagnosed with obstructive sleep apnoea ($n = 2350$) and SIDS ($n = 58$) between 1979 and 1998 were studied. The risk ratio for a first-degree relative of a patient with obstructive sleep apnoea was 2.0 (95% confidence interval [CI] = 1.7–2.8) ($P < 0.001$). The kinship coefficient, which determined the relatedness of the patients, was greater in the obstructive sleep apnoea group than in the control group of 1000 people. The risk ratio of the more severely affected patients with obstructive sleep apnoea/hypopnoea syndrome was slightly higher at 2.3 (95% CI = 1.2–3.2) ($P = 0.005$).

Comment

The authors concluded that there was a non-significant trend observed for relatedness between infants who died with SIDS and patients with severe obstructive sleep apnoea. These results are consistent with a familial component in sleep apnoea and suggest that infants who died of SIDS may have shared some of the same susceptibility factors with sleep apnoea.

Utility of non-invasive pharyngometry in epidemiologic studies of childhood sleep disordered breathing

Monahan KJ, Larkin EK, Rosen CL, Graham G, Redline S. *Am J Respir Crit Care Med* 2002; **165**: 1499–503

BACKGROUND. Excessive body weight has been hypothesized as affecting breathing in numerous ways, including alterations in upper airway structure (altered geometry) or function (increased collapsibility), disturbance of the relationship between respiratory drive and load compensation and by exacerbating obstructive sleep apnoea events via obesity-related reductions in functional residual capacity and increased whole-body oxygen demand |21|. These putative mechanisms suggest that specific anatomical locations of excess fat deposition leading to a small pharyngeal airway may be important in the aetiology of obstructive sleep apnoea. A variety of body habitus measures including neck morphology |22|, general obesity |22| and central obesity |23,24| have been cross-sectionally associated with obstructive sleep apnoea. However, there is no current consensus as to which body habitus phenotype is the most important in the pathophysiology of obstructive sleep apnoea. It is possible that different types of fat distribution are more important in specific subgroups defined by factors such as sex. Various methods of imaging the upper airway size are available including flow volume loops |25|, computed tomography |26| and magnetic resonance imaging scanning |27|, but none have proven diagnostically useful in differentiating obstructive sleep apnoea patients from normal subjects. This study looked at 203 children (aged 8–11 years) from a community-based cohort.

INTERPRETATION. The coefficient of variation for measurements of the minimum cross-sectional area of the pharynx was 11%. The minimum cross-sectional area was 1.17 cm^2 in children who rarely or never snored: the area was decreased by 10% in children with habitual snoring and by 18% in children with an apnoea/hypopnoea index of at least 5 events/h. The mean cross-sectional area did not differ between the groups.

Comment

The minimum cross-sectional area of the pharynx is reduced in children with sleep-disordered breathing. Acoustic pharyngometry appears to be a useful non-invasive technique for identifying risk factors for potential sleep-disordered breathing in pre-adolescent children.

Hormone replacement therapy and sleep-disordered breathing

Shahar E, Redline S, Young T, *et al.* for the Sleep Heart Health Study Research Group. *Am J Respir Crit Care Med* 2003: **167**: 1186–92

BACKGROUND. Sleep-disordered breathing is more common among post-menopausal women than among their pre-menopausal counterparts |28–30|, but it is not clearly understood why this should be so. Estimates of the prevalence of this disorder amongst women in their sixth decade range from 4 to 22% |31,32| depending on the definition used and the population studied. Along with the other biological sequelae of ageing, the transition to the post-menopausal period and the associated hormonal changes that ensue might increase the risk of developing sleep-disordered breathing or it may exacerbate a pre-existing disorder. This study examined the relationship between the use of replacement hormones and sleep-disordered breathing in a sample of 2852 non-institutionalized women aged 50 years or older who participated in a large community-based cohort study (Sleep Heart Study) in the USA (see Fig. 24.1).

INTERPRETATION. The frequency of apnoeas and hypopnoeas per hour (apnoea/hypopnoea index) slept was determined by an unattended, single night polysomnography at home. The prevalence of sleep-disordered breathing (apnoea/hypopnoea index >15 events/h) among hormone users (61 out of 907 or 7%) was approximately half that seen amongst non-hormone users (286 out of 1945 or 15%). Multivariate adjustment for known determinants of obstructive sleep apnoea/hypopnoea syndrome, including age, body mass index and neck circumference, modestly attenuated the association (adjusted odds ratio [OR] = 0.55 and 95% CI = 0.41–0.75). The inverse association between hormone use and sleep-disordered breathing was evident in various subgroups and was particularly strong amongst women of 50–59 years of age (adjusted OR = 0.36 and 95% CI = 0.21–0.60).

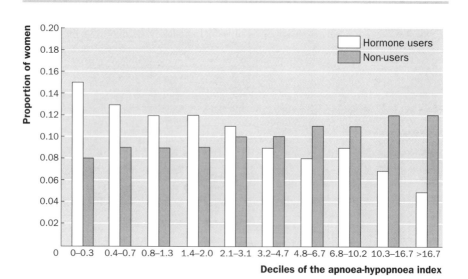

Fig. 24.1 Distribution of the apnoea/hypopnoea index according to the use of replacement hormones. Deciles correspond to the distribution of the index in the entire sample (users and non-users combined). Source: Shahar *et al.* (2003).

Comment

This interesting, large, community-based epidemiological study suggested that hormone replacement therapy may have a role in either preventing or modifying sleep-disordered breathing problems in post-menopausal women. Additional studies are needed in order to test this hypothesis.

Conclusion

There have been a number of studies looking at the prevalence of sleep apnoea in the general population and, although it is difficult to be certain due to methodological difficulties in many of these studies, it is likely that obstructive sleep apnoea has a prevalence of approximately 1–2% in middle-aged men and 0.5–1% in middle-aged women, thereby making this condition a significant public health problem and one that merits increased research funding. This condition is usually under-recognized and under-diagnosed and as such results in an increased level of behavioural and cardiovascular morbidity.

There appears to be a famililial component to the condition compounded by potentially modifiable factors such as upper airway geometry and function, obesity, nasal congestion and post-menopausal oestrogen depletion.

It is vital that there is a high clinical suspicion for the condition in both primary and secondary care so that potential sufferers can be diagnosed and treated speedily in an attempt to reduce the undoubted public health burden that this condition produces.

An excellent state-of-the-art review of the epidemiology of obstructive sleep apnoea was published in 2002 |**14**|.

References

1. Stradling JR, Crosby JH. Predictors and prevalence of obstructive sleep apnoea and snoring in 1001 middle aged men. *Thorax* 1991; **46**: 85–90.

2. Bearpark H, Elliot L, Grunstein R, Cullen S, Scheider H, Althaus W. Snoring and sleep apnoea. A population study in Australian men. *Am J Respir Crit Care Med* 1995; **151**: 1459–65.

3. Jennum P, Sjol A. Epidemiology of snoring and obstructive sleep apnoea in a Danish population, aged 30–60. *J Sleep Res* 1992; **1**: 240–4.

4. Engleman HM, Martin SE, Deary IJ, Douglas NJ. The effect of continuous positive airway pressure treatment and daytime function in sleep apnoea/hypopnoea syndrome. *Lancet* 1994; **343**: 572–5.

5. Ala KM, Young TB, Bidwell T, Palta M, Sketrue JB, Dempsey J. Sleep apnoea and hypertension. A population based study. *Ann Intern Med* 1994; **120**: 382–8.

6. Smith IE, Shneerson JM. Is the SF-36 sensitive to sleep disruption? A study in subjects with sleep apnoea. *J Sleep Res* 1995; **4**: 183–8.

7. Horne JA, Reyner LA. Sleep related vehicle accidents. *BMJ* 1995; **310**: 565–7.

8. Maycock G. Sleepiness and driving: The experience of UK car drivers. *J Sleep Res* 1996; **5**: 229–37.

9. Department of the Environment, Transport and the Regions 1999. *Valuations of the Benefits of Prevention of Road Traffic Accidents and Casualities.* London: The Department, 2000.

10. Horstmann S, Hess CW, Bassetti C, Gugger M, Mathis J. Sleepiness related accidents in sleep apnoea patients. *Sleep* 2000; **23**: 383–9.

11. Jennum P, Sjol A. Snoring, sleep apnoea and cardiovascular risk factors: The MONICA II Study. *Int J Epidemiol* 1993; **22**: 439–44.

12. Issa FG, Sullivan CE. Alcohol, snoring and sleep apnoea. *J Neurolsurg* 1992; **45**: 353–9.

13. Wetter DW, Young TB, Bidwell TR, Bader MS, Palta M. Smoking as a risk factor for sleep disordered breathing. *Arch Intern Med* 1994; **154**: 2219–24.

14. Young T, Peppard PE, Gottlieb I. Epidemology of obstructive sleep apnoea: a population health perspective. State of the art. *Am J Respir Crit Care Med* 2002; **165**: 1217–39.

15. Strohl KP, Saunders A, Feldman NT. Obstructive sleep apnoea in family members. *N Engl J Med* 1978; **299**: 969–73.

16. Redline S, Tishler PV, Tosteson TD, Kump K, Browner I, Ferrette V, Krejci P. The familial aggregation of obstructive sleep apnoea. *Am J Respir Crit Care Med* 1995; **151**: 682–7.

17. Redline S, Tishler PV. The genetics of sleep apnoea. *Sleep Med Rev* 2000; **4**: 583–602.

18. Kahn J, Groswasser J, Rebuffat E, Sottiaux M, Blum D, Foerst M, Franco P, Bochner A, Alexander M, Bachy A. Sleep and cardiorespiratory characteristics of infant victims of sudden death: a prospective case control study. *Sleep* 1992; **15**: 287–92.

19. Kato I, Groswasser J, Franco P, Scaliat S, Kelmanson I, Togari H, Kahn A. Developmental characteristics of apnoea infants who succumb to sudden infant death syndrome. *Am J Respir Crit Care Med* 2001; **164**: 346–57.

20. Gudmonson H, Gudbjardson DF, Kong A, Gudejartsson H, Frigge M, Gulchar JR, Stefanson K. The inheritance of human longevity in Iceland. *Eur J Human Genet* 2000; **8**: 743–9.

21. Barvaux VA, Aubert G, Rodenstein DO. Weight loss as a treatment for obstructive sleep apnoea. *Sleep Med Rev* 2000; **4**: 435–52.

22. Bearpark H, Elliott I, Grunstein R, Hedner J, Cullen S, Schneider H, Althaus W, Sullivan C. Snoring and sleep apnoea: a population study in Australian men. *Am J Respir Crit Care Med* 1995; **151**: 1459–65.

23. Levinson PD, McGarvey ST, Carlase CC, Eveloff SE, Herbert PN, Millman RP. Adiposity and cardiovascular risk factors in men with obstructive sleep medicine. *Chest* 1993; **103**: 1336–42.

24. Shinohara E, Kihara S, Yamashite S, Yamana M, Nishidie M, Kotani K, Nakamura T, Takemura K. Visceral fat accumulation. An important risk factor for obstructive sleep apnoea in obese subjects. *J Intern Med* 1997; **241**: 11–18.

25. Riley R, Guilleminault C, Herran J, Powell N. Cephalometric analyses and flow volume loops in obstructive sleep apnoea patients. *Sleep* 1993; **6**: 303–11.

26. Haponic EA, Thomas Smith PL, Bohlman ME, Allan RP, Goldman SM, Bleecker AR. Computerised tomography in obstructive sleep apnoea. Correlation of airway size with physiology wakefulness. *Am Rev Respir Dis* 1993; **27**: 221–6.

27. Martin SE, Marshall I, Douglas NJ. The effect of posture on airway calibre with the sleep apnoea/hypopnoea syndrome. *Am J Respir Crit Care Med* 1995; **125**: 721–4.

28. Block AJ, Boysen PG, Wynn AW. Sleep apnoea/hypopnoea and oxygen desaturation in normal subjects: a strong male predominance. *N Engl J Med* 1979; **300**: 513–17.

29. Redline S, Kump K, Tishler PV, Browner I, Ferrette V. Gender differences in sleep disordered breathing in a community based sample. *Am J Respir Crit Care Med* 1994; **149**: 722–6.

30. Bixler EO, Vgontzas AN, Lyn HM, TenHave T, Rein J, Vela-Bueno A, Kales A. Prevalence of sleep disordered breathing in women: the effects of gender. *Am J Respir Crit Care Med* 2001; **163**: 608–13.

31. Ancol-Israel S, Kripke DF, Klauber MR, MasonWJ, Fell R, Kaplan OJ. Sleep disordered breathing in the community dwelling elderly. *Sleep* 1991; **14**: 486–95.

32. Kripke DF, Ancol-Israel S, Klauber MR, Wingard DL, Mason WJ, Mullaney DJ. Prevalence of sleep disordered breathing in ages 40–64 years: a population based survey. *Sleep* 1997; **20**: 65–76.

25

Pathophysiology

Introduction

The pathophysiology of obstructive sleep apnoea is likely to be multifactorial, with contributions from airway anatomy, the state-dependent control of upper airway dilator muscles and ventilatory stability [1]. The production of a small or collapsible pharyngeal airway is crucial to the pathogenesis of this condition. During the wakeful state the pharyngeal airway remains patent due to high activity of the upper airway dilating muscles. However, at sleep onset this compensatory activation is reduced or lost resulting in partial or complete upper airway collapse and this may occur in association with a reduction in central respiratory drive and a decrease in lung volume.

As the pharyngeal airway size decreases hypoxemia and hypercapnia develop, which produce a progressive increase in respiratory drive to the upper airway muscles, but this increase in drive has to be accompanied by arousal from sleep in order to be effective. Following arousal hyperventilaton reverses the blood gas disturbance and the increase in respiratory drive then falls back to normal. The arousal terminates and the sufferer falls asleep again repeating the whole process thus producing un-refreshing fragmented sleep [1].

There is increasing evidence that obstructive sleep apnoea is linked to an increase in cardiovascular morbidity and mortality. Patients with untreated sleep apnoea have a higher nocturnal and daytime blood pressure [2] than control subjects and sub-sequent treatment with continuous positive airway pressure (CPAP) is beneficial [3,4]. Indeed, a recent guideline [5] has suggested that hypertension *per se* should be one factor that is assessed in addition to symptoms when the clinician is considering whether a patient with sleep apnoea warrants treatment or not.

Studies of random subjects from the general population have suggested that the existence of sleep apnoea constitutes a risk factor for cardiovascular disease inde-pendent of other known risk factors such as obesity [6]. However, the underlying mechanism of this risk is not well understood. There is evidence that repeated apnoeic-related hypoxic events in sleep apnoea can induce oxidative stress, which can affect energy metabolism, redox-sensitive gene expression and the expression of adhesion molecules similar to hypoxia-induced reperfusion injury. These processes may possibly lead to an increased atherogenic tendency in untreated sleep apnoea [7].

The basic pathophysiological processes underlying obstructive sleep apnoea/ hypopnoea syndrome may be classified as follows: (1) upper airway anatomy,

(2) upper airway muscular function, (3) ventilatory control, (4) inflammatory mechanisms and (5) endocrinological mechanisms. This list is not exhaustive and will be modified in future by ongoing research studies. Recent advances in each of these categories will be discussed in turn.

General review

Recent advances in understanding of the pathogenesis of obstructive sleep apnoea

Jordan A, White D, Fogel RB. *Curr Opin Pulmon Med* 2003; **9**(6): 459–64

B A C K G R O U N D . The pathogenesis of obstructive sleep apnoea is incompletely understood.

I N T E R P R E T A T I O N . This detailed review described the factors, such as upper airway anatomy, pharyngeal muscle control, unstable ventilatory control and the changes in lung volume during sleep, that may contribute to the pathogenesis of obstructive sleep apnoea. Additional factors such as pharyngeal surface tension and the ability to arouse from sleep may also independently influence the likelihood of developing obstructive sleep apnoea/hypopnoea syndrome. The exact contribution of each of these various factors in the pathogenesis of this condition may vary from individual to individual (see Fig. 25.1). The review recognized that sleep apnoea is an incompletely understood disorder, but that, if the apnoea pathogenesis can be understood in more detail, then therapeutic advances may be possible in the future.

Comment

This extensive review article discusses in detail the multiple factors that are involved in the pathogenesis of the obstructive sleep apnoea syndrome

Upper airway anatomy

Contribution of body habitus and craniofacial characteristics to segmental closing pressures of the passive pharynx in patients with sleep-disordered breathing

Watanabe T, Isono S, Tanaka A, Tanzawa H, Nishio T. *Am J Respir Crit Care Med* 2002; **165**: 260–5

B A C K G R O U N D . The site of the obstruction in sleep apnoea is at the level of the pharynx although exactly how factors such as cranial facial geometry and pharyngeal physiology interact to produce pharyngeal narrowing have still to be fully clarified. This

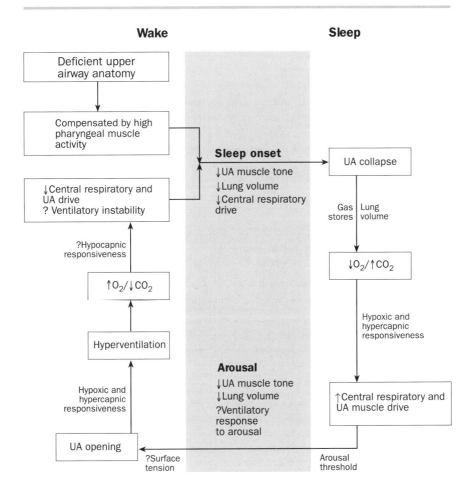

Wake   **Sleep**

Deficient upper
airway anatomy

Compensated by high
pharyngeal muscle
activity

Sleep onset   UA collapse
↓UA muscle tone
↓Lung volume
↓Central respiratory and   ↓Central respiratory
UA drive   drive   Gas | Lung
? Ventilatory instability   stores | volume

?Hypocapnic
responsiveness
                                                 ↓O$_2$/↑CO$_2$
↑O$_2$/↓CO$_2$

                                                 Hypoxic and
                                                 hypercapnic
Hyperventilation   responsiveness

Arousal
↓UA muscle tone
Hypoxic and   ↓Lung volume   ↑Central respiratory and
hypercapnic   ?Ventilatory   UA muscle drive
responsiveness   response
                         to arousal
UA opening
              ?Surface   Arousal
              tension   threshold

Fig. 25.1 The cyclical nature of obstructive sleep apnoea. UA, upper airway.
Source: Jordan *et al.* (2003).

**paper studied the effects of cranial facial characteristics and body habitus on the
collapsibility of the pharynx.**

INTERPRETATION. The authors measured the closing pressures of the passive pharynx
in 54 men with sleep-disordered breathing. Static pressure–volume relationships within
the velopharynx and oropharynx were measured endoscopically under general anaesthesia
and complete paralysis. The results were compared with 24 healthy subjects. Patients with
sleep apnoea had retrognathia, longer lower faces and downward development of the
mandible on lateral cephalometry. The closing pressure was positive at the velopharynx
level alone in 50% of the patients and at both the velopharynx and oropharynx levels in

44% of the patients. The patients who had positive closing pressures at both the velopharynx and the oropharynx had smaller maxillas and mandibles and less obesity than did the patients with positive closing pressure at the velopharynx alone.

Comment

The authors concluded that obesity and craniofacial abnormalities contribute synergistically to produce an increase in tissue pressure surrounding the pharynx leading to an increase in the collapsibility of the passive pharynx in patients with sleep apnoea.

Upper airway muscular function

Pharyngeal pressure and flow effects on genioglossal activation in normal subjects

Malhotra A, Pillar G, Fogel RB, *et al. Am J Respir Crit Care Med* 2002; **165**: 71–7

BACKGROUND. Twenty-five years ago Remmers *et al.* |8| demonstrated that inspiratory pharyngeal occlusion occurred in sleep apnoea and that this was associated with decreased electromyelographic (EMG) tone in the genioglossus, the main pharyngeal dilating muscle and that subsequent pharyngeal widening associated with arousal coincided with reactivation of this muscle. This paper studied genioglossus activity in 80 healthy volunteers during wakefulness.

INTERPRETATION. The subjects inhaled gases of different densities (helium–oxygen and air) to allow discrimination between the relative influences of airway pressure and airflow. The genioglossal EMG signal was correlated with pressure in the epiglottis (range of *r*-values 0.71–0.83) and the relationship did not change despite the variation in gas density or CO_2 tension. The correlations between genioglossal activity and both flow and resistance were weaker.

Comment

This was a well-designed and executed study demonstrating that negative pressure in the pharynx modulates activity of the genioglossus muscle independently of respiratory drive and adds further evidence to the principle that occlusion of the pharyngeal airway is in a large part a result of inadequate opposition through inspiratory suction of the upper airway by airway dilating muscle activity |9|.

An excellent review by Veasey |1| discussed the physiological basis of obstructive sleep apnoea/hypopnoea syndrome in detail (Fig. 25.2).

Ventilatory control

One of the features of obstructive sleep apnoea syndrome is that the ventilatory patterns and arterial oxygen levels may be completely normal when the patient is

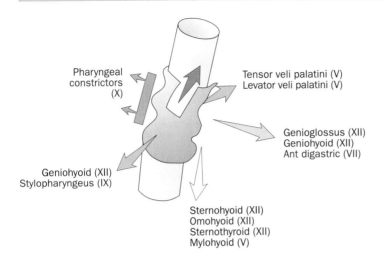

Fig. 25.2 Schematic of potential upper airway dilators in humans. Muscles surrounding the upper airway have the potential to dilate or stent the upper airway in many different directions. The force vectors for activation of specific muscle groups are represented. As a collapsible tube (grey), oropharyngeal patency is most effectively achieved by simultaneous activation of muscles with vectors in different directions. Elongation of the airway along with widening of the lateral walls may be most effective in rendering the airway less collapsible. Source: [1].

awake. During sleep, however, the upper airway collapses |8| resulting in large intra-thoracic and upper airway intraluminal pressure swings |8|. Hypoxia |9| and hyper-capnia |9| increase the sympathetic drive |10,11| and increase the upper airway dilator muscle activity which leads to a restoration of airway patency |12|.

This state dependency in upper airway patency and respiratory function suggests that state-dependent changes in neural drive to the upper airway dilator muscles prompt obstructive upper airway events. However, it is important to realize that these state-dependent changes in respiratory muscle activity are a normal phenom-enon of sleep |12|. The unique features in individuals with obstructive sleep apnoea compared with normal subjects are an over-reliance on upper airway dilator muscle activity and lung volume and a greater magnitude of sleep state-dependent reduc-tions in muscle activity.

Hypercapnia and ventilatory periodicity in obstructive sleep apnoea syndrome

Ayappa I, Berger KI, Norman RG, Oppenheimer BW, Rapoport DM, Goldran RM. *Am J Respir Crit Care Med* 2002; **166**: 1112–15

BACKGROUND. The aim of this study was to determine whether the daytime partial pressure of carbon dioxide (PCO_2) is related to the duration of ventilation between apnoeas.

INTERPRETATION. Eighteen patients with sleep apnoea (eight patients with a daytime PCO_2 of higher than 45 mmHg) were studied. The level of their daytime PCO_2 was not related to the average duration of their apnoeas nor to the average duration of ventilation between the apnoeas. However, their daytime PCO_2 was correlated with their ratio of apnoea duration to the duration of ventilation between the apnoeas ($r = 0.48$).

Commment

The relative balance between the duration of apnoeas and the duration of intervening ventilation is an important determinant of daytime hypercapnia in patients with obstructive sleep apnoea.

Inflammatory mechanisms

Elevated C-reactive protein in patients with obstructive sleep apnoea

Shamsuzzaman AS, Minnicki M, Lanfranchi P, *et al. Circulation* 2002; **105**(21): 2462–4

BACKGROUND. Inflammatory processes associated with obstructive sleep apnoea may act as potential mediators of cardiovasular morbidity and mortality. C-reactive protein is an important serum marker of inflammation. It is synthesized by the liver and regulated by cytokines. However, unlike cytokines it is stable for up to 24 h and may reflect the level of a given inflammatory response |13|. It can induce the production of adhesion molecules and monocyte chemoattractant protein in human endothelial cells. C-reactive protein may therefore be both a risk factor for and an active pathogenic agent in atherosclerosis. The relationship between C-reactive protein and cardiovascular disease is further strengthened by the finding that statins reduced plasma C-reactive protein levels and also decreased the incidence of cardiovascular events |14|.

INTERPRETATION. Twenty-two patients (18 males and four females) with newly diagnosed moderate to severe obstructive sleep apnoea (apnoea/hypopnoea index >20 events/h) and who were free of other diseases and were taking no medications were compared to 20 control subjects (15 males and five females) matched for age and body mass index (BMI) and in whom obstructive sleep was excluded. The plasma C-reactive protein levels were significantly higher in patients with obstructive sleep apnoea than the controls (median 0.33 mg/dl and range 0.09–2.73 mg/dl versus 0.09 mg/dl and 0.02–0.9 mg/dl) (P <0.003). The C-reactive protein levels in multivariate analysis were independently associated with obstructive sleep apnoea severity (F = 6.8; P = 0.032).

Comment

Obstructive sleep apnoea is associated with elevated levels of C-reactive, which is a marker of inflammation and cardiovascular risk. The severity of obstructive sleep apnoea appears to be proportional to the C-reactive level. This paper provided further evidence that intermittent hypoxia present in sleep apnoea may precipitate oxidative stress, which can in turn affect endothelial function and could be linked to increased vascular risk in these patients.

Elevated levels of C-reactive protein and interleukin-6 in patients with obstructive sleep apnoea syndrome are decreased by nasal continuous positive airway pressure

Yokoe T, Minoguchi K, Matsuo H, *et al. Circulation* 2003; **107**(8): 1129–34

BACKGROUND. Although C-reactive protein is a non-specific marker of inflammation it can directly induce the production of adhesion molecules on endothelial cells and up-regulate the cytokine interlukin-6 (IL-6) |15|.

INTERPRETATION. This study looked at the effect of nasal CPAP in 30 patients with obstructive sleep apnoea and 14 obese control subjects. The serum C-reactive protein and the production of IL-6 by monocytes were studied before and after 1 month's treatment using CPAP. Both the C-reactive protein and IL-6 levels were significantly higher in patients with sleep apnoea compared with the obese control subjects (P <0.01 and P <0.05, respectively). The IL-6 production by monocytes was higher in patients with sleep apnoea than in the obese control subjects (P <0.01). The major factors influencing the C-reactive protein levels in patients with sleep apnoea were the severity of their sleep apnoea and their BMI. The main factor influencing the IL-6 levels was the patients' BMI and the degree of nocturnal hypoxaemia. Nasal CPAP significantly decreased both the C-reactive protein (P <0.0001) and IL-6 values (P <0.001) and spontaneous IL-6 production by monocytes (P <0.01).

Comment

Obstructive sleep apnoea is associated with increased cardiovascular morbidity and mortality, but the underlying mechanism is not understood. It is known that sleep apnoea produces repeated hypoxic events overnight and this may initiate oxidative stress. This in turn may affect redox-sensitive gene expression and also the expression of adhesion molecules leading to endothelial damage and a subsequent rise in cardiovascular risk. The observation that treatment of sleep apnoea with nasal CPAP leads to a reduction in both C-reactive protein and IL-6 levels is interesting and deserves further investigation.

Increased adhesion molecules expression and production of reactive oxygen species in leukocytes of sleep apnoea patients

Dyugovskaya L, Lavie P, Lavie L. *Am J Respir Crit Care Med* 2002; **165**: 934–9

BACKGROUND. There are numerous levels of evidence linking oxidative stress in the pathogenesis of cardiovascular and cerebrovascular disease leading to an increased risk of hypertension, strokes, myocardial infarction and pulmonary hypertension |15–17|. Inflammatory leukocytes are one of the well-characterized pathways of free radical formation. Leukocyte accumulation and adhesion via appropriate receptors on the endothelium and initiation of leukocyte–endothelial cell interactions may critically impair endothelial cell function and propogate atherogenic processes. This study characterized the cellular phenotypes of peripheral whole-blood monocytes and granulocytes in 26 obstructive sleep apnoea patients compared to 31 healthy control subjects and studied their level of oxidative metabolism and the ability of monocytes for adhering to human endothelial cells in culture. In addition, the effect of CPAP treatment on cellular function was studied in the sleep apnoea group (*n* = 8).

INTERPRETATION. Obstructive sleep apnoea is associated with increased expression of two adhesion molecules, CD15 and CD11c, in monocytes. The monocytes of the patients adhered more avidly to endothelial cells in culture than did the monocytes of healthy subjects. Exposure of the monocytes from healthy subjects to hypoxia *in vitro* caused up-regulation of the expression of CD15 to levels comparable in the sleep apnoea patients. The patients displayed an increased production of reactive oxygen species in some subpopulations of monocytes and granulocytes. The treatment of eight patients with CPAP produced downregulation of CD15 and CD11c monocyte expression, decreased the basal production of reactive oxygen species by CD11+ monocytes and decreased the adherence of monocytes to the endothelium.

Comment

This well-designed study provided evidence that repeated hypoxic events cause endothelial and monocyte activation leading to increased intracellular production of reactive oxygen species and an alteration in adhesion molecule expression. This is important as it links the oxidative stress caused by recurrent apnoeic episodes to the pathogenesis of vascular disease.

Plasma vascular endothelial growth factor in the sleep apnoea syndrome: effects of nasal continuous positive airway pressure treatment

Lavi L, Kraiczi H, Hefetz A, *et al. Am J Respir Crit Care Med* 2002; **165**: 1624–8

BACKGROUND. Chronic hypoxic events can induce vascular remodelling. Vascular endothelial growth factor (EGF) is an angiogenic glycoprotein. This cytokine regulates many endothelial cell functions including mytogenesis, vascular permeability and vascular tone. Hypoxia is the major stimulus that regulates vascular EGF synthesis by controlling gene transcription and mRNA stabilization, although its synthesis is also stimulated when cells become deficient in glucose and in inflammatory reactions |16|. Patients with obstructive sleep apnoea have been reported as having raised vascular EGF concentrations correlating with the severity of their obstructive sleep apnoea.

INTERPRETATION. This study measured the plasma concentration of cytokines in three sets of experiments. The morning concentration of vascular EGF was increased in 85 men referred for investigation of suspected sleep apnoea (47 of whom subsequently had an apnoea/hypopnoea index of >20 events/h) in proportion to the apnoea/hypopnoea index. During sleep the hourly levels of vascular EGF were higher in five patients with sleep apnoea (129 pg/ml) than in six snorers (75 pg/ml) or six healthy subjects (33 pg/ml). After treatment with CPAP for 1 year nine patients experienced a decrease in vascular EGF from 57 to 40 pg/ml, whereas seven patients refusing CPAP therapy showed no changed in their vascular EGF values.

Comment

This study provided evidence of elevated levels of the cytokine vascular EGF in patients with obstructive sleep apnoea that could be reduced by CPAP treatment. Vascular EGF is a key mediator in angiogenesis and may contribute to the athero-genic process by inducing monocyte activation and migration |17|, modulating smooth muscle cell growth |18| and leading to the progression of coronary athero-sclerosis |19| and carotid artery stenosis |20|.

Endocrinological mechanisms

Obesity is an increasing public health problem in many Western societies. There has been a dramatic increase in the prevalence of obesity over the past 20 years in adult men and women of all ages and in all ethnic groups |21,22|. It is well recognized that many subjects with obstructive sleep apnoea have central obesity and may also have features of the metabolic syndrome |23,24|, which is a combination of hyperinsulin-aemia, glucose intolerance, dyslipidaemia, central obesity and hypertension |25,26|. These factors in the metabolic syndrome, which is also known as the insulin-resistant syndrome, have all been established as independent risk factors for vascular disease

|24|. There is therefore ongoing debate regarding the causal versus co-morbid relationship between obstructive sleep apnoea and cardiovascular disease.

Vgontzas *et al.* |27| recently reported that the fasting glucose and insulin levels were significantly higher in patients with sleep apnoea compared with weight-matched control subjects. Similarly a large population-based study in normo-glycaemic hypertensive men indicated a significant correlation between the variables of sleep-disordered breathing and indices of glucose metabolism after adjusting for measures of central obesity |28|. If these findings are confirmed the existence of a link between sleep-disordered breathing and insulin resistance would imply that respiratory dysfunction during sleep represents an independent risk factor for the metabolic syndrome.

Obstructive sleep apnoea is independently associated with insulin resistance

Ip SM, Lam B, Ng MMT, Lam WK, Tsang KWT. *Am J Respir Crit Care Med* 2002; **165**: 670–6

B ACKGROUND. Insulin resistance is a known risk factor for atherosclerosis and it is postulated that obstructive sleep apnoea syndrome represents a stress that promotes an insulin resistance. This study investigated the relationship between sleep-disordered breathing and insulin resistance indicated by fasting serum insulin levels and the insulin resistance index based on the homeostasis model assessment method.

INTERPRETATION. The study included 270 consecutive patients (197 males who were referred for polysomnography and who did not have known diabetes mellitus were included and 185 were documented subsequently to have obstructive sleep apnoea defined as an apnoea/hypopnoea index of >5 events/h). Obstructive sleep apnoea/hypopnoea syndrome subjects were more insulin resistant as indicated by their higher levels of fasting serum insulin ($P = 0.001$) and insulin resistance index ($P <0.001$). They were also older and more obese. Stepwise multiple linear regression analysis showed that obesity was the major determinant of insulin resistance, but the sleep-disordered breathing parameters (apnoea/hypopnoea index and minimum oxygen saturation) were also independent determinants of insulin resistance (fasting insulin:apnoea/hypopnoea index $P = 0.02$ and minimum O_2 $P = 0.041$ and insulin resistance index:apnoea/hypopnoea index $P = 0.044$ and minimum O_2 $P = 0.022$). This association between obstructive sleep apnoea and insulin resistance was seen in both obese and non-obese subjects. Each additional apnoea/hypopnoea event per hour slept increased the fasting insulin level and insulin resistance index by approximately 0.5%. Further analysis of the relationship of insulin resistance in hypertension confirmed that insulin resistance was a significant factor for hypertension in this cohort.

Sleep-disordered breathing and insulin resistance in middle aged and overweight men

Punjabi NM, Sorkin JD, Katzel LI, Goldberg P, Schwartz AR, Smith PL.
Am J Respir Crit Care Med 2002: **165**; 677–82

BACKGROUND. There is a general perception that obstructive sleep apnoea is associated with moderate to severe levels of obesity. This has resulted from earlier studies that were based on clinic examples of patients with BMIs >40 kg/m² |29|. The prevalence of sleep-disordered breathing in individuals with mild obesity is unknown. This study looked at the prevalence and metabolic consequences of obstructive sleep apnoea in a community-based population of overweight but otherwise healthy middle-aged men.

INTERPRETATION. One hundred and fifty mildly obese but otherwise healthy men were recruited from the community. The prevalence of sleep-disordered breathing ranged from 40 to 60% depending on the threshold apnoea/hypopnoea index. After adjusting for BMI and the percentage of body fat an apnoea/hypopnoea index of at least 5 events/h was associated with an increased risk of glucose tolerance (odds ratio [OR] = 2.15 and 95% confidence interval [CI] = 1.05–4.38). The OR for worsening glucose tolerance was 1.99 (95% CI = 1.11–3.56) for a 4% decrease in oxygen saturation. Multivariable linear regression analysis revealed that an increasing apnoea/hypopnoea index was associated with worsening insulin resistance independent of obesity.

Comment

Both the IP *et al.* and Punjabi *et al.* studies provide compelling evidence of an independent association between obstructive sleep apnoea and insulin resistance. This association is present even in non-obese sleep apnoea sufferers. These studies involved larger numbers of subjects than previous studies, which failed to show any such association |30| and it may be that these earlier studies were underpowered to show such an association.

Conclusion

Obstructive sleep apnoea/hypopnoea syndrome is a disorder characterized by recurring sleep-induced collapse of the pharyngeal airway. The principal daytime consequence of this syndrome is hypersomnolence, which results from the repeated arousals from sleep required to reopen the airway and restore normal breathing. This produces poor nocturnal sleeping quality. There are a wide variety of interacting physiological variables contributing to the maintenance of the patency of the upper airway during the state of being awake and sleep. The relative importance of each of these factors may differ from individual to individual. The recurrent episodes of hypoxia and hypercapnia that characterize obstructive sleep apnoea/hypopnoea syndrome may lead to an inflammatory response that ultimately results in the increased morbidity and mortality that is seen in this condition.

This field is evolving and in time a greater understanding of the basic pathophysiological mechanisms underlying this condition may lead to improved diagnostic and treatment modalities.

References

1. Veasey SC. Molecular and physiologic basis of obstructive sleep apnoea. *Clin Chest Med* 2003; **24**(2): 179–93.

2. Lavie P, Herar P, Hoffstein V. Obstructive sleep apnoea syndrome as a risk factor for hypertension: a population study. *BMJ* 2000; **320**: 479–482.

3. Faccenda JF, Mackay TW, Boon NA, Douglas NJ. A randomised placebo control trial of continuous positive airway pressure and blood pressure in the sleep apnoea/hypopnoea syndrome. *Am J Respir Crit Care Med* 2001; **163**: 344–8.

4. Pepperall JC, Ramdassingh-Dow S, Crosthwaite M, Mullins R, Jenkinson C, Stradling JR. Ambulatory blood pressure after therapeutic and subtherapeutic nasal continuous positive airway pressure for obstructive sleep apnoea: a randomised parallel trial. *Lancet* 2002; **359**: 204–10.

5. National Heart, Lung and Blood Institute (NHLBI). The National High Blood Pressure Education Program. *JNC* 7. Report available on-line at http://www.nhlbi.nih.gov

6. Nieto FJ, Young TB, Lind BK. Association of sleep disordered breathing, sleep apnoea and hypertension in a large community based study. *J Am Med Assoc* 2000; **283**: 1829–36.

7. Ohga E, Tomita T, Wada H, Yamamoto H, Nagase T, Ouchi Y. Effects of obstructive sleep apnea on circulating ICAM-1, IL-8 and MCP-1. *J Appl Physiol* 2003; **94**(1): 179–84.

8. Remmers JE, De Groot WJ, Saunderland EK, Anch AN. Pathogenesis of upper airway occlusion during sleep. *J Appl Physiol* 1978; **44**: 931–8.

9. Shepard Jr JW. Gas exchange in haemodynamics during sleep. *Med Clin North Am* 1985; **69**: 1243–64.

10. Tilkiam AG, Guilleminault C, Schroeder JS, Leahrman KL, Simmons FB, Dement WC. Haemodynamics in sleep induced apnoea: studies during wakefulness and sleep. *Ann Intern Med* 1976; **85**: 714–19.

11. Jennum P, Wildschiodtz G, Christenson NJ, Schwartz T. Blood pressure, catecholiamines and pancreatic polypetide in obstructive sleep apnoea with and without nasal continuous positive airway pressure (CPAP). *Am J Hypertens* 1989; **2**(11 Pt I): 847–52.

12. Wienged DA, Latz B, Zwillich CW, Wiegnd L. Geniohyoid muscle activity in normal men during wakefulness and sleep. *J Appl Physiol* 1990; **69**: 1262–9.

13. Meier-Ewert HK, Ridker PM, Rifai N. Absence of diurnal variation of C-reactive protein concentrations in healthy human subjects. *Clin Chem* 2001; **47**: 426–30.

14. Albert MA, Danielson E, Rifai N. Effect of statin therapy on C-reactive protein level: the pravastatin inflammation/CRP evaluation (PRINCE); a randomised trial and cohort study. *J Am Med Assoc* 2001; **286**: 64–70.

15. Lindmark E, Dinderholm E, Wallentin L. The relationship between interleukin 6 and mortality in patients with unstable coronary artery disease: the effects of an early invasive or non-invasive strategy. *J Am Med Assoc* 2001; **286**: 2107–13.

16. Leung DW, Cachianes G, Kuang WJ, Goeddel DV, Ferrara N. Vascular endothelial growth factor as a secreted angiogenic mytogen. *Science* 1989; **246**: 1306–9.

17. Clauss M, Gerlach M, Gerlach B, Brett J, Wang F, Familletti PC, Pan YC, Olander JV, Connolly DT, Stern D. Vascular permeability factor: a tumour derived polypeptide that induces endothelial cell and monocyte procoagulant activity, and promotes monocyte migration. *J Exp Med* 1990; **172**: 1535–45.

18. Doy K, Itoh H, Komatsu Y, Igaki T, Chun TH, Takaya K, Yamashita J, Inoue M, Yoshimasa T, Nakato K. Vascular endothelial growth factor suppresses C-type natriuretic peptide secretion. *Hypertension* 1996; **27**(3 Pt.II): 811–15.

19. Inoue M, Itoh H, Naruko T, Kojima A, Komatsu R, Doi K, Ogawa Y, Tamura N, Takaya K. Vascular endothelial growth factor (VEGF) expression in human coronary atherosclerotic lesions. Possible pathophysiological significance of VEGF in progression of atherosclerosis. *Circulation* 1998; **98**: 2108–16.

20. Lee SW, Jeong MH, Ba HR, Jeong SJ, Jang JY, Lim WJ, Kim SH, Kim JW, Cha JK. Circulating levels of interleukin-8 and vascular endothelial growth factor in patients with carotid stenosis. *J Korean Med Sci* 2001; **16**: 198–203.

21. National Institute of Health. Clinical guidelines on the identification, evaluation and treatment of overweight and obesity in adults – the evidence report. *Obesity Res* 1998; **6** (Suppl 2): 51S–209S.

22. Flegal KM, Carroll MD, Kuczmarski RJ, Johnson CL. Overweight and obesity in the United States: prevalence and trends, 1960–1994. *Int J Obesity Relat Metab Dis* 1998; **22**: 39–47.

23. Must A, Spedano J, Coakley EH, Field E, Colditz G, Dietz WH. The disease and burden associated with overweight and obesity. *J Am Med Assoc* 1999; **282**: 1523–9.

24. Pi-Sunyer FX. Medical hazards of obesity. *Ann Intern Med* 1993; **119**: 655–60.

25. Nieto FJ, Young TB, Lind BK, Shahar E, Samet JM, Redline S, D'Agostino RB, Newman AB, Lebowitz MD, Pickering TT. Association of sleep disordered breathing, sleep apnoea and hypertension in a large community based study. Sleep Heart Health Study. *J Am Med Assoc* 2000; **283**: 1829–36.

26. Peppard PE, Young T, Palta M, Skatrud J. A prospective study of the association between sleep disordered breathing and hypertension. *N Engl J Med* 2000; **342**: 1378–84.

27. Vgontzas AN, Papanicolaou DA, Bixler EO, Hopper K, Lotsiks A, Lin HM, Klaes A, Chrousos DP. Sleep apnoea and daytime sleepiness and fatigue: related to visceral obesity, insulin resistance and hypercytokinaemia. *J Clin Endocrinol Metab* 2000; **85**: 1151–8.

28. Elmasry A, Lindberg E, Berne C, Janson C, Gislason T, Awadtageldin M, Boman G. Sleep disordered breathing and glucose metabolism in hypertensive men: a population based study. *J Intern Med* 2001; **249**: 153–61.

29. Rajala R, Partinen M, Sane T, Pelkonen R, Huikuri K, Seppalainem AM. Obstructive sleep apnoea syndrome in morbidly obese patients. *J Intern Med* 1991; **230**: 125–9.

30. Davies RJ, Turner R, Crosby J, Stradling JR. Plasma insulin and lipid levels in untreated obstructive sleep apnoea and snoring: the comparison with matched controls and response to treatment. *J Sleep Res* 1994; **3**: 180–5.

26

Diagnosis

Introduction

Obstructive sleep apnoea represents one end of a spectrum, with normal quiet regular breathing at the mild end, moving through worsening levels of snoring to increased upper airways resistance and on to hypopnoeas and then apnoeas with ventilatory failure at the far end of the spectrum. Historical studies on unmatched normal studies have established an apparent narrow band of normality for the numbers of apnoeas per hour of sleep and the original definition of sleep apnoea (>5 apnoeas/h each of 10-seconds duration) has become internationally accepted |1|. However, it is unclear whether this is the best measure of the severity of sleep apnoea, but it is the one that is in most common usage and it does allow some comparison of disease severity between centres. Other measures including the oxygen desaturation index, electroencephalogram (EEG) analysis, autonomic arousal detection or body movement analysis may however be equally as good at characterizing the severity of sleep apnoea |2|, but these indices are defined in slightly different ways by different centres and, thus, intercentre comparisons may be extremely difficult. A recent international classification of the various indices used for defining sleep apnoea has recently been published and serves as a useful standard |3|.

Sleep apnoea may be usefully subdivided into varying degrees of severity based upon the apnoea/hypopnoea index: (1) mild sleep apnoea with an apnoea/hypopnoea index of 5–14/h, (2) moderate sleep apnoea with an apnoea/hypopnoea index of 15–30/h and (3) severe sleep apnoea with an apnoea/hypopnoea index of >30/h. It must be recognized, however, that any attempt to stratify the severity of sleep apnoea is arbitrary, although it is true that, in general, the more severe the breathing abnormality becomes the more symptomatic the patient actually is. It has to be recognized, however, that symptoms such as excessive daytime sleepiness do not always correlate with the degree of breathing abnormality recorded and that more research into the most appropriate measures of sleep apnoea severity is required.

Clinical assessment of patients with potential sleep apnoea usually involves investigating abnormalities occurring during sleep or occasionally investigations can be aimed at quantifying the magnitude of daytime sleepiness.

There are a variety of tests available for monitoring breathing patterns or the quality of sleep, ranging from simple oximetry and the measurement of a limited number of breathing and chest wall movement recordings through to complex polysomnography, which involves measuring a variety of electrophysiological signals as well as breathing and limb movement patterns. With increasing complexity more information is available, but this tends to be at the cost of increasing technical resources and expense.

There is a temptation to use the simplest possible technique for diagnosing obstructive sleep apnoea/hypopnoea syndrome and in this respect oximetry, which is cheap, easy to use, portable and readily available, is widely employed |**4**|. However, if oximetry is used alone it must be appreciated that it cannot definitely exclude a diagnosis of sleep apnoea, but it may be sufficient to confirm the presence of significant sleep apnoea if the result fits with the clinical suspicion.

The clinical value of performing full polysomnographic sleep studies on all patients with possible sleep apnoea has been questioned. Overnight polysomnography records were analysed in a prospective study of 200 patients with possible sleep apnoea in order to determine which signals contributed to diagnostic accuracy. Respiratory variables (thoraco-abdominal movement and oximetry) and leg movement censors were found to be helpful, but the neurophysiological signals did not contribute significantly to the diagnosis |**5**|. There is therefore an increasing tendency to use less complicated diagnostic techniques for determining whether or not sleep apnoea is present. These limited sleep studies measure more than the single channel of information recorded by oximetry and tend to measure a variety of respiratory signals, but give little or no information about sleep duration or quality: commonly measured combinations are oximetry, airflow, thoraco-abdominal movement and heart rate measurement. Snoring can also be measured using a microphone. There are lots of new machines emerging onto the market and this field is changing rapidly |**6–8**|.

Many of these limited sleep studies can be performed in the patient's home after adequate instruction. Studies performed in this way can be cost-effective |**9**|, convenient and accurate and can significantly speed up the investigation pathway. However, the limitations have to be appreciated and there is a need to move onto a hospital-based investigation in those patients whose home study result does not fit with the clinical suspicion of the doctor. There may also be significant problems with home-based equipment failure and night-to-night reproducibility and reliability, with sensitivity ranges from 32 to 100% and specificity from 33 to 100% compared with full polysomnography in a sleep centre |**4**|.

The individual clinician should examine the balance of the benefits associated with using a particular sleep study technique against the equipment available to them, the diagnostic algorithm used for aiding diagnosis and the resources available to the particular clinician.

There is no evidence base available to support the use of anthroprometric measurements, ear, nose and throat and dental assessments, radiological measurements or questionnaire studies for confidently confirming a diagnosis of sleep apnoea.

This chapter will look at (1) recent advances in diagnostic techniques in obstructive sleep apnoea/hypopnoea syndrome, (2) the factors influencing the accuracy of oximeters when used for investigating obstructive sleep apnoea/hypopnoea syndrome, (3) the trend towards greater use of limited sleep study devices in the home setting and (4) some of the different techniques that are available for measuring the airflow changes that characterize apnoeas and hypopnoeas in obstructive sleep apnoea/hypopnoea syndrome.

Oximetry

Oximeter's acquisition parameter influences the profile of respiratory disturbances

Davila D, Richards KC, Marshall BL, *et al. Sleep* 2003; **26**(1): 91–5

B A C K G R O U N D . Oximetry is a key variable monitor during both limited and full polysomnography-based sleep studies. One technical parameter that has been reported to influence the morphology of the oximetric signal (SpO_2: an assessment of the oxygen saturation of the arterial blood arriving at the fingertip or earlobe with each pulse beat) and the subsequent quantification of this data is the acquisition or recording setting of the oximeter. Oximeters can be manually set or default to specific recording settings that process signals over different averaging times. The aim of this study was to determine whether different oximetric recordings affect the profile of apnoeas/ hypopnoes scored on polysomnography and to assess the potential impact of these settings on subsequent clinical decision making.

I N T E R P R E T A T I O N . This was a prospective study performed in a sleep centre involving 30 patients. Each patient had three oximeters simultaneously attached to their digits during polysomnography. Each oximeter was programmed to record on a different setting: recording every 3, 6 or 12 s. Apnoeas and hypopnoeas were identified using polysomnography criteria. Significant differences in the mean frequency of respiratory events between each oximetry recording setting were noted ($P <0.001$).

Comment

The authors concluded that oximeters' acquisition settings do affect the saturation data recorded. This can impact upon the interpretation of respiratory events scored during polysomnography sleep studies. It is therefore important that the acquisition parameters of the oximeter should be disclosed whenever oximetric data are being published and indeed efforts should be made to standardize such settings when used during sleep studies. Faster oximetric settings that provide a less average assessment of oximetric data would appear to be the most accurate.

Limited sleep studies and their uses

Home diagnosis of obstructive sleep apnoea syndrome

Douglas NJ. *Sleep Med Rev* 2003; **7**(1): 53–9

B A C K G R O U N D . There is no evidence that the results of polysomnography more accurately identify patients with obstructive sleep apnoea than simpler investigative methods that may be performed in the patient's home and at a lower cost. This clinical review outlined the potential advantages and disadvantages of both polysomnography- and home-based sleep studies.

INTERPRETATION. This review article examined the evidence for and against home-based sleep studies. It concluded that home sleep studies have an important role to play in the speedy, cost-effective and accurate diagnosis of obstructive sleep apnoea. The exact role of such studies within an individual clinician's practice will depend on the financial and organizational structure of that practice.

Comment

This review helps to place the role of home-based sleep studies into context. It examines the evidence for and against home studies and concludes that home studies have a role to play in the investigation of subjects with potential sleep apnoea.

Home diagnosis of sleep apnoea: a systematic review of literature

An Evidence Review Co-sponsored by the American Academy of Sleep Medicine, the American College of Chest Physicians and the American Thoracic Society. *Chest* 2003; **124**: 1543–79

BACKGROUND. This study conducted a systematic review of the use of portable monitoring systems for the diagnosis of obstructive sleep apnoea. It highlighted the differences in sensitivity, specificity, mean differences/limits of agreement and correlation between portable monitoring devices and sleep laboratory-based polysomnography.

INTERPRETATION. The American Academy of Sleep Medicine, the American College of Chest Physicians and the American Thoracic Society Working Group reviewed the evidence regarding the use of portable diagnostic devices in the diagnosis of sleep apnoea. They felt that a formal meta-analysis of the research on this subject with summary receiver operating characteristic curves was not possible because of the marked heterogeneity of the methods, definitions, monitor types and signals measured. Fifty-one published studies were reviewed. Clinicians interested in using portable monitors for investigating patients with suspected sleep apnoea need to review carefully what they want the monitor to do (exclude/diagnose obstructive sleep apnoea), evaluate which signals the monitor should record, assess carefully the quality of the research that has been published regarding each individual monitor type and importantly consider whether the study or patient population that that particular monitor has been used with before is similar enough to their own population to allow a sensible acceptance of the published results using that particular type of monitor.

Comment

This extensive review article discusses the available evidence for the use of home-based sleep studies and offers advice to the reader regarding the pros and cons of such a diagnostic technique.

State of home sleep studies
Li CK, Ward Flemons W. *Clin Chest Med* 2003; **24**(2): 283–95

BACKGROUND. The technology for data acquisition and analysis of home monitors has evolved rapidly over recent years. This review article published by the American Academy of Sleep Medicine gives a classification system for portable monitors based upon the number and type of parameters recorded by each machine.

INTERPRETATION. This paper compared a variety of diagnostic devices in the diagnosis of potential sleep apnoea ranging from simple oximetry studies through to complicated polysomnography (see Table 26.1). It emphasized that increasing the complexity of the sleep study linked to improved analysis algorithms can improve the specificity of the monitor and, hence, the likelihood ratios for a positive result can be improved. It is emphasized that not all monitors record and analyse signals in the same way and it is therefore not possible to generalize the results from one monitor across all other monitors in that particular class of device. There is still only limited evidence available on the use of portable sleep study devices in the unattended setting in the patient's home and further research is required in this area in order to clarify the accuracy of such devices. It is important for a clinician to be able to review raw data emanated from the diagnostic device manually and not to rely upon computer-generated reports in order to check the validity of the result. Further research is needed in order to quantify the cost-effectiveness of home- versus hospital-based studies.

Comment

This review provided practical information for the clinician on the usefulness of the various types of sleep monitors that are available for allowing a diagnosis of obstructive sleep apnoea to be made in the home setting.

Lack of night-to-night variability of sleep-disordered breathing measured during home monitoring
Davidson TM, Gehrman P, Ferreyra H. *Ear Nose Throat J* 2003; **82**(2): 135–8

BACKGROUND. There has been some debate as to how accurate a single night's analysis of a sleeping pattern is in determining whether or not sleep apnoea is present. The conventional approach in many countries is to perform a single-night sleep study in order to confirm or refute the diagnosis of sleep apnoea. This study investigated whether there is significant night-to-night variability present in the recordings made during home monitoring.

Table 26.1 American Academy of Sleep Medicine classification system for sleep apnoea evaluation studies

	Type 1 Standard polysomnography	Type 2 Comprehensive portable polysomnography	Type 3 Modified portable sleep apnoea testing	Type 4 Continuous single or dual parameter recording
Parameters	Minimum of 7, including EEG, EOG, chin EMG, ECG, airflow, respiratory effort, oxygen saturation	Minimum of 7, including EEG, EOG, chin EMG, ECG, airflow, respiratory effort, oxygen saturation	Minimum of 4, including ventilation (at least 2 channels of respiratory movement, or respiratory movement and airflow), heart rate or ECG, oxygen saturation	Minimum of 1: oxygen saturation, flow or chest movement
Body position	Documented or objectively measured	Possible	Possible	No
Leg movement	EMG or motion sensor desirable but optional	Optional	Optional	No
Personnel in attendance	Yes	No	No	No
Interventions during the study	Possible	No	No	No

EEG, electroencephalography; EOG, electrooculography; EMG, electromyography; ECG, electrocardiograpy.
Source: Li *et al.* (2003).

INTERPRETATION. This single-centre study involved 44 patients with known sleep-disordered breathing. The authors used full polysomnographic techniques for determining whether the apnoea/hypopnoea index varied from night to night. Of the 44 patients studied 23 underwent a full sleep study for three consecutive nights and 21 patients were tested for two consecutive nights. There was no statistically significant change in the apnoea/hypopnoea index across the nights although there were a number of minor variations amongst individual patients.

Comment

The authors concluded that a single-night polysomnographic sleep study is representative of whether or not significant sleep apnoea is present using a home monitoring device incorporating EEG analysis.

Evaluation of a portable device for diagnosing the sleep apnoea/hypopnoea syndrome

Dingli K, Coleman EL, Vennelle M, *et al. Eur Respir J* 2003; **21**: 253–9

BACKGROUND. The waiting times for hospital-based monitoring of obstructive sleep apnoea syndrome continue to rise in this country. This study tested whether a new portable sleep diagnosis device (Embletta) may accurately diagnose the obstructive sleep apnoea syndrome at home. A synchronous comparison to polysomnography was performed in 40 patients and a comparison of home Embletta studies with laboratory-based polysomnography was performed in 61 patients.

INTERPRETATION. In this synchronous study, the mean difference (polysomnography–Embletta) in apnoeas/hypopnoeas per hour in bed was 2/h. In comparison to the apnoea/hypopnoea index per hour slept the Embletta (apnoea/hypopnoea) per hour in bed differed by 8 events/h. These data were used for constructing diagnostic categories in symptomatic patients from the Embletta results: 'probable sleep apnoea' ($\geq$20 apnoea/hypopnoea per hour in bed), 'possible sleep apnoea' (10–20 apnoea/hypopnoea per hour in bed) or 'not sleep apnoea' (<10 apnoea/hypopnoea per hour in bed). In the home study the mean difference in apnoea/hypopnoea per hour in bed was 3 events/h. In comparison to the polysomnographic apnoea/hypopnoea index per hour slept, the Embletta results for apnoea/hypopnoea per hour in bed differed by 6 $\pm$ 14 events/h. Using the above classification all nine patients characterized as not having obstructive sleep apnoea had an apnoea/hypopnoea index of <15 events/h slept on polysomnography and all 23 patients with obstructive sleep apnoea in the Embletta evaluation had an apnoea/hypopnoea index of $\geq$15 events/h on polysomnography, but 18 patients fell into the possible obstructive sleep apnoea category potentially requiring further investigations. Eleven home studies failed.

Comment

The home Embletta studies satisfactorily classified most patients, but 29 out of the 61 patients required further investigation in order to clarify whether or not they had sleep apnoea. Portable devices for diagnosing obstructive sleep apnoea are becoming increasingly available and allow the diagnosis of obstructive sleep apnoea to be made in the majority of cases as long as the limitations of the device are borne in mind by the clinician. If a limited sleep study result does not agree with the clinical suspicion a full sleep centre-based study should be considered. Home-based sleep studies do represent an opportunity for reducing diagnostic costs if used and interpreted correctly.

Polysomnography

Use of nasal cannula for detecting sleep apnoeas/hypopnoeas in infants and children

Trang H, Leske V, Gaultier C. *Am J Respir Crit Care Med* 2002; **166**: 465–8

B ackground . Breathing disturbances during polysomnography are generally identified by the detection of a clear reduction in airflow. The measurement of airflow at the nose can be performed using a thermistor, which detects the difference in temperature between inspired and expired air or by measurement of pressure at the nose with a cannula. Both of these techniques allow the detection of apnoeas/hypopnoeas.

I nterpretation . The tolerance of a nasal cannula by 14 infants (median age 2.6 months) and 16 children (median age 5.5 years) with suspected obstructive sleep apnoea was studied. The efficacy of the nasal cannula was compared with a nasobuccal thermistor in detecting apnoeas or hypopnoeas. All children tolerated the nasal cannula. A non-interpretable flow signal lasting more than 20% of the total sleep time occurred in five children using a cannula compared with only one child using the thermistor. A total of 465 obstructive apnoeas were identified: 43% of the apnoeas were detected by both techniques, 52% of the apnoeas missed by the thermistor were detected by nasal pressure monitoring and only 5% of the apnoeas missed by nasal pressure were detected by the thermistor. A total of 159 hypopnoeas were detected: nasal pressure detected 100% of these events, whereas the thermistor detected only 14%. Thermistors sense differences in temperature and do not have a linear relationship with true airflow.

Comment

A variety of techniques exist for allowing the non-invasive diagnosis of apnoeas and hypopnoeas. Every technique has limitations and in order to avoid misdiagnosis it is prudent to look for concomitant changes in other respiratory parameters or look for evidence of desaturation or arousal before making a diagnosis of obstructive sleep apnoea. When comparing different methods of recording airflow, measuring pressure at the nose with a nasal cannula appears to be a more reliable measurement of flow than the use of thermistors.

Validation of nasal pressure for identification of apnoeas/hypopnoeas during sleep

Heitman SJ, Atkar RS, Hajduk EA, Wanner RA, Ward Flemons W. *Am J Respir Crit Care Med* 2002; **166**: 386–91

BACKGROUND. The reference standard for identifying apnoeas/hypopnoeas is a pneumotachograph, but sleep can be disrupted whilst this device is being used. Nasal airflow estimation by measuring nasal pressure via nasal prongs is a non-invasive method of measuring breathing patterns during sleep and is well tolerated by patients. However, nasal pressure has not been validated for detecting apnoeas/hypopnoeas during sleep using an event analysis and this paper sought to validate this technique.

INTERPRETATION. Eleven patients undergoing polysomnography wore a nasal mask capable of measuring nasal airflow (via pneumotachograph and nasal pressures simultaneously). Each study was screened for respiratory disturbances and from these events 550 were randomly selected and blindly scored as an apnoea/hypopnoea or no such event each using the pneumotachograph, nasal pressure, square-root nasal pressure and respiratory inductance sum signals independently. The κ values for the inter-measurement agreement with the pneumotachograph were 0.76 for nasal pressure, 0.73 for square-root transformation of the nasal pressure and 0.50 for respiratory-inductive plethysmography. The inter-rater agreements were 0.68 for the pneumotachograph, 0.66 for nasal pressure, 0.61 for square-root transformation of the nasal pressure and 0.47 for respiratory-inductive plethysmography. The intra-rater agreements were 0.6 for the pneumotachograph, 0.82 for nasal pressure, 0.78 for square-root transformation of the nasal pressure and 0.76 for respiratory-inductive plethysomography.

Comment

Nasal pressure measurement provides a linear relationship of airflow except at the extremes of the range. The linear relationship can be improved with a mathematical square-root transformation of the signal. Pressure monitoring may not be as accurate as a thermistor in distinguishing hypopnoeas from apnoeas, but in routine use this distinction is not thought to be important |**10,11**|. Monitoring of nasal pressure is a reproducible method that closely agrees with pneumotachography in detecting apnoeas/hypopnoeas. It is well tolerated by patients, is non-invasive and, with the advent of commercially available, portable and affordable pressure transducers, it has the potential to be used widely.

Diagnosis of sleep apnoea by automatic analysis of nasal pressure and forced oscillation impedence

Steltner H, Stats R, Timmer J, *et al. Am J Respir Care Med* 2002; **165**: 940–4

BACKGROUND. Apnoeas and hypopnoeas recorded during polysomnography may be scored manually by sleep technicians or automatically using various computer programmes. This paper sought to validate a new algorithm for the automated detection and classification of apnoeas/hypopnoeas. The algorithm was based on time series analysis of nasal mask pressure and a forced oscillation signal related to respiratory input impedance.

INTERPRETATION. Polysomnography was performed in 19 subjects with suspected sleep apnoea and two independent observers scored the results. There was no discrepancy between automated scoring and manual scoring of the results.

Comment

The authors of this paper concluded that a newly developed algorithm for the automatic detection and classification of sleep apnoea correlated well with manually scored polysomnography results and this automated method may prove to be time saving and cost-effective in the analysis of sleep study data.

Conclusion

The above studies show that there are a variety of diagnostic techniques available for aiding the clinician in the diagnosis of potential sleep apnoea. These devices range in complexity and expense from simple channel oximeters that can be used portably both at home and in hospital to complex multichannel devices such as full polysomnography. These devices represent opposite ends of a spectrum of diagnostic complexity and many clinicians are now opting to use diagnostic machines that incorporate approximately four channels of information (oximetry, airflow, chest and abdominal movement and pulse rate) for investigating potential sleep apnoea. If the test result fits with the clinician's clinical suspicion as to whether or not sleep apnoea exists then a single night's study may be sufficient to allow a confident clinical assessment to take place, but it is vital that clinicians caring for patients with sleep disorders should be familiar with all of the limitations associated with the use of any individual sleep monitoring device, particularly if the potential diagnosis of sleep apnoea is refuted. However, it is vital to appreciate that the specific technology used for making the diagnosis is less important than the level of experience and training available for interpreting the results.

References

1. Guilleminault C, Tilkian A, Dement WC. Sleep apnoea syndromes. *Am Rev Med* 1976; **27**; 465–84.

2. Bennett LS, Langford BA, Stradling JR, Davies RJ. Sleep fragmentation indices as predictors of daytime sleepiness and nCPAP response in obstructive sleep apnoea. *Am J Respir Crit Care Med* 1998; **158**: 778–86.

3. The American Academy. Sleep related breathing disorders in adults: recommendations for syndrome definition and measurement techniques and clinical research. The Report of an American Academy of Sleep Medicine Task Force. *Sleep* 1999; **22**: 667–9.

4. Ross SD, Allan IE, Harrison KJ, Kvasz M, Connelly J, Sheinhait IA. *Systematic Review of Literature Regarding the Diagnosis of Sleep Apnoea*. Rockville, MD: Agency for Health Care Policy and Research, 1999.

5. Douglas NJ, Thomas S, Jan MA. Clinical value of polysomnography. *Lancet* 1992; **339**: 347–50.

6. Whittle AT, Finch SP, Mortimore IL, Mackay TW, Douglas NJ. Use of home sleep studies for the diagnosis of the sleep apnoea/hypopnoea syndrome. *Thorax* 1997; **52**: 1068–73.

7. Bradley PA, Mortimore IL, Douglas NJ. Comparison of polysomnography with ResCare Autoset in the diagnosis of the sleep apnoea/hypopnoea syndrome. *Thorax* 1995; **50**: 1201–3.

8. Rees K, Wraith PK, Berthon-Jones M, Douglas NJ. Detection of apnoeas, hypopnoeas and arousals by the Autoset in the sleep apnoea/hypopnoea syndrome. *Eur Respir J* 1998; **12**: 76–9.

9. Carrasco O, Montserrat JM, Loberas P, Ascasco C, Ballester E, Fornas C. Visual and different automatic scoring profiles of respiratory variable in the diagnosis of the sleep apnoea/hypopnoea syndrome. *Eur Respir J* 1996; **9**: 25–130.

10. Garcia Diaz EM, Capote Gil F, Cano Gomez S, Sanchez Armagol A, Carmona Bernal C, Soto Campos JG. Respiratory polygraphy in the diagnosis of obstructive sleep apnoea syndrome. *Arch Bronchopneumol* 1997; **33**: 69–73.

11. Montserrat JM, Farre R. Breathing flow disturbances during sleep. Can they be accurately assessed by nasal prongs? *Am J Respir Crit Care Med* 2002; **166**: 259–60.

27

Treatment

Introduction

Deciding which of the various treatment options is most appropriate for the management of sleep apnoea depends on both the severity of the condition and the preferences of the individual patient.

Current evidence from randomized, controlled trials indicates that those patients who respond best to treatment are those with objective evidence of significant sleep-disordered breathing in whom the daytime symptoms are most marked |**1,2**|. Treatment should be focused on trying to improve factors such as daytime sleepiness, poor driving performance, diminished quality of life and raised blood pressure rather than trying to treat asymptomatic patients |**3,4**|.

Weight loss should be encouraged in all patients with obesity contributing to their sleep apnoea, but attempts at weight loss should not delay the initiation of further treatment |**5–7**|.

The recommended treatment for moderate or severe obstructive sleep apnoea is continuous positive airway pressure (CPAP) |**8**|, but this treatment is not always easy for patients to accept. CPAP reverses upper airway obstruction during sleep |**1**| and reduces many of the consequences of severe sleep apnoea, most notably daytime sleepiness and psychological symptoms |**9–16**|.

Effective CPAP treatment on these outcomes in patients with mild sleep apnoea is less clear-cut. Three randomized, controlled trials |**9–11**| have indicated that there may be an improvement in some areas of neurobehavioural function in self-reported symptoms in this population, but improvements in objective measurements such as sleep latency in multiple sleep latency and maintenance of wakefulness tests and in cardiovascular function have not yet been shown. Various placebos including sham CPAP or tablets have been used as controls in these studies. The debate still exists as to which placebo offers the best form of control |**17,18**|.

CPAP functions as a pneumatic splint for maintaining upper airway patency throughout all phases of breathing during sleep. It operates by means of a flow generator that delivers pressure through air tubing to a nasal mask or full-face mask worn overnight.

An alternative form of treatment to CPAP in simple snorers or patients with mild obstructive sleep apnoea/hypopnoea syndrome is a mandibular repositioning splint device. These intra-oral devices hold the mandible forward during sleep thus enlarging the pharyngeal space. A recent controlled study showed that mandibular repositioning splints improve the apnoea/hypopnoea index, nocturnal saturations and arousal from sleep |**19**|. Uncontrolled intervention studies of mandibular repositioning splints have indicated that many patients obtain good results for objective efficacy and subjective effectiveness |**20–24**| and that efficacy for breathing pauses may be higher among patients with obstructive sleep apnoea/hypopnoea syndrome with lower levels of sleep-disordered breathing |**23–25**|. Follow-up studies have identified some drawbacks of mandibular repositioning splint therapy such as excessive salivation, occlusive changes and temporomandibular joint pain or toothache, but in general mandibular repositioning splints are tolerated well by the majority of patients in most case studies |**25**|.

Many different surgical approaches have also been used in the past for the treatment of obstructive sleep apnoea/hypopnoea syndrome: all of these operations had the intention of increasing the pharyngeal space during sleep. The commonest such operation was uvulopalatopharyngoplasty. There have been two systematic reviews that concluded there was no randomized, controlled trial evidence supporting the use of uvulopalatopharyngoplasty in obstructive sleep apnoea/hypopnoea syndrome |**26,27**|. Uncontrolled case series suggest at best a 50% improvement in 50% of patients |**24**|. The effects on objective measures of obstructive sleep apnoea/hypopnoea syndrome were poor and largely unpredictable, although statistically significant overall. A meta-analysis of laser-assisted uvulopalatopharynoplasty (LAUP) also concluded that LAUP and related procedures should not be used for any severity of obstructive sleep apnoea/hypopnoea syndrome |**28**|.

No matter which form of treatment is used for treating obstructive sleep apnoea/hypopnoea syndrome it should be appreciated that the treatment will be lifelong and requires adequate compliance in order to be effective.

This chapter will review some recent evidence on the use and benefits of CPAP and use and benefits of mandibular repositional splints.

Uses and benefits of continuous positive airway pressure

Continuous positive airway pressure treatment

A randomized control trial of continuous positive airway pressure (CPAP) in mild obstructive sleep apnoea
Barnes M, Houston D, Worsnop CJ, *et al. Am J Respir Crit Care Med* 2002;
165: 773–80

Background**.** This was a randomized, controlled trial into the efficacy of CPAP treatment in mild obstructive sleep apnoea.

Interpretation**.** Barnes *et al.* undertook a randomized, blinded, placebo-controlled, cross-over trial conducted in two Australian centres into the efficacy of CPAP for patients with mild sleep apnoea. They used a placebo tablet as the control. Each treatment period lasted for 2 months. Forty-two patients with apnoea/hypopnoea indices of 5–30 events/h (mean 13) were studied and 28 patients completed both treatment arms. CPAP produced improvement in self-reported snoring, restless sleep, daytime sleepiness and irritability. CPAP did not improve multiple sleep latency, the subjective sleepiness rating on the Epworth Sleepiness Scale, neurobehavioural function on question of life questionnaires or 24-hour blood pressure recordings. Placebo produced an improvement in many of the functional variables.

Comment

The authors concluded that CPAP failed to improve measures of objective or subjective daytime sleepiness in patients with mild obstructive sleep apnoea/hypopnoea syndrome despite adequate treatment, as documented by a fall in the apnoea/hypopnoea index and good compliance. A placebo effect may well account for some of the treatment responses reported with respect to the improvements in subjective sleepiness, mood and quality of life data.

This study emphasized that there is a need for adequate control comparison and baseline assessments in patients with mild disease in order to avoid placebo effects. Perhaps the most important contributing factor to the negative findings in this study was that the patients did not have to be symptomatically sleepy to be eligible for the study. It may well be that it is not enough simply to treat a given level of apnoeas or hypopnoeas per hour in a patient in order to achieve benefit from CPAP, but that the patient must be symptomatic in addition to having a sleep-disordered breathing pattern for treatment to be successful.

Practice parameters for the use of autotitrating continuous positive airway pressure devices for titrating pressures and treating adult patients with obstructive sleep apnoea syndrome

American Academy of Sleep Medicine Report, Standards of Practice Committee of the American Academy of Sleep Medicine. Littner M, Hirshkowitz M, Davila D, *et al. Sleep* 2002; **25**(2): 143–7

BACKGROUND. The current 'gold standard' for initiation of CPAP treatment is for a technician to titrate CPAP manually during a full hospital-based polysomnography in order to obtain a fixed single pressure that can subsequently be used at home. This review article from the American Academy of Sleep Medicine publishes a series of recommendations regarding the use of sophisticated autotitrating CPAP devices. These devices continually adjust pressure as needed for maintaining upper airway patency and can be used both in hospital and at home.

INTERPRETATION. The recommendations are as follows. (1) A diagnosis of the obstructive sleep apnoea must be established by an acceptable method. Initial titration and ongoing treatment with automatically adjustable CPAP devices are not currently recommended for patients with congestive cardiac failure, significant lung disease (e.g. chronic obstructive pulmonary disease [COPD]), daytime hypoxia and respiratory failure from any cause. In addition, patients who do not snore should not be titrated with an automatic device that relies on vibration or sound in the device algorithm for adjusting the pressure settings. (2) Automatic CPAP devices are not currently recommended for split night studies since none of the reviewed research studies examined this issue. (3) Certain automatic CPAP devices may be used during attended technician titration in order to identify using polysomnography which single pressure is needed with standard CPAP for the treatment of obstructive sleep apnoea. (4) Once an initial successful attended conventional CPAP or automatic CPAP titration has been determined by polysomnography certain automatic CPAP devices may be used in the self-adjusting mode for ongoing unattended treatment of patients with sleep apnoea at home. (5) The use of unattended automatic CPAP titration for either initially determining the pressures for fixed CPAP or for self-adjusting automatic CPAP treatment in CPAP-naïve patients is not currently established. (6) Patients being treated with fixed CPAP on the basis of prior automatic CPAP titration or continuing treatment with automatic CPAP must be followed up in order to determine the treatment effectiveness and safety. (7) Re-evaluation and if necessary a standard attended CPAP titration night should be performed if the symptoms do not resolve following initial automatic CPAP titration.

Comment

This extensive review article gives the reader useful and practical advice regarding the use of autotitrating CPAP devices.

The use of autotitrating continuous positive airway pressure for the treatment of adult obstructive sleep apnoea – American Academy of Sleep Medicine review
Berry RB, Parish JM, Hartse KM. *Sleep* 2002; **25**(2): 148–59

B A C K G R O U N D . This paper reviewed the efficacy of autotitrating CPAP in the treatment of obstructive sleep apnoea. It drew conclusions from 30 articles and stated a number of practice parameters for the use of these autotitrating CPAP devices in sleep apnoea treatment.

I N T E R P R E T A T I O N . Published data have indicated that automatic CPAP devices can be used for treating many patients with obstructive sleep apnoea and identifying an effective optimal fixed level of CPAP pressure.

Comment

Both of the previous two papers by the American Academy of Sleep Medicine published pragmatic recommendations regarding the use of these newly emerging sophisticated autotitrating CPAP devices both for the initial titration of CPAP pressure and in the subsequent treatment of sleep apnoea. This is a developing field that may prove to be extremely valuable and cost-effective. These devices also have a role in troubleshooting problems in patients who have difficulty complying with CPAP or in whom continuing daytime symptoms such as sleepiness are a problem despite good CPAP compliance and I am sure that their role will continue to expand in the future.

Can patients with obstructive sleep apnoea titrate their own continuous positive airway pressure?

Fitzpatrick MF, Alloway CED, Wakeford TM, MacLean AW, Munt PW, Day AG.
Am J Respir Crit Care Med 2003; **167**: 716–22

BACKGROUND. Manual CPAP titration in a sleep centre is costly and limits wide access for diagnostic studies. Many factors can affect CPAP compliance, but education and support rather than in-centre CPAP titration appear to be the most important in determining the long-term usage of CPAP. This study was designed for testing whether self-adjustment of CPAP pressure at home could provide equal or superior efficacy in the treatment of sleep apnoea compared to in-hospital initial CPAP titration.

INTERPRETATION. A randomized, single-blind, two-period, cross-over trial of CPAP treatment in the hospital setting for determining optimal CPAP pressure was compared to home self-adjustment of CPAP pressure (the starting pressure was based upon a prediction equation). Eighteen CPAP-naïve patients (16 males and two females aged 50 ± 15 years old with an apnoeic index of 40 ± 20) with newly diagnosed sleep apnoea were tested. Testing was performed both before and after CPAP treatment in each of two 5-week study limbs. CPAP compliance, the Sleep Apnoea Quality of Life Index, the Functional Outcomes of Sleep Questionnaire Score and the Epworth Sleepiness Score were studied together with polysomnographic assessment of sleep architecture, sleep apnoea severity and also an objective test of daytime sleepiness (a maintenance of wakefulness test). Both modes of CPAP treatment significantly improved objective and subjective measures of obstructive sleep apnoea severity and there was no difference in efficacy. The authors concluded that home self-titration of CPAP is as effective as in-hospital manual titration in the management of this group of patients with severe sleep apnoea.

Comment

This well-designed clinical study showed that home titration of initial CPAP pressure is possible in a selected patient population given adequate education and support. If confirmed with further studies then both routine home-based diagnosis and subsequent treatment of sleep apnoea patients may become the norm in the future.

Comparison between automatic and fixed airway pressure therapy in the home

Massie CA, McArdle N, Hart RW, *et al. Am J Respir Crit Care Med* 2003;
167: 20–3

B A C K G R O U N D . Long-term use of CPAP as treatment for sleep apnoea may be limited by side effects such as pressure intolerance, difficulty with exhalation, mask leakage, mask dislodgement or air leak through the mouth |29–32|. The factors that may influence CPAP compliance are a change in body weight, nasal patency or alcohol use. These factors, either singly or in combination, may result in suboptimal CPAP use and lead to less than optimal control of symptoms in patients with clinically significant sleep apnoea. In line with the advent of more sophisticated CPAP machines allowing the generation of varying pressures other than a fixed pressure an opportunity has arisen to study whether these autotitrating devices may produce improved compliance with CPAP use and, thus, lead to an improvement in daytime symptoms. This study was undertaken in order to look at treatment outcomes using such a device.

I N T E R P R E T A T I O N . Forty-four patients (mean age 49 ± 10 years) were randomized to 6 weeks' treatment at a laboratory-determined fixed pressure and 6 weeks on autotitrating CPAP. These patients required >10 cm of water CPAP pressure to control their sleep-disordered breathing. The average nightly use was greater in the automatic mode (306 versus 271 min) (P = 0.005), whereas the median and 95th centile pressures were lower in the automatic mode (P <0.002). Automatic CPAP resulted in better 36-item Short Form (SF-36) vitality scores (65 ± 20 versus 58 ± 23) (P <0.05) and mental health scores (80 ± 14 versus 75 ± 18) (P <0.05), but no significant differences in Epworth Sleepiness Scale score (P = 0.065). The patients noticed more restful sleep, better quality of sleep, less discomfort from pressure and less trouble getting to sleep for both the first week of therapy and for the average scores for weeks 2–6 (all P-values <0.006) when using the autotitrating device.

Comment

This study produced evidence that patients may both comply better and receive better treatment outcomes when using autotitrating CPAP devices. However, this particular group of patients required higher than average CPAP pressures and was limited by being a single-blind study and also being performed over a short time period. Nonetheless, it does suggest that troubleshooting problems using the more sophisticated form of CPAP machines available nowadays is useful in those patients in whom compliance is a problem.

Response of automatic continuous positive airway pressure (CPAP) devices to different sleep breathing patterns: a bench study

Farre R, Montserrat JM, Rigau J, Trepat X, Pinto P, Navajas D. *Am J Respir Crit Care Med* 2002; **166**: 469–73

BACKGROUND. Over recent years more sophisticated CPAP devices have become available to allow the provision of automatic adjustment of applied pressure. The pressure treatment algorithms employed by individual devices vary from device to device and this present study was designed for studying the responses of difference devices to the different patterns of breathing that are present in patients with sleep apnoea.

INTERPRETATION. Five different CPAP devices (Autoset Portable II plus, Autoset T, Goodnight 418P, Virtuoso – LX and DeVilbis Auto Adjust LT) were studied in detail in terms of their responses to various breathing patterns commonly seen in patients with sleep apnoea. The breathing patterns were reproduced from a waveform generator in the laboratory. The various breathing patterns were either normal, apnoeas, hypopnoeas, snoring or flow limitation. The responses of each machine to differing airflow patterns varied considerably. Two devices did not modify their CPAP response when subjected to repetitive apnoeas and the other three devices developed increases in pressures at different rates. Responses to air leaks were also different between the devices.

Comment

Regardless of the algorithm used for automatically adjusting CPAP pressure, subjecting various CPAP devices to reference breathing patterns in the laboratory is an extremely useful way of evaluating the performance of these individual machines. However, further clinical studies are necessary in order to determine which type of autotitrating CPAP device is useful in treating different subpopulations of patients with sleep apnoea.

Cost-effectiveness of nCPAP treatment in patients with moderate to severe obstructive sleep apnoea

Mar J, Rueda JR, Duran-Cantolla J, Schechter C, Chilcott J. *Eur Respir J* 2003; **21**: 511–22

BACKGROUND. Patients with undiagnosed obstructive sleep apnoea are heavy users of the healthcare system. Expenditure on undiagnosed patients is approximately twice that of age- and gender-matched controls. This difference extends back over 10 years prior to the diagnosis of obstructive sleep apnoea being made |33|. Treatment with CPAP reduces these costs with evidence of decreased hospitalization due to cardiovascular and pulmonary disease |34|. Hospitalization and other costs associated with road traffic accidents are also reduced in those using CPAP therapy |35–37|. The overall mean hospitalization days per year decrease with CPAP use |38|. This paper studied the cost-effectiveness of CPAP treatment in moderate to severe obstructive sleep apnoea.

INTERPRETATION. Fifty-one patients with moderate to severe symptomatic sleep apnoea (apnoea/hypopnoea index ≥30 events/h) were studied using a Markov model of health economic profiling. The study population was from Spain. The incremental cost-effectiveness of this ratio of CPAP treatment was less than 6000 Euros per quality-adjusted life year. On disaggregated analysis, CPAP treatment accounted for 86% of incremental costs, while 84% of incremental effectiveness was attributable to improved quality of life.

Comment

Treatment of patients with symptomatic obstructive sleep apnoea syndrome with CPAP has a cost-effectiveness that is broadly equivalent to that of other commonly funded treatments such as antihypertensive medication. The key clinical benefit of CPAP treatment is improvement in the quality of life of patients with symptomatic sleep apnoea. This benefit is also precisely that for which the evidence base for treatment is strongest. However, further studies are needed in order to confirm these data.

Improving CPAP use by patients with the sleep apnoea/hypopnoea syndrome (SAHS)
Engleman HM, Wild MR. *Sleep Med Rev* 2003; **7**(1); 81–9

BACKGROUND. CPAP is the treatment of choice for moderate to severe sleep apnoea, but suboptimal adherence to CPAP treatment is a problem. Between 5 and 50% of sleep apnoea patients who are recommended for CPAP use either reject this treatment option or discontinue the treatment within the first week and 12–25% of remaining patients have discontinued CPAP treatment by 3 years. This clinical review looked at the factors that favour continued CPAP use and strategies that can be developed to try to improve adherence to treatment.

INTERPRETATION. The authors reviewed the currently available evidence on CPAP use and the factors that influence adherence and then provided a model of escalating interventions that can be used in those patients in whom CPAP use appears low. This model incorporates educational and behavioural support and the use of low-technological interventions (e.g. chin straps or mask refitting) as well as exploring the role of relatively more expensive higher technological interventions for increasing CPAP usage (e.g. humidification devices and the use of automatically titrating CPAP devices).

Comment

This review emphasized that initial patient preparation for subsequent CPAP treatment using verbal, written and video education on diagnosis and treatment is important. It is also vital to establish realistic expectations of potential CPAP benefit and to reassess the patient in terms of symptom control at an early stage. Compliance with CPAP use from time clocks is appropriate and important and the short-term substitution of automatically adjusting intelligent CPAP units for troubleshooting problems is valuable.

Further research into the psychological determinants of CPAP usage and the effect of structured cognitive behavioural therapy interventions on the long-term adherence of CPAP are required as well as further economic cost-effectiveness studies of differing CPAP service provision models for determining the optimal resource allocation.

Measurement properties of the Calgary Sleep Apnoea Quality of Life Index

Flemons WW, Reimer MA. *Am J Respir Crit Care Med* 2002; **165**: 159–64

BACKGROUND. Untreated symptomatic sleep apnoea has been shown to affect a patient's quality of life adversely. This has been studied using such generic health status measures as the Nottingham Health Profile and Medical Outcome Survey SF–36 |39–41|. However, these questionnaires are relatively non-specific and are not designed for testing questions specifically related to sleep quality. The Calgary Sleep Apnoea Quality of Life Index was developed as an instrument for measuring within-subject change in response to treatment in obstructive sleep apnoea/hypopnoea syndrome. It studies four domains: normal daily routine, social interactions, emotional functioning and symptoms. The questionnaire was developed according to published guidelines that had been successfully used in the past for producing validated disease-specific quality of life questionnaires for diseases such as asthma and COPD |42,43|. This study measured quality of life before and after treatment with CPAP in 90 patients with sleep apnoea.

INTERPRETATION. A Calgary Index responsiveness index of 1.9 and an effect size of 1.1 were obtained and these responses were much greater than the domains on the SF-36 questionnaire. At baseline the Calgary Index was correlated with the SF-36, the Epworth Sleepiness Scale and a global rating of the quality of life. The Calgary Index had a high reliability coefficient of 0.92 on testing and re-testing 2 weeks later.

Comment

This paper concluded that the Calgary Sleep Apnoea Quality of Life Index displays excellent responsiveness in patients being treated with CPAP and it also shows evidence of the validity discriminative and deserves to be used in the future when quality of life issues are being assessed in patients with sleep apnoea.

The use of this index is also discussed in the review published by Reimer and Ward-Flemons in 2003 |44|.

Effect of nasal continuous positive airway pressure treatment on blood pressure in patients with obstructive sleep apnoea

Becker HF, Jerrenturp A, Ploch T, *et al. Circulation* 2003; **107**: 68–73

BACKGROUND. There is increasing evidence that obstructive sleep apnoea is an independent risk factor for arterial hypertension. There have only been a small number of studies published thus far |17,18| showing any effect of CPAP treatment on hypertension in patients with obstructive sleep apnoea and the measured impact has been modest. This paper sought to improve the currently available data on the effect of CPAP treatment on hypertension in patients with significant sleep apnoea.

INTERPRETATION. Sixty patients with moderate to severe obstructive sleep apnoea were randomly assigned to receive either effective or subtherapeutic CPAP for 9 weeks. Nocturnal polysomnography and continuous non-invasive blood pressure recording for 19 h was performed both before and after treatment with CPAP. Thirty-two patients (16 in each group) completed this study. Apnoeas/hypopnoeas were reduced by 95 and 50%, respectively, in the therapeutic and subtherapeutic groups. The mean arterial pressure decreased by 9.9 ± 11.4 mmHg with effective CPAP treatment, whereas no relevant change occurred with subtherapeutic CPAP ($P = 0.01$). The mean diastolic and systolic blood pressures all decreased significantly by approximately 10 mmHg both at night and during the day in the effectively treated CPAP group.

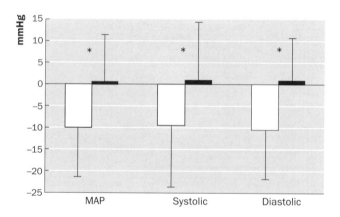

Fig. 27.1 Changes in blood pressure with effective (closed bars) and subtherapeutic (open bars) CPAP. *Significant difference. MAP, mean arterial blood pressure; systolic, systolic blood pressure; diastolic, diastolic blood pressure. MAP, $P = 0.01$; systolic blood pressure, $P = 0.04$; diastolic blood pressure, $P < 0.005$. Source: Becker *et al.* (2003).

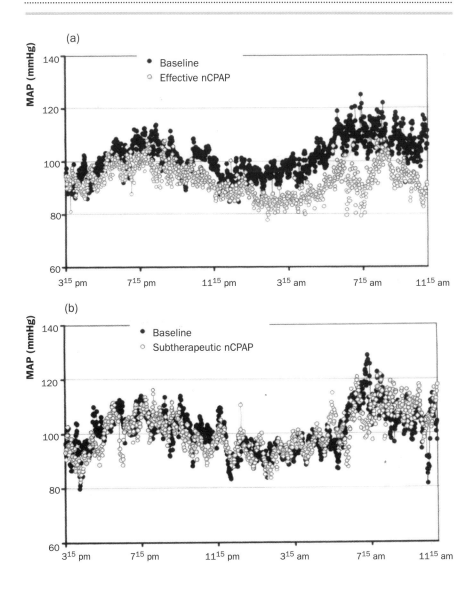

Fig. 27.2 (a) Time course of mean arterial blood pressure (MAP) before (closed circles) and on treatment (open circles) with therapeutic continuous positive airways pressure (CPAP). On average, 7.2 ± 1 hours were recorded during the night. (b) Time course of MAP before (closed circles) and on treatment (open circles) with subtherapeutic CPAP. On average, 7.1 ± 1 hours were recorded during the night. Source: Becker *et al.* (2003).

Comment

This paper adds further valuable evidence to the hypothesis that effective CPAP treatment in patients with moderate to severe sleep apnoea leads to a substantial reduction in both daytime and night-time arterial blood pressure (Figs 27.1 and 27.2). This drop of 10 mmHg in the mean blood pressure in the effective treatment group would be predicted to reduce coronary heart disease risk by 37% and stroke risk by 56% thus potentially producing enormous public health benefit.

Ambulatory blood pressure after therapeutic and subtherapeutic nasal continuous positive airway for obstructive sleep apnoea: a randomized parallel trial
Pepperell JCT, Ramdassingh-Dow S, Crosthwaite N, *et al. Lancet* 2001; **359**: 204–10

B A C K G R O U N D . If blood pressure can be reduced by CPAP this may lead to a reduction in cardiovascular risk in patients with significant sleep apnoea. This study aimed to see whether therapeutic versus subtherapeutic CPAP reduced blood pressure.

I N T E R P R E T A T I O N . This study described a randomized, parallel trial for comparing the effect of therapeutic (*n* = 59) and subtherapeutic (*n* = 59) CPAP (approximately 1 cmH$_2$0 pressure) for 1 month in 118 men with obstructive sleep apnoea (Epworth Sleepiness Scale score more than 9 and a greater than 4% oxygen desaturation index of greater than 10 events/h). The primary outcome measure was the change in the 24-hour mean blood pressure recorded. The secondary outcome measures were changes in systolic, diastolic, sleep and wake blood pressures and relations between blood pressure changes, baseline blood pressure and the severity of sleep apnoea. CPAP reduced the mean arterial ambulatory blood pressure by 2.5 mmHg (standard error [SE] 0.8) whereas subtherapeutic CPAP increased the blood pressure by 0.8 mmHg (SE 0.7) (difference –3.3 and 95% confidence interval –5.3 to –1.3) (*P* = 0.0013, unpaired test. The benefit in the blood pressure response was seen in both systolic and diastolic blood pressures and both during sleep and wakefulness. The benefit was most marked in patients with more severe sleep apnoea and was independent of the baseline blood pressure. The benefit was also particularly large in those patients who were receiving prior drug treatment for hypertension.

Comment

This paper using sham CPAP as a control adds to the evidence that treatment of patients with moderate to severe sleep apnoea with CPAP is of benefit in terms of blood pressure response. A previous study from Edinburgh |**17**| using tablets as a placebo also suggested that blood pressure falls in patients with sleep apnoea treated with CPAP and that this benefit was again most marked in those patients with most marked sleep-disordered breathing. The Edinburgh paper together with this paper and the Becker paper also suggest that CPAP treatment confers significant benefits in terms of blood pressure response in the most severe group of patients.

Continuous positive airway pressure treatment improves pulmonary haemodynamics in patients with obstructive sleep apnoea

Sajkov D, Wang T, Saunders MA, Bune AJ, McEvoy RD. *Am J Respir Crit Care Med* 2002; **165**: 152–8

BACKGROUND. Pulmonary hypertension is a common complication in patients with moderate to severe obstructive sleep apnoea |45,46|. This can occur in the absence of any co-existing pulmonary or heart disease |47–49|. The potential mechanisms producing daytime pulmonary hypertension in sleep apnoea are elevated daytime pulmonary vascular tone secondary to hypoxic pulmonary vasoconstriction, hypoxia-induced endothelial dysfunction |50| and pulmonary vascular remodelling |49|. It is unknown whether pulmonary hypertension is reversible once it becomes established in humans, although a number of animal models have suggested that, if hypoxia can be abolished, then the pulmonary vascular remodelling is potentially reversible |51|. Patients with significant sleep apnoea have repeated episodes of nocturnal hypoxia and this can lead to pulmonary hypertension. The purpose of this study was to determine whether pulmonary hypertension associated with sleep apnoea without lung or cardiac disease is reversible with CPAP treatment and whether any change was associated with ventilation perfusion imbalance reversal, altered responsiveness to hypoxia or improved pulmonary vascular compliance.

INTERPRETATION. Twenty patients (average apnoea/hypopnoea index 49 events/h) were studied before and after 4 months of CPAP treatment. Treatment with CPAP decreased the pulmonary artery pressure from 17 to 14 mmHg and the total pulmonary vascular resistance fell from 231 to 186 dyn/s/cm^5. The pulmonary vascular response to hypoxia (assessed at inspired oxygen concentrations of 11, 21 and 50%) decreased by 37%, a plot of pulmonary artery pressure versus cardiac output (measured during infusions of dobutamine) moved downwards and arterial diastolic pressure also fell. These improvements were not related to changes in left ventricular diastolic pressure or oxygen tension.

Comment

This paper suggested that CPAP treatment reduces pulmonary vascular response and hypoxic pulmonary vascular reactivity in obstructive sleep apnoea and this may be due to an improvement in pulmonary endothelial function in response to the improvement in the hypoxia.

Uses and benefits of mandibular repositioning splints

 ### Control of oral appliance therapy in the treatment of obstructive sleep apnoea
Ferguson KA. *Clin Chest Med* 2003; **24**(2): 355–64

B ACKGROUND. Oral appliances (mandibular repositioning splints) are a useful treatment option for simple snoring and mild cases of obstructive sleep apnoea. They are appealing, as they are simple to use, silent, portable, improve pharyngeal patency and have a relatively low complication rate. They may also be used in patients who have failed other treatment options, but they are not as effective as CPAP therapy in more severe cases of sleep apnoea |52|. The short-term side effects are generally minor and are related to excessive salivation, jaw and tooth discomfort and occasional temporomandibular joint discomfort. These symptoms usually improve over time, but may lead to discontinuation of usage. However, more severe occlusal changes can occasionally occur when the device is used.

I NTERPRETATION. This review discussed the mechanism of action of these devices. They reposition the tongue, lift the soft palate and improve upper airway patency (see Figs. 27.3 (a), (b) and (c)).The effect does depend upon body position. The American

(a)

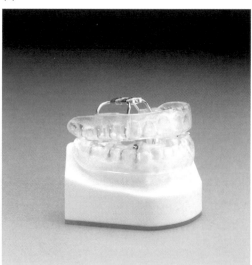

Fig. 27.3 (a), (b) and (c) Some of the various oral appliances that are available for the treatment of obstructive sleep apnoea.
Source: Ferguson (2003).

(b)

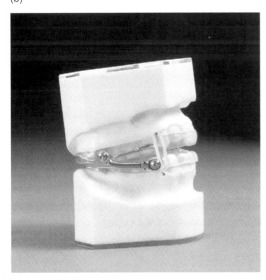

(c)

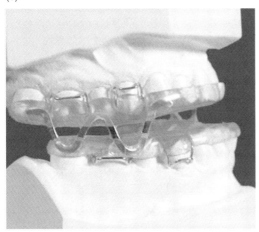

Academy of Sleep Medicine has published guidelines about the use of oral appliances in the treatment of sleep apnoea |53|. These guidelines state that oral appliances are indicated as first-line therapy in patients with simple snoring and mild sleep apnoea and as second-line therapy for patients with moderate to severe sleep apnoea when other therapies have failed. As more randomized, controlled trials of their usage are performed it may well be that their indications for use will expand.

Comment

This article outlines the benefits and complications of various types of oral devices in the treatment of obstructive sleep apnoea.

Randomized cross-over trial of two treatments for sleep apnoea/hypopnoea syndrome. Continuous positive airway pressure and mandibular repositioning splint

Engleman HM, McDonald JP, Graham D, *et al. Am J Respir Crit Care Med* 2002; **166**: 855–9

BACKGROUND. Systematic reviews of treatment for sleep apnoea have found high-level, randomized, controlled trial evidence confirming CPAP as the best evaluated treatment for the symptomatic patient. However, CPAP is only tolerated in approximately 80% of patients |54| and, thus, there is a need for alternative treatment options. Previous controlled studies have shown that mandibular repositioning splints improved the apnoea/hypopnoea index, nocturnal saturation and arousals from sleep in sleep apnoea patients. Systematic reviews |55,56| have also included three recent trials of mandibular repositioning splint treatment against CPAP in sleep apnoea |57–59|. All were cross-over trials, but only two were randomized |58,59|. These reported greater patient satisfaction preference and lower side effects for mandibular repositioning splints over CPAP despite the inferior effectiveness of the mandibular splint devices in correcting the apnoea/hypopnoea index and improving both nocturnal and daytime symptoms. These studies used a small amount of patients and they were influenced by the withdrawal of some of the patients. This current study was designed in order to allow a direct prospective comparison of the clinical effectiveness of long-term home treatment with CPAP and mandibular splint devices analysed on an intention-to-treat basis in a mixed-severity group of patients with sleep apnoea. Assessments included validated objective and subjective measures where available. A subanalysis was planned in patients with lower apnoea/hypopnoea indices in order to assess any differential treatment response amongst this particular group of patients. Patients' preferences for either CPAP or mandibular repositioning splint treatment were also studied.

INTERPRETATION. A randomized, cross-over trial of 8 weeks of CPAP versus 8 weeks of treatment with a mandibular repositioning splint was performed in consecutive new outpatients with obstructive sleep apnoea/hypopnoea syndrome (apnoea/hypopnoea index ≥5/h and two symptoms including sleepiness). Assessments at the end of both arms included a home sleep study, subjective ratings of treatment value, sleepiness, symptoms, well-being and objective tests of sleepiness and cognition. Forty-eight out of

51 recruits completed the trial (twelve women, mean age 46 ± 9 years, Epworth Sleepiness Scale score 14 ± 4 and median apnoea/hypopnoea index 22/h with interquartile ratio 11–43/h). Seven out of 21 measured variables improved to a significantly greater extent with CPAP than with the mandibular splints: the apnoea/hypopnoea index (8 versus 15 events), the Epworth Sleepiness Scale (8 versus 12), effectiveness rating and functional outcomes of sleepiness on a questionnaire, mental component on Short-Form 36 Health Survey and Health Transition scores. No differences between the two treatments were seen for objective sleepiness, cognitive performance or preference for treatment. Patients with mild sleep apnoea (apnoea/hypopnoea index <15 events/h) also had a better response to CPAP than with the splint device.

Comment

This comprehensive study showed that a mandibular repositioning splint is not as effective as CPAP in the treatment of any severity of sleep apnoea. As such CPAP should remain the first-line treatment for symptomatically sleepy patients with sleep apnoea even those with mild sleep apnoea (apnoea/hypopnoea index <15 events/h). Nonetheless, a mandibular splint device does offer a useful treatment option in simple snorers or mild sleep apnoea patients who are intolerant of CPAP |**60**|. Indications for mandibular splint devices may well vary in the future as further studies are performed.

Oral appliance therapy improves symptoms in obstructive sleep apnoea: a randomized controlled trial

Gotsopoulos H, Chen C, Qian J, Cistulli PA. *Am J Respir Crit Care Med* 2002; **166**: 743–8

BACKGROUND. This study was designed to test the effectiveness of a mandibular splint device in patients with mild sleep apnoea versus a placebo. A randomized, controlled trial of 73 patients and a respiratory disturbance index of 27 events/h was performed comparing a mandibular splint device to an inactive oral appliance.

INTERPRETATION. The active splint produced improvements in the sleep latency on a multiple sleep latency test (10.3 versus 9.1 min) and on Epworth Sleepiness Scale scores (7 versus 9 min) over a 4-week period. The proportion of patients with normal subjective sleepiness was higher in the active splint group (82 versus 60%), although objective sleepiness did not differ between the two groups.

Comment

This study concluded that 4 weeks of treatment with a mandibular splint device improves daytime sleepiness and a range of other symptoms in patients with sleep apnoea compared to placebo.

Mandibular advancement devices: rate of contra-indications in 100 consecutive obstructive sleep apnoea patients

Petit FX, Pepin JL, Bettega G, Sadek H, Raphael B, Lave P. *Am J Respir Crit Care Med* 2002; **166**: 274–8

BACKGROUND. It is important to determine the proportion of patients who may have a contra-indication to the use of a mandibular repositioning splint device as they are becoming more commonly used.

INTERPRETATION. Commonly described contra-indications to the use of mandibular repositioning splints are a lack of a significant number of teeth in each arch (there is a particular need for posterior teeth to be present in order to obtain good fixation of the device within the mouth), existence of peri-odontal disease or significant tooth mobility, active temporomandibular joint dysfunction or the presence of limited maximal protrusive distance. It has been estimated that at least 6 mm of anterior movement of the mandible is required for allowing a sufficient increase in the pharyngeal area with use of a mandibular splint device for the treatment to be effective. One hundred unselected patients with sleep apnoea were studied in order to determine the proportion of patients with contra-indications to the use of mandibular repositioning splints. Case notes and X-rays were analysed by two expert maxillo-facial surgeons (each blinded to the other). The surgeons agreed on absolute contra-indications in 96 of the 100 patients. Contra-indications were found in 34% of the patients and these included insufficient remaining teeth, peri-odontal abnormalities in 50% of the patients and temporomandibular joint dysfunction in two patients. Sixteen patients required dental and peri-odontal treatment before a mandibular splint device could be considered, but overall it was estimated that one-third of the patients with sleep apnoea had contra-indications to the use of mandibular splint devices.

Comment

Although it seems attractive to use mandibular splint devices in preference to CPAP in patients with sleep apnoea, as they are cheap, portable, silent and easy to use, there are a significant number of drawbacks to their usage. They are not as effective a treatment option as CPAP if CPAP can be tolerated in the symptomatic patient. If an oral appliance is contemplated a careful assessment prior to use of the device is required and long-term follow-up is essential.

Conclusion

Various treatment options are available once the diagnosis of sleep apnoea is made and the individual management approach depends on both the severity of the underlying condition and the characteristics of the individual patient.

The Scottish Intercollegiate Guidelines Network's *Management of Obstructive Sleep Apnoea/Hypopnoea Syndrome in Adults – A National Clinical Guideline* |**53**|, which is an evidence-based publication, was published in 2003 and lists a number of recommendations regarding the treatment of obstructive sleep apnoea/hypopnoea syndrome.

1. Whilst weight loss should be encouraged in all patients with obesity contributing to their obstructive sleep apnoea/hypopnoea syndrome, initiation of further treatment should not be delayed.

2. CPAP is the first-choice therapy for patients with moderate or severe obstructive sleep apnoea/hypopnoea syndrome that is sufficiently symptomatic to require intervention.

3. Persistent low CPAP use (less than 2 h per night) over 6 months, following efforts to improve patient comfort, should lead to a review of treatment.

4. Intra-oral devices are an appropriate therapy for snorers and for patients with mild obstructive sleep apnoea/hypopnoea syndrome with normal daytime alertness.

5. Intra-oral devices are an appropriate alternative therapy for patients who are unable to tolerate CPAP.

6. The use of intra-oral devices should be monitored following initiation of therapy in order to allow device adjustment and assessment of obstructive sleep apnoea/hypopnoea syndrome control and symptoms.

7. Pharmacological therapy should not be used as first-line therapy for obstructive sleep apnoea/hypopnoea syndrome.

8. The use of uvulopalatopharyngoplasty or LAUP is not recommended.

Both the general public and the medical profession are becoming more aware of obstructive sleep apnoea/hypopnoea syndrome and as such an increasing number of patients are being referred for investigation and possible treatment. This will hopefully lead to an improvement in the quality of life of many patients with obstructive sleep apnoea/hypopnoea syndrome and a reduction in the morbidity and mortality attributable to this condition in the future.

References

1. The National Health and Medical Research Council. *The Effectiveness of Nasal Continuous Positive Airway Pressure (CPAP) in Obstructive Sleep Apnoea in Adults.* Canberra. The Council; 2000 cited April 2003, available on-line from http://www.health.gov.au/nhmrc/publication/pdf/hpr21.pdf Reference 2.

2. Jenkinson C, Davies RJ, Mullins R, Stradling JR. Comparison of therapeutic and sub-therapeutic continuous positive airway pressure for obstructive sleep apnoea: a random-ised prospective parallel trial. *Lancet* 1999; **353**: 2100–5.

3. Hack M, Davies RJ, Mullins R, Choy SJ, Ramdassingh-Dow S, Jenkinson C. A randomised prospective parallel trial of therapeutic versus subtherapeutic nasal continuous positive airway pressure on simulated steering performance in patients with obstructive sleep apnoea. *Thorax* 2000; **55**: 224–31.

4. Barbe F, Mayoralas LR, Duran J, Masa JD, Maimo A, Monserrat JM. Treatment with con-tinuous positive airway pressure is not effective in patients with sleep apnoea but no day-time sleepiness. A randomised, controlled trial. *Ann Intern Med* 2001; **134**: 1015–23.

5. Harvey EL, Glenny A-M, Kirk SFL, Summberbell CD. Improving health professionals management and the organisation of care for overweight and obese people (Cochrane Review). In: *The Cochrane Library*, Issue 1. Oxford: Update Software, 2002.

6. Smith PL, Gold AR, Meyers DA, Happonik EF, Bleecker ER. Weight loss in mild to mod-erately obese patients with obstructive sleep apnoea. *Ann Intern Med* 1985; **103**: 850–5.

7. Dhabuwalla A, Cannan RJ, Stubbs RS. Improvement in co-morbidity following weight loss from gastric bypass surgery. *Obesity Surg* 2000; **10**: 428–35.

8. Wright J, White J, Ducharme F. Continuous positive airway pressure for obstructive sleep apnoea (Cochrane Review). In: *The Cochrane Library*, Issue 1. Oxford: Update Software, 2002.

9. Engleman HM, Martin SC, Deary IJ, Douglas NJ. Effect of CPAP therapy on daytime function in patients with mild sleep apnoea/hypopnoea syndrome. *Thorax* 1997; **52**: 114–19.

10. Redline S, Adams N, Strauss ME, Roebuck T, Winters M, Rosenberg C. Improvement of mild sleep disordered breathing with CPAP compared with therapy. *Am J Respir Crit Care Med* 1998; **157**: 858–65.

11. Ballester E, Badia JR, Hernandez L, Carrasco E, De Pablo J, Fornas C. Evidence of the effectiveness of continuous positive airway pressure in the treatment of sleep apnoea/hypopnoea syndrome. *Am J Respir Crit Care Med* 1999; **159**: 495–501.

12. Engleman HM, Martin SC, Kingshott RN, Mackay TW, Deary IJ, Douglas NJ. Random-ised placebo controlled trial of daytime function after continuous positive airway pressure (CPAP) therapy for the sleep apnoea/hypopnoea syndrome. *Thorax* 1998; **53**: 341–5.

13. Loberas P, Ballester E, Monserrat JM, Botifilly E, Ramirez A. Comparison between manual and automatic CPAP titration in patients with sleep apnoea/hypopnoea syn-drome. *Am J Respir Crit Care Med* 1996; **154**: 1755–8.

14. Teschler H, Berthon-Jones M, Thompson AB, Henkel A, Henry J, Konietzko N. Auto-mated continuous positive airway pressure titration for obstructive sleep apnoea syn-drome. *Am J Respir Crit Care Med* 1996; **154**: 734–40.

15. Meurice JC, Marc I, Series F. Efficacy of auto-CPAP in the treatment of obstructive sleep apnoea/hypopnoea syndrome. *Am J Respir Crit Care Med* 1996; **153**: 794–8.

16. McArdle N, Grove A, Devereux I, Brown IT, Douglas NJ. Split night versus full night studies for sleep apnoea/hypopnoea syndrome. *Respir J* 2000; **15**: 670–5.

17. Faccenda JF, Mackay TW, Boon NA, Douglas NJ. A randomised placebo controlled trial of continuous positive airway pressure on blood pressure in the sleep apnoea/hypopnoea syndrome. *Am J Respir Crit Care Med* 2001; **163**: 344–8.

18. Pepperell J, Ramdassingh-Dow S, Crossthwaite N, Mullins R, Jenkinson C, Stradling JR, Davies RJ. Ambulatory blood pressure after therapeutic and subtherapeutic nasal continuous positive airway pressure for obstructive sleep apnoea: a randomised parallel trial. *Lancet* 2001; **359**: 204–10.

19. Mehta A, Qian J, Petocz P, Darendeliler MA, Sistulli PA. A randomised controlled study of a mandibular advancement splint for obstructive sleep apnoea. *Am J Respir Crit Care Med* 2002; **163**: 1457–61.

20. Schmidt-Nowara WW, Wiegand L, Cartwright R, Perz-Gurra F, Menn S. Oral appliances for the treatment of snoring and obstructive sleep apnoea: a review. *Sleep* 1995; **18**: 501–510.

21. Marklund M, Franklin KA, Sahlan C, Lundgren R. The effect of a mandibular advancement device on apnoeas and sleep in patients with obstructive sleep apnoea. *Chest* 1998; **113**: 707–13.

22. Schmidt-Nowara WW, Mead T, Hays MB. Treatment of snoring and obstructive sleep apnoea with a dental orthosis. *Chest* 1991; **99**: 1378–85.

23. Pancer J, Al-Faifi S, Al-Faifi M, Hoffstein V. Evaluation of a variable mandibular advancement appliance for the treatment of snoring and sleep apnoea. *Chest* 1999; **116**: 1511–18.

24. Clark GT, Blumenfeld I, Joffe M, Peled E, Lavi P. A crossover study comparing the efficacy of continuous positive airway pressure with anterior mandibular positioning devices in patients with obstructive sleep apnoea. *Chest* 1996; **109**: 1477–83.

25. Pantin CC, Hillman DR, Tennant M. Dental side-effects of an oral device to treat snoring and sleep apnoea. *Sleep* 1999; **22**: 237–40.

26. Sher AE, Schechtman KB, Piccirillo JF. The efficacy of surgical modification of the upper airway in adults with obstructive sleep apnoea syndrome. *Sleep* 1996; **19**: 156–7.

27. Bridgman SA, Dunn KM, Ducharme F. Surgery for obstructive sleep apnoea (Cochrane Review). In: *The Cochrane Library*, Issue 1. Oxford: Update Software, 2002.

28. Verse T, Pirsig W. Meta-analysis of laser-assisted uvulopalatopharyngoplasty. What is clinically relevant up to now? *Laryngorhinootologie* 2000; **79**: 273–84.

29. McArdle N, Devereux G, Heidarnejad H, Engleman HM, Mackay TW, Douglas NJ. Longterm use of CPAP therapy for sleep apnoea/hypopnoea syndrome. *Am J Respir Crit Care Med* 1999; **159**: 1108–14.

30. Engleman HM, Asgari-Jirhandh N, McLeod AL, Ramsay CF, Deary IJ, Douglas NJ. Self-reported use of CPAP and benefit of CPAP therapy on a patient survey. *Chest* 1996; **109**: 1470–6.

31. Weaver T, Kribbs MB, Pack AI, Kline LR, Cheugh DK, Maisland G. Night-to-night variability in CPAP used over the first 3 months of treatment. *Sleep* 1997; **20**: 278–83.

32. Massie CA, Hart RW, Peralaz K, Richards GN. Effects of humidification on nasal symptoms and compliance in sleep apnoea patients using continuous positive airway pressure. *Chest* 1999; **116**: 403–8.

33. Hoy CJ, Vennelle M, Kingshott RM, Engleman HM, Douglas NJ. Can intensive support improve continuous positive airway pressure use in patients with the sleep apnoea/hypopnoea syndrome? *Am J Respir Crit Care Med* 1999; **159**: 1096–100.

34. Kappur V, Blough DK, Sandblom RM, Hert R, De Maine JB, Sullivan SD. The medical cost of undiagnosed sleep apnoea. *Sleep* 1999; **22**: 749–55.

35. Peker Y, Hedner J, Johansson A, Bend M. Reduced hospitalisation with cardiovascular and pulmonary disease in obstructive sleep apnoea patients on nasal CPAP treatment. *Sleep* 1997; **20**: 645–53.

36. Krieger N, Meslier N, Lebrun T, Levy P, Phillip-Joet F, Sailly JC. Accidents in obstructive sleep apnoea patients using nasal continuous positive airway pressure: a prospective study. The Working Group ANTADIR, Paris and CRESGE, Lille, France. Association Nationale de Traitement a Domicile des Insuffisants Respiratoires. *Chest* 1997; **112**: 1561–6.

37. George CF. Reduction in motor vehicle collisions following treatment of sleep apnoea with nasal CPAP. *Thorax* 2001; **26**: 508–12.

38. Douglas NJ, George CF. Treating sleep apnoea is cost effective. *Thorax* 2002; **27**: 93.

39. Bahaman A, Delaive K, Ronald J, Manfreda J, Roos L, Kryger MH. Health care utilisation in males with obstructive sleep apnoea syndrome 2 years after diagnosis and treatment. *Sleep* 1999; **22**: 740–7.

40. Jenkinson C, Stradling J, Petersen S. Comparison of three measures of quality of life outcome in the evaluation of continuous positive airway pressure therapy for sleep apnoea. *J Sleep Res* 1997; **6**: 199–204.

41. Engleman HM, Martin SC, Douglas NJ. Compliance with CPAP therapy in patients with sleep apnoea/hypopoea syndrome. *Thorax* 1994; **49**: 263–6.

42. Juniper EF, Guyatt GH. Development and testing of a new measure of health status for clinical trials in rhinoconjunctivitis. *Clin Exp Allergy* 1991; **21**: 77–83.

43. Guyatt JA, Berman LB, Townsend M, Pugsley O, Chambers LW. A measure of quality of life for clinical trials including lung disease. *J Clin Epidemiol* 1997; **42**: 773–8.

44. Reimer MA, Ward-Flemons W. Quality of life in sleep disorders. A clinical review. *Sleep Med Rev* 2003; **7**(4): 335–49.

45. Podszus T, Bauer W, Mayer J, Penzel T, Peter JH, Wichart P. Sleep apnoea and pulmonary hypertension. *Clin Wochenschr* 1986; **65**: 131–4.

46. Fletcher AC, Schaf JM, Miller J, Fletcher JG. Longterm cardiopulmonary sequela in patients with sleep apnoea and chronic lung disease. *Am Rev Respir Dis* 1987; **135**: 525–33.

47. Krieger J, Sforza E, Apprill M, Lampert E, Weitzembloom E, Ratomaharo J. Pulmonary hypertension, hypoxaemia and hypercapnia in obstructive sleep apnoea patients. *Chest* 1999; **96**: 729–37.

48. Sajkov D, Cowie RJ, Thornton AT, Espinoza HA, McEvoy RD. Pulmonary hypertension and hypoxaemia in obstructive sleep apnoea syndrome. *Am J Respir Crit Care Med* 1994; **149**: 416–22.

49. Sannar BM, Doberauer C, Conerman M, Sturm A, Zidek W. Pulmonary hypertension in patients with obstructive sleep apnoea syndrome. *Arch Intern Med* 1997; **157**: 2483–7.

50. Sagquove D, Wang T, Saunders NA, Bune AJ, Neil AM, McEvoy RD. Daytime pulmonary haemodynamics in patients with obstructive sleep apnoea without lung disease. *Am J Respir Crit Care Med* 1999; **159**: 1518–26.

51. Faller DV. Endothelial cell responses to hypoxia stress. *Clin Exp Pharmacol Physiol* 1999; **26**: 74–84.

52. Kolar F, Ostadal B. Right ventricular function in rats with hypoxic pulmonary hypertension. *Pflugers Arch* 1991; **419**: 121–6.

53. Scottish Intercollegiate Guidelines Network. *Management of Obstructive Sleep Apnoea/ Hypopnoea Syndrome in Adults – A National Clinical Guideline.* Scottish Intercollegiate Guidelines Network (SIGN73), available on-line at http://www.sign.ac.uk.

54. American Sleep Disorders Association. Practice parameters for the treatment of snoring and obstructive sleep apnoea with oral appliances. *Sleep* 1995; **18**: 511–13.

55. Krieger J. Longterm compliance with CPAP therapy in obstructive sleep apnoea patients and in snorers. *Sleep* 1996; **19**: S136–43.

56. Australian National and Medical Research Council. *Effectiveness of Nasal Continuous Positive Airway Pressure (nCPAP) in Obstructive Sleep Apnoea Adults.* Canberra: Ausinfo, 2000.

57. Wright J, White J. Continuous positive airway pressure for obstructive sleep apnoea. *Cochrane Database Syst Rev* 2000; **2**.

58. Clark GT, Blumenfeld I, Yoffe N, Peled E, Lavie P. A crossover study comparing the efficacy of continuous positive airway pressure with anterior mandibular positioning devices in patients with obstructive sleep apnoea. *Chest* 1996; **109**: 1477–83.

59. Ferguson KA, Ono T, Lowe AA, Keenan SP, Fleetham JA. A randomised crossover study of an oral appliance versus nasal continuous positive airway pressure in the treatment of mild–moderate obstructive sleep apnoea. *Chest* 1996; **109**: 1269–75.

60. Ferguson KA, Ono T, Lowe AA, Al-Majed S, Love LL, Fleetham JA. A short term controlled trial of an adjustable oral appliance for the treatment of mild–moderate obstructive sleep apnoea. *Thorax* 1997; **52**: 362–8.

Abbreviations

ACCESS	A Case Control Etiology of Sarcoidosis Study	EGF	epidermal growth factor
ACRN	Asthma Clinical Research Network	ELISA	enzyme-linked immunosorbent assay
AMP	adenosine monophosphate	EMG	electromyelographic
APACHE	Acute Physiology and Chronic Health Evaluation	ENFUMOSA	European Network for Understanding Mechanisms of Severe Asthma
AQLQ	Asthma Quality of Life Questionnaire	ERS	European Respiratory Society
ATS	American Thoracic Society	ECRHS	European Community Respiratory Health Survey
AUC	area under the curve		
BAL	bronchoalveolar lavage	ECOG	European Cooperative Oncology Group
BMI	body mass index		
BTS	British Thoracic Society	FACT-L	Functional Assessment of Cancer Therapy – Lung
CAPS	Childhood Asthma Prevention Study	FEV_1	forced expiratory volume in 1 s
CCR2	C-C chemokine receptor 2		
CFA	cryptogenic fibrosing alveolitis	FF	fibroblastic foci
		FVC	forced vital capacity
CFU	colony forming unit	G-CSF	granulocyte colony-stimulating factor
CHD	coronary heart disease		
CI	confidence interval	GOLD	Global Initiative for Chronic Obstructive Lung Disease
COPD	chronic obstructive pulmonary disease		
		GP	general practitioner
CPAP	continuous positive airway pressure	HAART	highly active antiretroviral therapy
CPI	composite physiologic index	HIV	human immunodeficiency virus
CRDQ	Chronic Respiratory Disease Questionnaire	HLA	human leukocyte antigen
		hMPV	human metapneumovirus
CRQ	Chronic Respiratory Questionnaire	HR	hazard ratio
		HRCT	high-resolution computed tomography
CT	computed tomography		
CVD	collagen vascular disease	HRT	hormone replacement therapy
DIP	desquamative interstitial pneumonia		
		HVS	hyperventilation syndrome
D_{Lco}	diffusing capacity for carbon monoxide	ICU	intensive care unit
		IDEAL	IRESSA Dose Evaluation in Advanced Lung cancer
DPLD	diffuse parenchymal lung disease		
		IFN	interferon
EEG	electroencephalogram	Ig	immunoglobulin

IIP	idiopathic interstitial pneumonia	PEF	peak expiratory flow
IL	interleukin	PD_{20}	provocating dose that causes a 20% drop in FEV_1
ILD	interstitial lung disease	PET	positron emission
IPF	idiopathic pulmonary fibrosis		tomography
IQR	interquartile range	PIAMA	Prevention and Incidence of
ISAAC	International Study of		Asthma and Mite Allergy
	Asthma and Allergies in	PS	pulse steroids
	Childhood	QALY	quality-adjusted life year
ISOLDE	Inhaled Steroids in	ROC	receiver operating
	Obstructive Lung Disease in		characteristics
	Europe	RR	relative risk
K_{co}	gas transfer coefficient	RT-PCR	reverse transcriptase
LAUP	laser-assisted		polymerase chain reaction
	uvulopalatopharynoplasty	RV	residual volume
LPS	lipopolysaccharide	SaO_2	oxygen saturation of arterial
MAP	mean arterial blood pressure		blood
MHC	major histocompatibility	SARS	severe acute respiratory
	complex		syndrome
MRC	Medical Research Council	SARS-CoV	SARS-associated coronavirus
MRI	magnetic resonance imaging	SD	standard deviation
nCPAP	nasal continuous positive	SE	standard error
	airway pressure	SIDS	sudden infant death
NSIP	non-specific interstitial		syndrome
	pneumonia	SIRS	systemic inflammatory
OR	odds ratio		response syndrome
$(P(A–a)O_2)$	alveolar–arterial oxygen	SNP	single nucleotide
	tension difference		polymorphisms
$PaCO_2$	partial pressure of carbon	TB	tuberculosis
	dioxide in arterial blood	TGF	transforming growth factor
PaO_2	partial pressure of oxygen in	TLC	total lung capacity
	arterial blood	TNF	tumour necrosing factor
PCO_2	partial pressure of carbon	Th	T helper
	dioxide	UIP	usual interstitial pneumonia
PCR	polymerase chain reaction	*YIRM*	*Year in Respiratory Medicine*

Index of Papers Reviewed

Aaron SD, Vandemheen KL, Hebert P, Dales R, Stiell IG, Ahuja J, Dickinson G, Brison R, Rowe BH, Dreyer J, Yetisir E, Cass D, Wells G. Out-patient oral prednisone after emergency treatment of chronic obstructive pulmonary disease. *N Engl J Med* 2003; 348(26): 2618–25. **139**

American Academy of Chest Physicians. Diagnosis and management of lung cancer. ACCP evidence-based guidelines. *Chest* 2003; 123 (Suppl 1): 1–338. **349**

American Academy of Sleep Medicine Report, Standards of Practice Committee of the American Academy of Sleep Medicine. Littner M, Hirshkowitz M, Davila D, WM, Kushida CA, Woodson BT, Johnson SF, Merrill SW. Practice parameters for the use of autotitrating continuous positive airway pressure devices for titrating pressures and treating adult patients with obstructive sleep apnoea syndrome. *Sleep* 2002; 25(2): 143–7. **391**

An Evidence Review Co-sponsored by the American Academy of Sleep Medicine, the American College of Chest Physicians and the American Thoracic Society. Home diagnosis of sleep apnoea: a systematic review of literature. *Chest* 2003; 124: 1543–79. **380**

Antures G, Neville E, Duffy J, Ali N on behalf of the BTS Pleural Disease Group, a subgroup of the BTS Standards of Care Committee. BTS guidelines for the management of malignant pleural effusion. *Thorax* 2003; 58 (Suppl 2): ii29–38. **331**

Ayappa I, Berger KI, Norman RG, Oppenheimer BW, Rapoport DM, Goldran RM. Hypercapnia and ventilatory periodicity in obstructive sleep apnoea syndrome. *Am J Respir Crit Care Med* 2002; 166: 1112–15. **368**

Bakhshandeh A, Bruns I, Traynor A, Robins HI, Eberhardt K, Demedts A, Kaukel E, Koschel G, Gatzemeier U, Kohlmann T, Dalhoff K, Ehlers EM, Gruber Y, Zumschlinge R, Hegewisch-Becker S, Peters SO, Wiedemann GJ. Ifosfamide, carboplatin and etoposide combined with 41.8°C whole-body hyperthermia for malignant pleural mesothelioma. *Lung Cancer* 2003; 39: 339–45. **327**

Baldi A, Groeger AM, Esposito V, Cassandro R, Tonini G, Battista T, Di Marino MP, Vincenzi B, Santini M, Angelini A, Rossiello R, Baldi F, Paggi MG. Expression of p21 in SV40 large T antigen-positive human pleural mesothelioma: relationship with survival. *Thorax* 2002; 57(4): 353–6. **307**

Barnes M, Houston D, Worsnop CJ, Neill AM, Mykytyn IJ, Kay A, Trinder J, Saunders NA, Douglas McEvoy R, Pierce RJ. A randomized control trial of continuous positive airway pressure (CPAP) in mild obstructive sleep apnoea. *Am J Respir Crit Care Med* 2002; 165: 773–80. **390**

Barr RG, Rowe BH, Camargo Jr CA. Methylxanthines for exacerbations of chronic obstructive pulmonary disease: meta-analysis of randomized trials. *BMJ* 2003; 327(7416): 643. **138**

Cooper S, Osborne J, Newton S, Harrison V, Thompson Coon J, Lewis S, Tattersfield A. Effect of two breathing exercises (Buteyko and pranayama) in asthma: a randomized controlled trial. *Thorax* 2003; 59: 674–9. **64**

Cox LS, Clark MM, Jett JR, Patten CA, Schroeder DR, Nirelli LM, Swensen SJ, Hurt RD. Change in smoking status after spiral chest computed tomography scan screening. *Cancer* 2003; 98(11): 2495–501. **337**

Davidson TM, Gehrman P, Ferreyra H. Lack of night-to-night variability of sleep-disordered breathing measured during home monitoring. *Ear Nose Throat J* 2003; 82(2): 135–8. **381**

Davila D, Richards KC, Marshall BL, O'Sullivan PS, Osbahr LA, Huddleston RB, Jordan JC. Oximeter's acquisition parameter influences the profile of respiratory disturbances. *Sleep* 2003; 26(1): 91–5. **379**

De Ruysscher D, Slotman B. Treatment of intervention sites of malignant pleural mesothelioma with radiotherapy: a Dutch–Belgian survey. *Radiother Oncol* 2003; 68: 299–302. **317**

Dingli K, Coleman EL, Vennelle M, Finch SP, Wraith PK, Mackay TW, Douglas NJ. Evaluation of a portable device for diagnosing the sleep apnoea/hypopnoea syndrome. *Eur Respir J* 2003; 21: 253–9. **383**

Douglas NJ. Home diagnosis of obstructive sleep apnoea syndrome. *Sleep Med Rev* 2003; 7(1): 53–9. **379**

Ducharme FM. Inhaled glucocorticoids versus leukotriene receptor antagonists as single-agent asthma treatment: systematic review of current evidence. *BMJ* 2003 326: 621–3. **56**

Dyugovskaya L, Lavie P, Lavie L. Increased adhesion molecules expression and production of reactive oxygen species in leukocytes of sleep apnoea patients.

Am J Respir Crit Care Med 2002; 165: 934–9. **370**

El-Solh AA, Pietrantoni C, Bhat A, Aquilina AT, Okada M, Grover V, Gifford N. Microbiology of severe aspiration pneumonia in institutionalized elderly. *Am J Respir Crit Care Med* 2003; 167: 1650–4. **294**

Engels EA, Katki HA, Nielsen NM, Winther JF, Hjalgrim H, Gjerris F, Rosenberg PS, Frisch M. Cancer incidence in Denmark following exposure to poliovirus vaccine contained with simian virus 40. *J Natl Cancer Inst* 2003; 95(7): 532–9. **306**

Engleman HM, McDonald JP, Graham D, Lello GE, Kingshott RN, Coleman EL, Mackay TW, Douglas NJ. Randomized cross-over trial of two treatments for sleep apnoea/hypopnoea syndrome. Continuous positive airway pressure and mandibular repositioning splint. *Am J Respir Crit Care Med* 2002; 166: 855–9. **404**

Engleman HM, Wild MR. Improving CPAP use by patients with the sleep apnoea syndrome (SAHS). *Sleep Med Rev* 2003; 7(1): 81–9. **396**

European Network for Understanding Mechanisms of Severe Asthma Study Group. The ENFUMOSA cross-sectional European multicentre study of the clinical phenotype of chronic severe asthma. The European Network for Understanding Mechanisms of Severe Asthma. *Eur Respirat J* 2003; 22: 470–7. **30**

Farre R, Montserrat JM, Rigau J, Trepat X, Pinto P, Navajas D. Response of automatic continuous positive airway pressure (CPAP) devices to different sleep breathing patterns: a bench study. *Am J Respir Crit Care Med* 2002; 166: 469–73. **395**

Favaretto AG, Aversa SML, Paccagnella A, Manzini Vde P, Palmisano V, Oniga F, Stefani M, Rea F, Bortolotti L, Loreggian L, Monfardini S. Gemcitabine combined with carboplatin in patients with malignant pleural mesothelioma. A multicentre phase II study. *Cancer* 2003; 97: 2791–8. **319**

Ferguson KA. Control of oral appliance therapy in the treatment of obstructive sleep apnoea. *Clin Chest Med* 2003; 24(2): 355–64. **402**

Fine MJ, Stone RA, Lave JR, Hough LJ, Obrosky DS, Mor MK, Kapoor WN. Implementation of an evidence-based guideline to reduce duration of intravenous antibiotic therapy and length of stay for patients hospitalized with community-acquired pneumonia: a randomized controlled trial. *Am J Med* 2003; 115: 343–51. **281**

Fishman A, Martinez F, Naunheim K, Piantadosi S, Wise R, Ries A, Weinmann G, Wood DE; National Emphysema Treatment Trial Research Group. A randomized trial comparing lung volume reduction surgery with medical therapy for severe emphysema. *N Engl J Med* 2003; 348(21): 2059–73. **125**

Fitzpatrick MF, Alloway CED, Wakeford TM, MacLean AW, Munt PW, Day AG. Can patients with obstructive sleep apnoea titrate their own continuous positive airway pressure? *Am J Respir Crit Care Med* 2003; 167: 716–22. **393**

Fizazi K, Doubre H, Le Chevalier T, Riviere A, Viala J, Daniel C, Robert L, Barthelemy P, Fandi A, Ruffie P. Combination of raltitrexed and oxaliplatin is an active regimen in malignant mesothelioma: results of a phase II study. *J Clin Oncol* 2003; 21(2): 349–54. **323**

Flaherty KR, Colby TV, Travis WD, Toews GB, Mumford J, Murray S, Thannickal VJ, Kazerooni EA, Gross BH, Lynch JP III, Martinez FJ. Fibroblastic foci in usual interstitial pneumonia. Idiopathic versus collagen vascular disease. *Am J Respir Crit Care Med* 2003; 167: 1410–15. **175**

Flaherty KR, Mumford JA, Murray S, Kazerooni EA, Gross BH, Colby TV, Travis WD, Flint A, Toews GB,

Lynch JP III, Martinez FJ. Prognostic implications of physiologic and radiographic changes in idiopathic interstitial pneumonia. *Am J Respir Crit Care Med* 2003; 168: 543–8. **180**

Flaherty KR, Thwaite EL, Kazerooni EA, Gross BH, Toews GB, Colby TV, Travis WD, Mumford JA, Murray S, Flint A, Lynch JP III, Martinez FJ. Radiological versus histological diagnosis in UIP and NSIP: survival implications. *Thorax* 2003; 58: 143–8. **189**

Flemons WW, Reimer MA. Measurement properties of the Calgary Sleep Apnoea Quality of Life Index. *Am J Respir Crit Care Med* 2002; 165: 159–64. **397**

Flores RM, Akhurst T, Gonen M, Larson SM, Rusch VW. Positron emission tomography defines metastatic disease but not locoregional disease in patients with malignant pleural mesothelioma. *J Thorac Cardiovasc Surg* 2003; 126(1): 11–16. **314**

Fritscher-Ravens A, Davidson BL, Hauber H-P, Bohuslavizki KH, Bobrowski C, Lund C, Knofel WT, Soehendra N, Brandt L, Pepe MS, Pforte A. Endoscopic ultrasound, positron emission tomography and computerized tomography for lung cancer. *Am J Respir Crit Care Med* 2003; 168: 1293–7. **338**

Gallagher PM, Lowe G, Fitzgerald T, Bella A, Greene CM, McElvaney NG, O'Neill SJ. Association of IL-10 polymorphism with severity of illness in community-acquired pneumonia. *Thorax* 2003; 58: 154–6. **273**

Gamble E, Grootendorst DC, Brightling CE, Troy S, Qiu Y, Zhu J, Parker D, Matin D, Majumdar S, Vignola AM, Kroegel C, Morell F, Hansel TT, Rennard SI, Compton C, Amit O, Tat T, Edelson J, Pavord ID, Rabe KF, Barnes NC, Jeffery PK. Anti-inflammatory effects of the phosphodiesterase-4 inhibitor cilomilast

Hirsch FR, Varrella-Garcia M, Bunn PA Jr, Di Maria MV, Veve R, Bremmes RM, Baron AE, Zeng C, Franklin WA. Epidermal growth factor receptor in non-small cell lung carcinoma: correlation between gene copy number and protein expression and impact on prognosis. *J Clin Oncol* 2003; 21(20): 3798–807.   **347**

Ho JC, Ooi GC, Mok TY, Chan JW, Hung I, Lam B, Wong PC, Li PC, Ho PL, Lam WK, Ng CK, Ip MS, Lai KN, Chan-Yeung M, Tsang KW. High-dose pulse versus non-pulse corticosteroid regimens in severe acute respiratory syndrome. *Am J Respir Crit Care Med* 2003; 168: 1449–56.   **269**

Horak E, Lanigan A, Roberts M, Welsh L, Wilson J, Carlin JB, Olinsky A, Robertson CF. Longitudinal study of childhood wheezy bronchitis and asthma: outcome at age 42. *BMJ* 2003; 326: 422–3.   **21**

Hughes R, Goldkorn A, Masoli M, Weatherall M, Burgess C, Beasley R. Use of isotonic nebulized magnesium sulphate as an adjuvant to salbutamol in treatment of severe asthma in adults: randomized, placebo-controlled trial. *Lancet* 2003; 361: 2114–17.   **80**

Ichinose Y, Genka K, Koike T, Kato H, Watanabe Y, Mori T, Iioka S, Sakuma A, Ohta M; NK421 Lung Cancer Surgery Group. Randomized, double-blind, placebo-controlled trial of bestatin in patients with resected stage I squamous-cell lung carcinoma. *J Natl Cancer Inst* 2003; 95: 605–10.   **342**

Innes NJ, Stocking JA, Daynes TJ, Harrison BDW. Randomized pragmatic comparison of UK and US treatment of acute asthma presenting to hospital. *Thorax* 2002; 12: 1040–4.   **78**

Inoue A, Saijo Y, Maemondo M, Gomi K, Tokue Y, Kimura Y, Ebina M, Kikuchi T, Moriya T, Nukiwa T. Severe acute interstitial pneumonia and gefitinib. *Lancet* 2003; 361: 137–9.   **348**

Ip SM, Lam B, Ng MMT, Lam WK, Tsang KWT. Obstructive sleep apnoea is independently associated with insulin resistance. *Am J Respir Crit Care Med* 2002; 165: 670–6.   **372**

Jackson LA, Neuzil KM, Yu O, Benson P, Barlow WE, Adams AL, Hanson CA, Mahoney LD, Shay DK, Thompson WW; Vaccine Safety Datalink. Effectiveness of pneumococcal polysaccharide vaccine in older adults. *N Engl J Med* 2003; 348: 1747–55.   **258**

Johnson JL, Ssekasanvu E, Okwera A, Mayanja H, Hirsch CS, Nakibali JG, Jankus DD, Eisenach KD, Boom WH, Ellner JJ, Mugerwa RD; Uganda–Case Western Reserve University Research Collaboration. Randomized trial of adjunctive interleukin-2 in adults with pulmonary tuberculosis. *Am J Respir Crit Care Med* 2003; 168(2): 185–91.   **229**

Jordan A, White D, Fogel RB. Recent advances in understanding of the pathogenesis of obstructive sleep apnoea. *Curr Opin Pulmon Med* 2003; 9(6): 459–64.   **364**

Judson MA, Thompson BW, Rabin DL, Steimel J, Knattereud GL, Lackland DT, Rose C, Rand CS, Baughman RP, Teirstein AS for the ACCESS Research Group. The diagnostic pathway to sarcoidosis. *Chest* 2003; 123: 406–12.   **199**

Kaiser L, Wat C, Mills T, Mahoney P, Ward P, Hayden F. Impact of oseltamivir treatment on influenza-related lower respiratory tract complications and hospitalizations. *Arch Intern Med* 2003; 163: 1667–72.   **265**

Kalra S, Utz JP, Ryu JH. Interferon gamma-1b therapy for advanced idiopathic pulmonary fibrosis. *Mayo Clin Proc* 2003; 78: 1082–7.   **193**

Katzenstein ALA, Zisman DA, Litzky LA, Nguyen BT, Kotloff RM. Usual interstitial pneumonia; histologic study of biopsy and

Lightowler JV, Wedzicha JA, Elliott MW, Ram FS. Non-invasive positive pressure ventilation to treat respiratory failure resulting from exacerbations of chronic obstructive pulmonary disease: Cochrane systematic review and meta-analysis. *BMJ* 2003; 326(7382): 185. **143**

LoBue PA, Moser KS. Use of isoniazid for latent tuberculosis infection in a public health clinic. *Am J Respir Crit Care Med* 2003; 168(4): 443–7. **211**

Macaubas C, de Klerk NH, Holt BJ, Wee C, Kendall G, Firth M, Sly PD, Holt PG. Association between antenatal cytokine production and the development of atopy and asthma at age 6 years. *Lancet* 2003; 362: 1192–7. **6**

Mahadevua PJ, Fleisher LA, Frick KD, Eng J, Goodman SN, Powe NR. Lung cancer screening with helical computed tomography in older adult smokers: a decision and cost-effectiveness analysis. *J Am Med Assoc* 2003; 289: 313–22. **336**

Malhotra A, Pillar G, Fogel RB, Edwards JK, Ayas N, Akahoshi T, Hess D, White DP. Pharyngeal pressure and flow effects on genioglossal activation in normal subjects. *Am J Respir Crit Care Med* 2002; 165: 71–7. **366**

Mar J, Rueda JR, Duran-Cantolla J, Schechter C, Chilcott J. Cost-effectiveness of nCPAP treatment in patients with moderate to severe obstructive sleep apnoea. *Eur Respir J* 2003; 21: 511–22. **395**

Massie CA, McArdle N, Hart RW, Schmidt-Nowara WW, Lankford A, Hudgel DW, Gordon N, Douglas NJ. Comparison between automatic and fixed airway pressure therapy in the home. *Am J Respir Crit Care Med* 2003; 167: 20–3. **394**

McNeill L, Allen M, Estrada C, Cook P. Pyrazinamide and rifampin versus isoniazid for the treatment of latent tuberculosis: improved completion rates but more

hepatotoxicity. *Chest* 2003; 123(1): 102–6. **214**

McWilliams T, Wells AU, Harrison AC, Lindstrom S, Cameron RJ, Foskin E. Induced sputum and bronchoscopy in the diagnosis of pulmonary tuberculosis. *Thorax* 2002; 57(12): 1010–14. **225**

Mendes R, O'Brien MER, Mitra A, Norton A, Gregory RK, Padhani AR, Bromelow KV, Winkley AR, Ashley S, Smith IE, Souberbielle BE. Clinical and immunological assessment of *Mycobacterium vaccae* (SRL172) with chemotherapy in patients with malignant mesothelioma. *Br J Cancer* 2002; 86: 336–41. **326**

Mihrshahi S, Peat JK, Marks GB, Mellis CM, Tovey ER, Webb K, Britton WJ, Leeder SR for the Childhood Asthma Prevention Study Team. Eighteen-month outcomes of house dust mite avoidance and dietary fatty acid modification in the Childhood Asthma Prevention Study (CAPS). *J Allergy Clin Immunol* 2003; 111: 162–8. **45**

Mitnick C, Bayona J, Palacios E, Shin S, Furin J, Alcantara F, Sanchez E, Sarria M, Becerra M, Fawzi MC, Kapiga S, Neuberg D, Maguire JH, Kim JY, Farmer P. Community-based therapy for multidrug-resistant tuberculosis in Lima, Peru. *N Engl J Med* 2003; 348(2): 119–28. **232**

Monahan KJ, Larkin EK, Rosen CL, Graham G, Redline S. Utility of non-invasive pharyngometry in epidemiologic studies of childhood sleep disordered breathing. *Am J Respir Crit Care Med* 2002; 165: 1499–503. **357**

Mussini C, Pezzotti P, Antinori A, Borghi V, Monforte A, Govoni A, De Luca A, Ammassari A, Mongiardo N, Cerri MC, Bedini A, Beltrami C, Ursitti MA, Bini T, Cossarizza A, Esposito R for the Changes in Opportunistic Prophylaxis Study Group. Discontinuation of secondary prophylaxis

Price DB, Hernandez D, Magyar P, Fiterman J, Beeh KM, James IG, Konstantopoulos S, Rojas R, van Noord JA, Pons M, Gilles L, Leff JA for the Clinical Outcomes with Montelukast as a Partner Agent to Corticosteroid Therapy International Study Group. Randomized, controlled trial of montelukast plus inhaled budesonide versus double-dose inhaled budesonide in adult patients with asthma. *Thorax* 2003; 58: 211–16.   **57**

Punjabi NM, Sorkin JD, Katzel LI, Goldberg P, Schwartz AR, Smith PL. Sleep-disordered breathing and insulin resistance in middle aged and overweight men. *Am J Respir Crit Care Med* 2002; 165: 677–82.   **373**

Ramsey SD, Berry K, Etzioni R, Kaplan RM, Sullivan SD, Wood DE; National Emphysema Treatment Trial Research Group. Cost-effectiveness of lung volume reduction surgery for patients with severe emphysema. *N Engl J Med* 2003; 348(21): 2092–102.   **128**

Rello J, Bodi M, Mariscal D, Navarro M, Diaz E, Gallego M, Valles J. Microbiological testing and outcome of patients with severe community-acquired pneumonia. *Chest* 2003; 123: 174–80.   **276**

Rello J, Ollendorf DA, Oster G, Vera-Llonch M, Bellm L, Redman R, Kollef MH for the VAP Outcomes Scientific Advisory Group. Epidemiology and outcomes of ventilator-associated pneumonia in a large US database. *Chest* 2002; 122: 2115–21.   **291**

Research Committee of the British Thoracic Society. Pulmonary disease caused by *Mycobacterium malmoense* in HIV-negative patients: 5-year follow-up of patients receiving standardized treatment. *Eur Respir J* 2003; 21(3): 478–82.   **233**

Ries AL, Kaplan RM, Myers R, Prewitt LM. Maintenance after pulmonary rehabilitation in chronic lung disease: a randomized trial.

Am J Respir Crit Care Med 2003; 167(6): 880–8.   **119**

Robinson DR, Campbell DA, Durham SR, Pfeffer J, Barnes PJ, Chung KF. Systematic assessment of difficult to treat asthma. *Eur Respir J* 2003; 22: 478–83.   **36**

Root RK, Lodato RF, Patrick W, Cade JF, Fotheringham N, Milwee S, Vincent JL, Torres A, Rello J, Nelson S for the Pneumonia Sepsis Study Group. Multicenter, double-blind, placebo-controlled study of the use of filgrastim in patients hospitalized with pneumonia and severe sepsis. *Crit Care Med* 2003; 31: 367–73.   **286**

Sajkov D, Wang T, Saunders MA, Bune AJ, McEvoy RD. Continuous positive airway pressure treatment improves pulmonary haemodynamics in patients with obstructive sleep apnoea. *Am J Respir Crit Care Med* 2002; 165: 152–8.   **401**

Salman GF, Mosier MC, Beasley BW, Calkins DR. Rehabilitation for patients with chronic obstructive pulmonary disease: meta-analysis of randomized controlled trials. *J Gen Intern Med* 2003; 18(3): 213–21.   **117**

Saydain G, Islam A, Afessa B, Ryu J, Scott JP, Peters SG. Outcome of patients with idiopathic pulmonary fibrosis admitted to the intensive care unit. *Am J Respir Crit Care Med* 2002; 166: 839–42.   **191**

Scagliotti GV, Shin D-M, Kindler HL, Vasconcelles MJ, Keppler U, Manegold C, Burris H, Gatzemeier U, Blatter J, Symanowski JT, Rusthoven JJ. Phase II study of Pemetrexed with and without folic acid and vitamin B_{12} as front-line therapy in malignant pleural mesothelioma. *J Clin Oncol* 2003; 21(8): 1556–61.   **320**

Schaaf BM, Boehmke F, Esnaashari H, Seitzer U, Kothe H, Maass M, Zabel P, Dalhaff K. Pneumococcal septic shock is associated with the interleukin-10–1082 gene promoter polymorphism. *Am J Respir Crit Care Med* 2003; 168(3): 476–80.   **273**

Szafranski W, Cukier A, Ramirez A, Menga G, Sansores R, Nahabedian S, Peterson S, Olsson H. Efficacy and safety of budesonide/formoterol in the management of chronic obstructive pulmonary disease. *Eur Respir J* 2003; 21(1): 74–81. **103**

Thomas M, McKinley RK, Freeman E, Foy C, Prodger P, Price D. Breathing retraining for dysfunctional breathing in asthma: a randomized controlled trial. *Thorax* 2003; 58: 110–15. **65**

Torres A, Muir JF, Corris P, Kubin R, Duprat-Lomon I, Sagnier PP, Hoffken G. Effectiveness of oral moxifloxacin in standard first-line therapy in community-acquired pneumonia. *Eur Respir J* 2003; 21: 135–43. **284**

Trang H, Leske V, Gaultier C. Use of nasal cannula for detecting sleep apnoeas/hypopnoeas in infants and children. *Am J Respir Crit Care Med* 2002; 166: 465–8. **384**

Van der Valk P, Monninkhof E, Van der Palen J, Zielhuis G, Van Herwaarden C. Effect of discontinuation of inhaled corticosteroids in patients with chronic obstructive pulmonary disease: the COPE study. *Am J Respir Crit Care Med* 2002; 166(10): 1358–63. **98**

Van Haarst JMW, Baas P, Manegold Ch, Schouwink JH, Burgers JA, de Bruin HG, Mooi WJ, van Klaveren RJ, de Jonge MJ, van Meerbeeck JP. Multicentre phase II study of gemcitabine and cisplatin in malignant pleural mesothelioma. *Br J Cancer* 2002; 86: 342–5. **318**

Vaqueriza MJ, Casan P, Castillo J, Perpina M, Sanchis J, Sobradillo V, Valencia A, Verea H, Viejo JL, Villasante C, Gonzalez-Esteban J, Picado C for the Capacidad de Singular Oral en la Prevncion de Exacerbaiones Asmaticas Study Group. Effect of montelukast added

to inhaled budesonide on control of mild to moderate asthma. *Thorax* 2003; 58: 204–11. **57**

Veeraraghavan S, Latsi PI, Wells AU, Pantelidis P, Nicholson AG, Colby TV, Haslam PL, Renzoni EA, du Bois RM. BAL findings in idiopathic nonspecific interstitial pneumonia and usual interstitial pneumonia. *Eur Respir J* 2003; 22: 239–44. **186**

Villena V, Lopez-Encuentra A, Pozo F, Echave-Sustaeta J, Ortuno-de-Solo B, Estenoz-Alfaro J, Martin-Escribano P. Interferon gamma levels in pleural fluid for the diagnosis of tuberculosis. *Am J Med* 2003; 115(5): 365–70. **240**

Vogelzang NJ, Rusthoven JJ, Symanowski J, Denham C, Kaukel E, Ruffie P, Gatzemeier U, Boyer M, Emri S, Manegold C, Niyikiza C, Paoletti P. Phase III study of Pemetrexed in combination with cisplatin versus cisplatin alone in patients with malignant pleural mesothelioma. *J Clin Oncol* 2003; 21(14): 2636–44. **321**

Vonbank K, Ziesche R, Higenbottam TW, Stiebellehner L, Petkov V, Schenk P, Germann P, Block LH. Controlled prospective randomized trial on the effects on pulmonary haemodynamics of the ambulatory long-term use of nitric oxide and oxygen in patients with severe COPD. *Thorax* 2003; 58(4): 289–93. **115**

Wagenaar M, Vos PJ, Heijdra YF, Teppema LJ, Folgering HT. Combined treatment with acetazolamide and medroxyprogesterone in chronic obstructive pulmonary disease patients. *Eur Respir J* 2002; 20(5): 1130–7. **113**

Wang Y, Zhao R, Chattopadhyay S, Goldman ID. A novel folate transport activity in human mesothelioma cell lines with high affinity and specificity for the new-generation antifolate, Pemetrexed. *Cancer Res* 2002; 62: 6434–7. **322**

General index

KEEPING UP TO DATE IN ONE VOLUME

Subject matters dealt with in previous volume

The Year in Respiratory Medicine 2003

Asthma

Incidence and prevalence of asthma; epidemiology; genetics of asthma; clinical course of asthma; airway wall remodelling; investigations; pathology of asthma; treatment

Chronic obstructive pulmonary disease (COPD)

Important observations derived from epidemiological studies; advances in 'stable' COPD, exacerbations of COPD and their management

Respiratory infection

Tuberculosis; community acquired pneumonia; ventilator associated pneumonia; bronchiectasis

Lung cancer

Early detection and prevention of lung cancer; diagnosis and staging of lung cancer; treatment of lung cancer

---

Atlas Medical Publishing Ltd
Oxford Centre for Innovation
Mill Street
Oxford OX2 0JX, UK

T: +44 1865 811116
F: +44 1865 251550
E: info@clinicalpublishing.co.uk
W: www.clinicalpublishing.co.uk

KEEPING UP TO DATE IN ONE SERIES

"The Year in ..."

EXISTING AND FUTURE VOLUMES

To receive more information about these books and future volumes,
or to order copies, please contact the address below:

Atlas Medical Publishing Ltd
Oxford Centre for Innovation
Mill Street
Oxford OX2 0JX, UK

T: +44 1865 811116
F: +44 1865 251550
E: info@clinicalpublishing.co.uk
W: www.clinicalpublishing.co.uk